AF695038

This unique volume provides fascinating insights on the state of assisted reproduction across Europe, where an uneven legal terrain and diverse religious regimes have produced various feminist and biopolitical responses. But the book also takes readers across borders, showing how ARTs, now firmly entrenched in the global South, have brought new movements of people, capital, and ideas of family and citizenship. Featuring both original social science scholarship and trenchant critical analysis, this book is a must read for scholars interested in the global spread of biotechnology and its repercussions.

Marcia C. Inhorn, *PhD, MPH, is the William K. Lanman, Jr. Professor of Anthropology and International Affairs in the Department of Anthropology and The Whitney and Betty MacMillan Center for International and Area Studies at Yale University, USA*

This is the new book we have been waiting for! ART – assisted reproduction – is now "the new normal." Yet until now, no study has examined in detail what that acutally means. Lie and Lykke's volume examines the post-normalization world of assisted reproduction in a global context, revealing how ART plays out differently from nation to nation, reflecting and accommodating the specific local pressures of politics, gender roles, economic pressures, and biopolitical expectations. The essays in this volume are surprising and illuminating in the variety of practices, assumptions, economic and social impacts and dilemmas they uncover and analyze. An essential text for scholars and advances students in sociology, political science, history, anthropology and literature, as well as women's gender and sexuality studies.

Susan Squier *is a professor at Penn State University, Pennsylvania, USA*

Assisted Reproduction Across Borders

Today, it often seems as though Assisted Reproductive Technologies (ARTs) have reached a stage of normalization, at least in some countries and among certain social groups. Apparently some practices – for example in vitro fertilization (IVF) – have become standard worldwide. The contributors to *Assisted Reproduction Across Borders* argue against normalization as an uncontested overall trend.

This volume reflects on the state of the art of ARTs. From feminist perspectives, the contributors focus on contemporary political debates triggered by ARTs. They examine the varying ways in which ARTs are interpreted and practised in different contexts, depending on religious, moral and political approaches. *Assisted Reproduction Across Borders* embeds feminist analysis of ARTs across a wide variety of countries and cultural contexts, discussing controversial practices such as surrogacy from the perspective of the global South as well as the global North as well as inequalities in terms of access to IVF.

This volume will appeal to scholars and students of anthropology, ethnography, philosophy, political science, history, sociology, film studies, media studies, literature, art history, area studies, and interdisciplinary areas such as gender studies, cultural studies, and postcolonial studies.

Merete Lie is Professor in the Department of Interdisciplinary Studies of Culture and leader of the Centre for Gender Research at the Norwegian University of Science and Technology (NTNU), Norway.

Nina Lykke is Professor of Gender Studies at Linköping University, Sweden, co-director of GEXcel International Collegium for Advanced Transdisciplinary Gender Studies, and director of InterGender International Research School, Sweden.

Routledge Advances in Feminist Studies and Intersectionality

Core editorial group: Dr. Kathy Davis (Institute for History and Culture, Utrecht, The Netherlands), Professor Jeff Hearn (Managing Editor; Örebro University, Sweden; Hanken School of Economics, Finland; University of Huddersfield, UK), Professor Anna G. Jónasdóttir (Örebro University, Sweden), Professor Nina Lykke (Managing Editor; Linköping University, Sweden), Professor Elżbieta H. Oleksy (University of Łódź, Poland), Dr. Andrea Petö (Central European University, Hungary), Professor Ann Phoenix (Institute of Education, University of London, UK), Professor Chandra Talpade Mohanty (Syracuse University, USA)

Routledge Advances in Feminist Studies and Intersectionality is committed to the development of new feminist and profeminist perspectives on changing gender relations, with special attention to:

- Intersections between gender and power differentials based on age, class, dis/abilities, ethnicity, nationality, racialisation, sexuality, violence, and other social divisions.
- Intersections of societal dimensions and processes of continuity and change: culture, economy, generativity, polity, sexuality, science and technology.
- Embodiment: Intersections of discourse and materiality, and of sex and gender.
- Transdisciplinarity: intersections of humanities, social sciences, medical, technical and natural sciences.
- Intersections of different branches of feminist theorizing, including: historical materialist feminisms, postcolonial and anti-racist feminisms, radical feminisms, sexual difference feminisms, queerfeminisms, cyberfeminisms, posthuman feminisms, critical studies on men and masculinities.
- A critical analysis of the travelling of ideas, theories and concepts.
- A politics of location, reflexivity and transnational contextualising that reflects the basis of the Series framed within European diversity and transnational power relations.

16 Writing Academic Texts Differently
Intersectional Feminist Methodologies and the Playful Art of Writing
Edited by Nina Lykke

17 Gender, Globalization, and Violence
Postcolonial Conflict Zones
Edited by Sandra Ponzanesi

18 Gendered Tropes in War Photography
Mothers, Mourners, Soldiers
Marta Zarzycka

19 Assisted Reproduction Across Borders
Feminist Perspectives on Normalizations, Disruptions and Transmissions
Edited by Merete Lie and Nina Lykke

Assisted Reproduction Across Borders

Feminist Perspectives on Normalizations, Disruptions and Transmissions

Edited by Merete Lie and Nina Lykke

Routledge
Taylor & Francis Group
LONDON AND NEW YORK

First published 2017 by Routledge

2 Park Square, Milton Park, Abingdon, Oxfordshire OX14 4RN
52 Vanderbilt Avenue, New York, NY 10017

Routledge is an imprint of the Taylor & Francis Group, an informa business

First issued in paperback 2019

Copyright © 2017 by Taylor & Francis

The right of the Merete Lie and Nina Lykke to be identified as the authors of the editorial matter, and of the authors for their individual chapters, has been asserted in accordance with sections 77 and 78 of the Copyright, Designs and Patents Act 1988.

All rights reserved. No part of this book may be reprinted or reproduced or utilized in any form or by any electronic, mechanical, or other means, now known or hereafter invented, including photocopying and recording, or in any information storage or retrieval system, without permission in writing from the publishers.

Notice:
Product or corporate names may be trademarks or registered trademarks, and are used only for identification and explanation without intent to infringe.

Library of Congress Cataloging in Publication Data
Names: Lie, Merete, editor. | Lykke, Nina, editor.
Title: Assisted reproduction across borders : feminist perspectives on normalizations, disruptions and transmissions / edited by Merete Lie and Nina Lykke.
Description: New York, NY : Routledge, 2017. | Series: Routledge advances in feminist studies and intersectionality ; 19
Identifiers: LCCN 2016014922| ISBN 9781138674646 (hardback) | ISBN 9781315561219 (e-book)
Subjects: LCSH: Human reproductive technology–Social aspects. | Surrogate motherhood. | Feminist theory.
Classification: LCC HQ761 .A87 2017 | DDC 305.4201–dc23
LC record available at https://lccn.loc.gov/2016014922

ISBN: 978-1-138-67464-6 (hbk)
ISBN: 978-0-367-35082-6 (pbk)

Typeset in Times New Roman
by Wearset Ltd, Boldon, Tyne and Wear

Contents

Contributors

Stine Willum Adrian is an Associate Professor in Techno-Anthropology at Aalborg University in Copenhagen, Denmark. Adrian's research interests lie in questions concerning gender, medical technology, science and technology studies, intersectional analysis, practice theory, ethics, and material feminisms. She has previously conducted a comprehensive ethnographic study of fertility clinics and sperm banks in Denmark and Sweden. Her current work explores the globalization of Danish sperm due to the expansion of Danish sperm banking, and Denmark's situation as a European destination for donor insemination. Together with Charlotte Kroløkke, Lene Myong and Tine Tjørnhøj-Thomsen she co-edited the book *Critical Kinship Studies* (Rowman and Littlefield 2015).

Bettina Bock von Wülfingen is a cultural historian of the life sciences. Since completing her PhD dissertation on changes in the notion of health under the influence of assisted reproductive technologies (Genetisierung der Zeugung, 2007), funded by diverse international fellowships, she has been based at the Institute for Cultural History and Theory, Humboldt-Universität zu Berlin. She is currently preparing her second book, entitled *Economies and the Cell: Conception and Heredity 1900 to 2000*, for publication. As a member of the Cluster of Excellence Image Knowledge Gestaltung at the Humboldt-Universität zu Berlin, her current focus is on the transition from reproduction and production to (re-)generation in the life sciences on the basis of a case study on neuro-regeneration and, additionally, on the cultural history of visual evidence and image production in the life sciences during the long nineteenth century.

Isabelle Engeli is Reader at the Department of Politics, Language, and International Relations at the University of Bath. She specializes in comparative public policy, human biotechnology and reproductive rights, and the politics of gendering policy attention and action. She has recently co-led an international project on party competition and morality politics in Western Europe. She is co-editor of *Morality Politics in Western Europe: Parties, Agenda and Policy Choice* (Palgrave Macmillan 2013) and co-editor of *Comparative Policy Studies: Conceptual and Methodological Challenges* (Palgrave 2014).

Her work was awarded the 2012 APSA Best Paper in Comparative Policy Analysis and the 2011 Carrie Chapman Catt Prize. Engeli is co-convener of the ECPR Standing Group on Gender and Politics and the European Conference in Politics and Gender.

Lise Eriksson is a postdoctoral researcher in Sociology at Åbo Akademi University, Finland. Her research interests include reproductive technologies, surrogacy, family politics, and the sociology of religion. Her current research project studies surrogacy in the Nordic countries. Her PhD thesis is an analysis of debates on assisted reproduction in the Parliament of Finland during the 2000s (*Barnets bästa i politikens främsta rum* [The Best Interests of the Child in the Main Chamber of Politics], Åbo Akademi University 2012). Eriksson was a Visiting Scholar at Uppsala University in 2010, and at the Norwegian University of Science and Technology (NTNU) in 2013–14.

Kristin Engh Førde is an anthropologist and PhD candidate at the Institute of Health and Society at the University of Oslo and a researcher at the Norwegian Centre for Violence and Traumatic Stress Studies. Her PhD project is an ethnographic study of transnational, commercial surrogacy in India, and is expected to be finalized and published in 2016.

Malathi Michelle Iyengar is a former public school teacher and a current PhD candidate in Ethnic Studies at the University of California, San Diego, USA. She also serves as the San Diego unit chair for the UAW 2865, the labor union representing more than 13,000 teaching assistants, readers, graders, and tutors across the University of California system.

Edyta Just is Assistant Professor and coordinator of the InterGender Consortium and Research School in Interdisciplinary Gender Studies at the Unit of Gender Studies, Linköping University. She holds degrees in political science from the University of Lodz, Poland, and gender studies from Utrecht University, the Netherlands. Her fields of expertise include: gender studies, pedagogy, philosophy, and cultural studies of science and technology, in particular of neuroscience. Her recent publications include: *Quilting Stories* (2012, edited volume with M. M. Wojtaszek), *Esthetic Experiments* (2013, edited volume with M. M. Wojtaszek) and "Computing and Affective Body-Brain: A Critically-Creative Reflection on Affect, in Gendered Neurocultures" (eds. Sigrid Schmitz and Grit Höppner, 2014).

Maria Kirpichenko has completed her masters degree at the Department of Interdisciplinary Studies of Culture, Norwegian University of Science and Technology (NTNU). She was previously awarded a master's degree in visual anthropology at the University of Tromsø, Norway, and a master's degree in history with a focus on modern European history at the Petrozavodsk State University, Russia. Her current research interests include feminist theory, queer theory, postcolonial theory, visual anthropology, and documentary film making.

Charlotte Kroløkke is Professor with special responsibility for cultural analyses of reproductive medicine at the Department for the Study of Culture at the University of Southern Denmark. She is head of research projects involving reproductive medicine and mobility and her academic interests concern the ways in which ARTs are debated, experienced, and constructed by egg donors, fertility travelers, elective freezers, and in public debates.

Merete Lie is Professor at the Department of Interdisciplinary Studies of Culture and head of the Centre for Gender Research at the Norwegian University of Science and Technology (NTNU). She is a social anthropologist and her main fields of research are: gender, science and technology, including biotechnologies, biopolitics and ICT; and globalization, including fieldwork in China and Southeast Asia. She is the coordinator of research projects on assisted reproductive technologies, medical imaging, and welfare technologies. Previous publications: *Making Technology our Own? Domesticating Technology into Everyday Life* (co-editor) and *He, She and IT Revisited: New Perspectives on Gender in the Information Society*, and on biopolitics they incude: *The Social Meaning of Children and Fertility Change in Europe* (co-editor, Routledge 2013). Her current research is medical imagining and bioart.

Nina Lykke is Professor of Gender Studies, Linköping University, Sweden. She is co-director of GEXcel International Collegium for Advanced Transdisciplinary Gender Studies as well as scientific leader of the Swedish-International Research School, InterGender. She has been scientific director of the Nordic Research School in Interdisciplinary Gender Studies, and managing director of the European Feminist Studies Association, AOIFE. She has published extensively within the areas of feminist theory, intersectionality studies, feminist cultural studies, and feminist technoscience studies, including the following books and edited volumes: *Between Monsters, Goddesses and Cyborgs* (1996, with Rosi Braidotti), *Cosmodolphins* (2000, with Mette Bryld), *Bits of Life* (2008, with Anneke Smelik), *Feminist Studies* (2010), *Theories and Methodologies in Postgraduate Feminist Research* (2011, with Rosemarie Buikema and Gabriele Griffin), and *Writing Academic Texts Differently* (2014). Her current research is a queerfeminist, autophenomenographic, and poetic exploration of cancer cultures, death, and mourning.

Orla McDonnell is a lecturer in the Department of Sociology at the University of Limerick, Ireland. Her research interests are in the areas of social theory and health, and the interfaces between medical technologies, reproductive politics, and society. She is co-author of *Social Theory, Health and Healthcare* (Palgrave 2009), and author of "Striving towards a Normative Identity: The Social Production of Meaning of Assisted Reproductive Technology in Ireland" (in A. C. Bastos, *et al.* (eds.) *Cultural Dynamics of Women's Lives*) and co-author of "The Veto of Moral Politics: The Catholic Church and ART in Ireland" (in DeVies *et al.* (eds.) *The View from Here: Bioethics and the Social Sciences*).

Tara Mehrabi is a doctoral student at the Unit of Gender Studies, Linköping University, Sweden. She holds a master's degree in Science, Technology, and Society (STS) from the same university, where she graduated in 2010 with a thesis on the co-construction of family structure and egg donation in Iran. In her PhD research, she is focusing on knowledge production practices in an Alzheimer's science laboratory, in which she discusses human and animal relationalities, death, and the ethics of killability. Her current research interests include: gender, medicine, and technology; feminist technoscience studies; human–animal studies; new materialisms; and feminist post-humanities.

Marit Melhuus is Professor of Social Anthropology at the University of Oslo. Over the past few years she has been working in Norway, addressing issues of kinship, biotechnology, and law, publishing widely on these interlinked themes, including the book *Problems of Conception: Issues of Law, Biotechnology, Individuals and Kinship* (Berghahn 2012). Tangentially, she has addressed the theme of the transnational flow of concepts and substances and is co-editor of the volume *Holding Worlds Together: Ethnographies of Knowing and Belonging* (Berghahn 2007). She has previously worked in Argentina and Mexico, focusing on economic anthropology, gender, and morality. She co-edited the volume *Machos, Mistresses, Madonnas* (Verso 1996). She is currently involved in the project "Anthropos and the Material," with a particular interest in labor.

Verena Namberger is a doctoral student at the Center for Transdisciplinary Gender Studies, Humboldt University Berlin, Germany. She holds a Diploma in Political Sciences from the Free University of Berlin, graduating in 2012 with a thesis on critical race theory and the materiality of the body. In her PhD research, she uses the South African economy of egg donation as a site to understand the commodification of the (re)productive body in the life sciences, tracing the different bodily assemblages that are constructed, materialized, and experienced in this bioeconomy. In addition, she is active in anti-racist groups in Berlin and a member of the political publishing collective Edition Assemblage. Her current research interests include: feminist theory, feminist science and technology studies, new materialisms, body studies, cultural studies of ARTs, biopolitics, philosophy, and history of the life sciences.

Manuela Perrotta is a lecturer in Technology and Organization at the School of Business and Management at Queen Mary University of London. Her research focuses on reproductive technologies as culturally embedded socio-technical products entangled in a network of professional, political, economic, and moral considerations. Her current research interests focus on professional learning and visual enskillment in the field of IVF imaging. She has published numerous articles and book chapters and has presented her work at many international conferences. In 2013 she edited a special issue of the journal *Tecnoscienza: Italian Journal of Science and Technology Studies* on "Re-conceiving Life in the Labs: The Emerging Meanings of Cells in the Italian Reproductive Biomedicine and Beyond."

Julianne Pidduck is Associate Professor in the Department of Communication at the Université de Montréal, Canada. A specialist in feminist and queer analysis of the moving image, she is the author of *Contemporary Costume Film: Space, Place and the Past* (2004), and has published widely in journals, including: *Camera Obscura, GLQ, Studies in French Cinema, Screen, Media Culture & Society, Cinémas*, and the *Canadian Journal of Film Studies*. Her chapter in this volume is drawn from a larger study entitled "Queer Kinship, Audiovisual Relations," an exploration of kinship, intimacy, and family in LGBTQ-authored film, video, and television productions.

Malin Noem Ravn is a coordinator for research and development at the intermunicipal company Fosen Helse. Previously she worked as a social anthropologist and gender researcher at the Norwegian University of Science and Technology (NTNU). Ravn's main fields of interest are: cultural conceptions of the body, reproduction, biotechnologies, health care, kinship studies, and qualitative research methods. Her recent publications include the co-authored "The Voices Heard and the Voices Silenced: Recruitment Processes in Qualitative Interview Studies" (*Qualitative Research* 2015). She is one of the editors of the Norwegian anthology *Det skapende mennesket. Antropologiske dialoger om tegn, ting og tolkning* [Homo Faber: Anthropological Dialogues on Signs, Objects, and Interpretation] (2015), and of the anthology *Reproduksjon, kjønn og likestilling: Familieplanlegging i det samtidige Norge* [Reproduction, Gender, and Gender Equality: Family Planning in Contemporary Norway] (2016).

Christine Rothmayr Allison is a Professor in the Political Science Department at the University of Montreal, Canada. Her two main fields of interest are: comparative public policy, focusing on the fields of biotechnology and biomedicine; and courts and politics, in particular, the impact of court decisions on public policy-making in North America and Europe. Her current projects include "Comparative Policy Agendas: The Supreme Court of Canada." Her latest book (edited with Isabelle Engeli) is entitled *Comparative Policy Studies: Conceptual and Methodological Challenges* (Palgrave 2014).

Marcin Smietana is a postdoctoral scholar within the Marie Curie IOF scheme of the European Union, at the University of California, Berkeley (Department of Gender & Women's Studies) and the University of Cambridge, UK (Reproductive Sociology Research Group), for his research project "SurrogARTs: Transition to Parenthood and Negotiating Relatedness in Families Created through Transnational Surrogacy." He is also a member of the AFIN (Adoptions, Families, Infancies) research group at the Autonomous University of Barcelona (Spain). His PhD in sociology from the University of Barcelona was based on his research with Spanish gay father families created through adoption and surrogacy and their children's schools. He received his MA in sociology from the Jagiellonian University in his native Cracow (Poland).

The late **Kristin H. Spilker** was a social anthropologist and gender researcher at the Norwegian University of Science and Technology (NTNU). Her research fields were: ARTs, biopolitics, and gender directed at cultural studies of changing kinship relations and untraditional families. Her very original research employs multisite ethnographies and situational analyses. Her publications include her PhD thesis: *Assisted Kinship: Biopolitics in the Age of Assisted Reproduction* (in Norwegian), "Reproductive Imaginations: Stories of Egg and Sperm" (*NORA* 2011), and "Gender and Bioethics Intertwined: Egg Donation in the Context of Equal Opportunities" (*The European Journal of Women's Studies* 2007).

Sigrid Vertommen is an assistant to the Middle East and North Africa Research Group of the Department of Conflict and Development Studies at Ghent University in Belgium. She is on the verge of finalizing her doctoral research on the political economy of assisted reproduction in Palestine/Israel.

Polina Vlasenko is a PhD student in the Department of Anthropology at Indiana University, Bloomington, USA. Her current research is focused on the experiences of egg donors in Ukraine and the role that the transnational travel of gametes, reproductive migrants, and medical laborers to and from Ukraine play in the global politics, economies, and technologies of life. She has previously explored how gender normalization is achieved through the governance of freedom in IVF treatment in Ukraine.

Kalindi Vora is Associate Professor of Ethnic Studies and affiliate faculty of the Critical Gender and Science Studies Programs at the University of California, San Diego, USA. Her book, *Life Support: Biocapital and the New History of Outsourced Labor* (University of Minnesota Press 2015), examines domestic work, customer care, the commodification of human organs, gestational surrogacy, and knowledge work as representing a global economy of vitality that relies on the affective and biological labor of feminized workers. Her research and publications have focused on gendered labor, globalization, the South Asian area and diaspora studies, postcolonial studies, and feminist theory.

Lucy van de Wiel is a Research Associate at the Reproductive Sociology Research Group (ReproSoc), University of Cambridge. Her research interests include: egg freezing, time-lapse embryo imaging, cross-border reproductive care, feminist visual culture studies, and critical gerontology. In November 2015, she successfully defended her PhD thesis *Freezing Fertility: Oocyte Cryopreservation and the Gender Politics of Ageing* at the University of Amsterdam. This study critically examined how the possibility of egg freezing both triggers the articulation of existing age normativities and reconfigures the temporal logic of reproductive ageing. Her research has appeared in various international peer-reviewed journals, including *Maternal Studies*, *International Journal of Feminist Approaches to Bioethics*, and *Women's Studies International Forum*.

Acknowledgments

This book has been a very long time in the making – mainly due to personal reasons. We thank all the contributors for their patience and trust, and we are happy that almost everybody was still able to participate when we initiated the finalizing process. Everyone did a great job.

We also warmly thank Liz Sourbut for her very careful and creative language editing, and Magdalena Górska for putting so much energy and thoughtful work into the general editing process, despite being in the middle of the very last phase of finalizing her PhD dissertation. Thanks also to Tetyana Bureychak for help with Russian–English translations.

We would like to warmly thank the anonymous Routledge reviewers of the manuscript for their commitment and insightful comments. Many thanks also to our always very supportive Routledge editor, Max Novick.

We also thank each other and all the participants for stimulating discussions and the excellent cooperation we have had throughout this long process. We acknowledge each other as equally committed editors/authors, and we note that our names on the cover and on the editorial introductory chapter are mentioned in alphabetical order, and do not refer to a first or second editor/author.

Sadly, Kristin H. Spilker passed away in 2014. She was a key person in the research team at NTNU, from the beginning of her research on ARTs for her PhD in 2002 onwards. Kristin was a gifted and original researcher and a person we will never forget.

During work on the book (2014), one of us (Nina) lost her life partner, Mette Bryld. I (Nina) began my research on assisted reproduction together with Mette. This was in 1997, when Danish law excluded lesbian couples and single women from accessing medically monitored assisted reproduction. Thank you, Mette, for your lifelong commitment to feminist politics and your sophisticated cultural analyses.

Merete Lie and Nina Lykke
December 13, 2015
Trondheim and Linköping

Permissions

Chapter 20

Chapter 20 is an abbreviated, updated and revised version of the article:
Adrian, Stine Willum. 2010. "Sperm Stories: Policies and Practices of Sperm Banking in Denmark and Sweden." *European Journal of Women's Studies* 17 (4): 393–411. © The Author(s) 2010.
Reprinted by Permission of SAGE Publications Ltd.

Chapter 21

Figures 21.1 and 21.2. Stills from video "Baby Eeva Video – Eeva."
Kbhandal 2013. *Early Embryo Viability Assessment Test.* June 14, 2013. www.eevaivf.com/video-of-eeva-conception/.
Reprinted with permission of the Glasgow Centre for Reproductive Medicine (GCRM).
Figure 21.3. Still from "Eeva In Action (ASRM 2013)."
Auxogyn 2014. YouTube video, 2:06. Posted by "The Eeva Test,"
January 8, 2014. www.youtube.com/watch?v=hdL0kY5rPbM.
Reprinted with permission of Progyny, Inc.

Editorial Introduction

Assisted Reproduction Across Borders: Feminist Perspectives on Normalizations, Disruptions and Transmissions

Merete Lie and Nina Lykke[1]

After the birth of the first "test-tube baby" in the UK in 1978, assisted reproductive technologies (ARTs) attracted a great deal of interest from researchers within the cultural and social sciences, particularly those with feminist research perspectives. From feminist viewpoints, the introduction of ARTs has posed new questions and dilemmas. A decade earlier, Shulamith Firestone had envisioned a feminist future where,

> The reproduction of the species by one sex for the benefit of both would be replaced by (at least the option of) artificial reproduction: children would be born to both sexes equally, or independently of either, however one chooses to look at it.
>
> (Firestone 1971, 11)

But Firestone's radical assertion of the necessity for technologies to liberate women from childbirth was not generally accepted back then and, during the 1980s, the network FINRRAGE[2] articulated feminist voices against what it saw as a male-dominated technoscience taking control of women's bodies through ARTs. Over time, however, there has been a growing demand for more ARTs and opposition to restrictions on access; in other words, ARTs are now positioned as a means to achieve the "democratization" of childbirth and queer family-building, including same-sex and single-parent families. In some countries, predominantly secular western democracies, it has been politically possible for queer, feminist, and different sexual political movements to raise demands for equal access to ARTs, regardless of gender or sexual identities, even though exclusionary policies and practices of assisted reproduction are still very much on the agenda in these contexts as well. Still, it is an inevitable paradox of the contemporary, neoliberal, and globalized world in which ART policies and practices are performed, that ARTs have created new possibilities for some people as recipients of gametes, cures, and gestational labor, whereas others, in particular women in precarious situations, have become the providers. Generally, this takes place in contexts where intersections between gendered and geopolitical inequalities and power differentials have mutually reinforced each other.

ARTs are technologies that concern very intimate aspects of people's lives while also being public matters of vital concern – this is encapsulated in the notion of biopolitics (Foucault 1979). This term implies public policies governing the vital processes of life: sexuality; conjugal, parental, and familial relations; health and disease; birth and death (Rose 2001, 1). The aim of these policies is not only regulation through restrictions but also individual and collective self-governance. In order to appreciate the interweaving of private and public matters, global outreach and local diversity, emotions, economy, and legal constraints, we have included a wide variety of research in this volume, with the aim of demonstrating cultural variation. The various chapters give insights into local variations related to vital matters like religion, family and gender norms, sexualities, demography, and legalization and, moreover, how access is framed and interpreted, both on a global scale and also from local perspectives.

Against this background, *one major aim* of this volume is to throw light on the wide variance in perceptions, acceptance, in/exclusion, and legalization of technologies that are basically the same. ARTs are accessible worldwide, but in very different ways and definitely not by everyone. Access to ARTs includes many different elements; among them are the legal regulation that takes place on a national level, a rapidly developing fertility industry in a global marketplace and, not least, the cultural norms and traditions that are vital to varying practices worldwide. These elements are intricately interwoven as well as rapidly shifting and enter into ever-new co-constructions and configurations with bodies and technologies. Thus, while we started working on this volume with the idea that we needed to study the phase in which ARTs had become normalized and the procedures standardized, what we saw were endless processes of political negotiations around both new and established procedures. We also began with the aim of grasping the wide variation in ART practices in Europe, but we quickly realized that these practices have no borders. Thus, one point of departure was that ARTs are no longer "new technology" or cutting-edge science but are regarded, in large parts of the world, as mundane practices. This can be exemplified by how, in Norway, the general understanding of involuntary childlessness is that this definition only applies *after* you have tried IVF, whereas previously, you were perceived as involuntarily childless when accessing a fertility clinic (Lie, Ravn, and Spilker 2013). In other words, in some contexts, some ART procedures are now included in the normal repertoire of getting pregnant. The broad term "ARTs" includes a wide spectrum of techniques, of which some have been working successfully for many years and are available globally, while new or refined techniques are continuously emerging. Whereas ARTs attracted much interest when they were new, we find that normalization processes and new procedures call for new research questions and empirical investigations; among other things, of the different and continuously changing policies and practices which are the focus of this volume.

In addition to demonstrating how ART policies and practices constitute a political minefield which casts legislators and individual users in different national and global contexts into unexpected dilemmas and stirs up a wide variety of different responses, a *second major aim* of this volume is to widen the scope of investigation, nationally and globally. Standard references within feminist studies of ARTs have predominantly been based on empirical studies from the UK and the USA, most notably Sarah Franklin's *Embodied Progress: A Cultural Account of Reproduction* (1997) and Charis Thompson's *Making Parents: The Ontological Choreography of Reproductive Technologies* (2005), but also a considerable number of other studies.[3] A starting point for this volume is instead a diverse European and global outlook through which we aim to provide a culturally grounded framework for reworking the perspectives that emerged out of the UK/US context, which formed the point of reference for much former theorizing about ARTs. This volume also distinguishes itself from previous cultural analyses of assisted reproduction beyond the US/UK context, which have had specific regional foci: on the Middle East and the Muslim world (Inhorn 2012), on Russia, Switzerland and Germany (de Jong and Tkach 2009), or on the non-western world more generally (Inhorn and van Balen 2002; Birenbaum-Carmeli and Inhorn 2009). While our book undoubtedly builds on the perspectives developed in previous research on ARTs, this volume differs from these predecessors in taking a diverse European perspective as its regional point of departure, and at the same time balancing this with a more global outlook. Our idea is that data gathered from this wide array of social, cultural, and geopolitical contexts are likely to generate different questions and issues than those to which previous research has drawn attention. We are searching for new perspectives on contemporary ART practices, looking for both local diversity and more general, global trends in how these technologies work at the societal, cultural, and personal levels.

When the introduction of and access to ARTs become topics of public debate, this generally concerns medical practice and ethics. The importance of cultural aspects, such as religion, myths, and origin stories in the domestication of reproductive technologies is seldom mentioned (Squier 1994). The studies in this volume display a wide variety of cultural differences in terms of access to ARTs, such as traditions relating to religion, kinship, gender relations, and sexualities. These are matters that both affect ART practices and are affected by them. This volume therefore focuses on how practices of ARTs vary in relation to the sociocultural context within which they are introduced, and discusses how power and normativity are both reproduced and undermined differently in different national and regional contexts. Moreover, the contributors demonstrate the adaptability of ART practices to varying national situations; for example, the different roles that ARTs may play in different kinds of religious fundamentalist societies as well as more secularized ones. Intersections of postcolonial, transnational, and queer feminist theories are mobilized to account for the complex interactions between local and global aspects of ARTs.

It is a challenge, though, to include both global and local perspectives and, to accomplish this, a multi-faceted approach is pertinent. We emphasize that ARTs need to be studied within their social and cultural contexts, but it is just as important to take into account the fact that they function within a global market, embedded in transnational geopolitics and post/colonial power structures. Moreover, the different legal frameworks regulating access to ARTs may be considered as cultural markers emphasizing distinctions that a nation may want to make visible. Some European countries, for example Germany, have comparatively strict laws on ARTs that have been supported by strong arguments against eugenics, as a counter-reaction to the country's Nazi past (Bock von Wülfingen, this volume). Jasanoff (2005) also argues that policies regulating the life sciences (in more general terms) have been incorporated into nation-building projects in order to symbolically illustrate what a nation stands for and contribute to the cultural image of a country. Ireland's anti-abortion laws spilling over into strong prolife attitudes – and a "moral veto" (McDonnell, this volume) of ART practices – may serve as an example.

The volume thus casts light upon the importance of the social and cultural contexts of ARTs within national contexts and, at the same time, it considers how these differences affect transnational transmissions. This includes ideas and values associated with notions of kinship and family, motherhood and fatherhood, nationhood and citizenship, geopolitical positioning and transnational mobility – i.e., ideas and values that resonate forcefully with ideas and values related to gender, ethnicity, race, and sexuality. Nation states have enacted legal regulations that vary across the globe and consequently a technique that is not legal in one country is accessible once borders are crossed. For example, both India and South Africa have become much-sought-after destinations for western middle-class people seeking egg donation and surrogacy (see Vora and Iyengar, Førde, and Namberger, this volume). However, the destinations of fertility travelers have shifted over time and, as this volume shows, such travelers have taken diverse routes. For example, Iran, as the first Islamic country to allow third-party gamete donation, has become a destination for fertility travelers in the Muslim world (see Mehrabi, this volume). The mechanisms that shape the foundations of a "donation" business[4] in a particular country are not uni-directional, and the reason why people in search of donors choose a particular country is not only the legal access to a specific treatment and its costs, but is also related to people's cultural perceptions of the country in question and its population (see Førde, Smietana, and Kroløkke, this volume).

Against this background, it is pertinent to reflect on the biopolitics of ARTs through the lens of a variety of policies, as well as considering legal and cultural frameworks from global, regional, and national perspectives. Europe makes an interesting case study here, because of the diversity of policies amongst its nations, varying in degree from restrictive regulations to practically no national legal frameworks at all. Still, the relationships between different countries are as important as their differences. National policies of regulating access to ARTs create points of reference for others as "good" or "immoral" examples. Furthermore, restrictive regulations in some countries are actively used as a market opportunity in others, generally initiated by private entrepreneurs. These relations between a commercial market and the most intimate areas of individuals' lives call for research across established academic boundaries. ARTs involve matters that, traditionally, have been considered culturally exempt from the monetary sphere, such as a child and a womb. Illicit trading of children has of course always existed, but today the many steps toward "making a baby" are specified in price-lists as a new repro-economics (Waldby and Mitchell 2006; Almeling 2011). This requires a perspective that combines local and cultural particularities with the realities of a global market, for instance asking how the global market for ARTs looks from a particular local perspective. In other words, what is considered to be within or out of reach – be it in moral, cultural, ethnic, racialized, or economic terms. It is thus pertinent to study these matters from the consumer's and the provider's side respectively, not seeking a kind of "unified" perspective (like the popular win-win model) but precisely to reveal the importance of situated knowledges. Within this local–global framework, the authors of this volume seek to find lenses through which to focus on the situation from different perspectives.

As ARTs have "matured," the medical procedures, legal regulations, and patterns of acceptance/rejection by different publics have changed over time, along with how ARTs are understood and integrated into the general perceptions of human reproduction. Over time, ever-new methods are introduced, meaning that more obstacles to fertility – sociocultural as well as biological – can be overcome and evermore people are able to conceive, personally or by surrogacy, a baby that carries their own genetic inheritance. This has resulted in changing policies and laws, and processes of "maturation" and "normalization," including evermore ARTs and new groups of users. But, as this volume shows, it has also given rise to new kinds of exclusion.

In Norway, for example, a few years ago a chief of police was exposed in the media because he and his male partner became parents through a surrogacy arrangement abroad. This caused a stir because surrogacy is forbidden in Norway, but at the same time, due to the support he received, the story was used to demonstrate Norwegian exceptionalism in terms of tolerance vis-à-vis gay fatherhood, what Jasbir Puar has aptly pinpointed as characteristic of western homonationalism (i.e., the showcasing of "modern tolerance and humanism" versus "more backwards others," Puar 2007; Petersen, Myong and Kroløkke, forthcoming). On the other hand, as discussed by Melhuus (this volume), Norwegian women who intend to become parents through surrogacy arrangements abroad, but without either using their own genetic material or teaming up with a man to act as the intending father, can easily find themselves in rather precarious and troubled situations when seeking to obtain Norwegian citizenship for the children. Mechanisms of exclusion, will affect the children who are born out of these particular surrogacy arrangements. Moreover, the Indian women who carry out the reproductive labor for a new citizen in another country, as pointed out by Vora and Iyengar (this volume), are entirely ineligible for citizenship in the same country and the benefits following from it.

We may well ask whether fertility travel and ART practices such as surrogacy are in the process of becoming included in what are considered to be normal and morally acceptable ways of having a baby, at least amongst parts of an affluent, transnationally oriented, urban middle class. We may also ask whether a "normalization" of diversity in terms of a broadening of the notion of the family to include new queer family types – celebrated as well as deplored as a consequence of ARTs – is occurring, at least in some more secular countries and contexts. But we find it just as important to ask whether ART practices are embedded in processes of exclusion and othering that reinforce global inequalities, colonial legacies and the stigmatization of non-normative lifestyles and sexualities, reminiscent of the notion of "stratified reproduction," "...an idea developed by Shellee Colen, to describe the power relations by which some categories of people are empowered to nurture and reproduce, while others are disempowered" (Ginsburg and Rapp 1995, 3). This illuminates the question with which we began; namely, whether these technologies are liberating or not, from feminist perspectives. Going back to Firestone's ideas from 1971, she argued in favor of technologies that would liberate women from childbirth. The ways in which ARTs are put into practice today, rather than freeing women from childbirth, have made it a possibility for more women. Moreover, ARTs have opened the way for fatherhood without a female partner, but a "body with a womb" is still needed to bear the children. Today, the negotiations taking place around who will have access to ARTs have replaced previous feminist struggles against technoscience gaining control over women's bodies, and the unequal power relations that characterize the transnational trafficking in gametes and gestational labor have erased all claims of reproduction being a common ground for women worldwide.

Contents of the Volume

To accomplish the aims we have outlined, the research contributions gathered in this volume scrutinize the ways in which ARTs have given rise to an expanding global market for intensive transnational traffic in human gametes, embryos, and gestational labor and how this reflects unequal global power relations. Moreover, the volume focuses on the functions, regulations, and discourses of ARTs in different national and regional contexts, in Europe and beyond. The volume covers countries with more liberal or "permissive" laws, policies, and approaches to ARTs (Denmark, Finland) as well as more conservative ones (Norway, Germany). This includes countries where various kinds of religious fundamentalism (Christian, e.g., Poland and Ireland, as well as Muslim, e.g., Iran) influence state policies and mainstream public opinion. The ways in which ART practices and policies can become entangled in different ways with nationalist projects and demographic agendas are also highlighted, demonstrating, for example, how ARTs are mobilized as part of the conflict between Israel and Palestine, or in paradoxical ways are both affirmed and denied as means to overcome demographic crises in Russia and Ukraine.

The chapters in this volume provide empirical material from a range of countries, giving evidence of how differently ARTs are interpreted and practiced, and often bringing together different perspectives on the very same matters; for example, by discussing surrogacy practices from the perspective of the global South as well as the global North. Some chapters in the volume approach these exchanges and what they involve in historical, racial, and legal terms. Other chapters use personal stories to illuminate what is taken into consideration and what factors are out of bounds, so to speak, or perhaps considered too difficult to involve at the individual level.

Even though all the contributions highlight perspectives that are situated in specific national, regional, or transnational contexts, the overall ambition of the volume is to reflect on and theorize general trends in contemporary ART practices, policies, and discourses. In this sense, it is intended neither to give an exhaustive country-by-country account, nor to present a mere report on the state of the art of ARTs in various countries. All the contributions combine the presentation of specific contexts with theoretical reflections on the shifting meanings, materialities, and (bio)politics of ARTs in the contemporary world. Through these reflections, the volume will emphasize that, even though ARTs today are solidly founded in standardized and routinized biomedical procedures and practices, their performative effects, their entanglement in global and local power relations, and their way of reinforcing or deconstructing intersecting power differentials are by no means clear or given. As theorized by Kristin Spilker (this volume), ARTs are tricksters and, as Donna Haraway taught us, when tricksters break loose, "there are always more things going on than you thought" (Haraway 2004, 321).

In line with these overall reflections on the content of the volume, it is organized into five main parts corresponding to five themes: transnational reproflows, national constraints and conditions, religious and other kinds of fundamentalism, demographic agendas and biopolitics, and the "new normals" and their discontents.

Transnational Reproflows

Part I, "ARTs in a Neoliberal World of Transnational Reproflows", focuses on overall global perspectives: the expanding transnational traffic in human gametes, embryos, and gestational labor – what Marcia Inhorn has termed "reproflows" to capture the transnational movements of "reproductive exiles," i.e., people crossing borders in search of reproductive "assistance" or as reproductive "assistors" (Inhorn 2010, 184). From different angles and locations, the contributors scrutinize this traffic and the ways in which it is governed by the entangled logics of geopolitical inequalities, global neoliberal markets, and exclusionary national regulations. For example, in recent years, India has become a global hotspot for surrogacy arrangements between low-income Indian women and people from a long list of countries in North America and Europe as well as Australia, Israel, Taiwan, Japan, Pakistan, Bangladesh, Tanzania, Nigeria, and Ethiopia (see Vora and Iyengar, this volume). These arrangements have become a profitable business for local Indian companies. The chapters contribute with ethnographic material from North and South and with different perspectives on the negotiations and accommodations that are taking place. The relations between US citizens and Indian surrogacy are analyzed in the light of a history of racialization, slavery, and access to citizenship, whereas the approach utilized in studying those who travel *to* India is to investigate how they negotiate understandings of ethics in this field. Research on those who are on the receiving side reveals how ethics is balanced against feelings of being victimized, and how ethics is negotiated primarily in terms of kin and neighbors – related to the situation of coming home with a baby – and less to the situation in the country where the exchange takes place. However, it is not only citizenship, politics, and ethics that are vital in these exchanges, but also economics, for the countries receiving the fertility travelers, and for the choice of where to go. This is an aspect which is often overlooked in debates on ARTs where, for example, the issue of the donation of gametes, eggs in particular, is usually embedded in discourses of altruism. Instead of under-communicating the commercial aspects, it is of vital importance to take bioeconomic frameworks into account in analyses of ARTs. This is spelled out in the case of South Africa, which over the last decade has become a global hub for fertility travel and a thriving market for the provision of donor eggs and embryos. Cultural perceptions of donors and surrogates are also vital for the choices made by prospective parents, and so are matters of racialization and stereotypes – from the gratified "a baby that looks like us" to the overt grading of prices for gametes according to the provider's skin color and national background.

Chapter 1, "Citizen, Subject, Property: Indian Surrogacy and the Global Fertility Market," by Kalindi Vora and Malathi Michelle Iyengar, University of California, San Diego, USA, casts a critical eye over the way in which India has become one of the central nodes for transnational surrogacy arrangements. The focus of the chapter is relations with US clients, framed as a discussion of the ways in which the exploitation of the gestational labor of poor Indian women in precarious situations is related in terms of genealogies to the history of slavery and structural racism in the USA. In this context, Vora and Iyengar draw on Marx's labor theory, Aihwa Ong's (1999) discussion of "flexible," i.e., unstable and context-dependent, citizenship, and engage in a discussion of the long-term effects of the historical institutionalization of property rights in the USA along racialized lines, that is, "whiteness as property" (Harris 1993). These concepts are mobilized in order to critically examine how Indian surrogate mothers are producing citizenship for others, but not for themselves.

Chapter 2, "Fair Play in a Dirty Field? The Ethical Work of Commissioning Surrogacy in India," by Kristin Engh Førde, University of Oslo, Norway, turns her gaze in the opposite direction to look at western couples, in this case heterosexual and (male) same-sex Scandinavian couples, who have engaged in surrogacy arrangements with Indian companies. The chapter highlights the moral dilemmas which these arrangements force open for the middle-class couples from Scandinavian welfare states, with their high stakes in egalitarian values. The main focus for these couples is to negotiate self-images that live up to what they consider to be decent moral standards of equality and humaneness, when confronted with situations of deep structural inequality. The author employs recent anthropological theories of ethics in trying to grasp how the couples construct an understanding of themselves as morally "good" subjects by displacing the problems of inequality, viewing them as internal Indian ones, and thus avoiding any need to address the historical and geopolitical power relations outlined in the previous chapter.

Chapter 3, "'Families Like We'd Always Known'? Spanish Gay Fathers' Normalization Narratives in Transnational Surrogacy," by Marcin Smietana, University of California, Berkeley, USA, and University of Cambridge, UK, focuses on gay fathers from Spain, who perceive it as morally and culturally preferable to engage in surrogacy arrangements in the USA rather than, for example, India. Smietana discusses the normalizing discourses of the interviewees, their wish to build families like the ones "we'd always known" versus the ways in which the interviewees feel that they are being singled out and discriminated against by Spanish legislation. Since 2005, Spain has allowed same-sex couples to marry, but has provided no legal regulations for gay fatherhood. This means that surrogacy arrangements are in principle declared legally non-valid, with far-reaching implications for both parents and children.

Chapter 4, "Destination Spain: Negotiating Nationality and Fertility when Traveling for Eggs," by Charlotte Kroløkke, University of Southern Denmark, shifts the focus from surrogacy to transnational traffic in human eggs and embryos. With an intra-European focus on Danish fertility travel to Spain, Kroløkke shows that in both countries egg donation is handled through a dominant discourse of altruism. However, there is a difference between the Danish and Spanish contexts, in that equality in terms of the right to have a child plays a big role in Denmark, while maternal rights are highlighted in the Spanish context. A key point of the chapter is to emphasize the essentialized understandings of the ways in which eggs are supposed to embody intersections of femininity with national and ethnic stereotypes. In the discourses of the interviewees, for example, exoticized and essentializing notions of Spanish hyper-femininity are constructed as a basis for empowerment and compared to less empowered and "exploited" "eastern European" femininities.

Chapter 5, "The South African Economy of Egg Donation: Looking at the BioEconomic Side of Normalization," by Verena Namberger, Humboldt University, Berlin, turns to South Africa, another global hotspot for fertility travel. The focus is on South African egg provision agencies and the expanding online market for human eggs and embryos. Based on ethnographic fieldwork, the author argues that the "success story" and maturation of a thriving egg provision business in South Africa needs to be understood as a complex interplay of sociocultural and economic aspects, because not only technologies but also business models travel. The chapter explores the characteristics of the South African market – advertising its "racially diverse donor pool" and "first-world medical standards" – by unraveling the industry's logic(s) of value based on strategies of discursive naturalization, consumerism, and a politics of normalization. Namberger sketches the egg provision business as a "normalized," bioeconomic realm where new relations of reproduction co-emerge and existing norms of (paid) labor related to gender, race, and kinship are renegotiated as part of the process.

National Constraints and Conditions

Part II: "Perplexed State Regulations, Legal Inconsistencies and Cultural Tricksters." While Part I deals with the transnational reproflows that are emerging due to national constraints and conditions, Part II scrutinizes these constraints and conditions with a special focus on legal issues, shifting regimes of regulation, and the paradoxes they often seem to generate. Contributors explore how different kinds of national regulations, embedded in institutionalized discursive regimes, are implemented in order to come to terms with the diversity of new reproductive practices made possible by ARTs. The authors discuss the specifics of different national situations, while also making it clear that the expanding spectrum of new reproductive and family-building practices, which ARTs at least potentially sustain and make possible, share an ability to cause perplexity and uncertainty among national-level legislators, and can give rise to powerful legal inconsistencies and contradictions, as well as political disruptions and U-turns.

Reproduction, in addition to "making children" and "making parents," also creates bonds between people. These bonds transform the parents (regardless of their sex) from a couple into a family, connect relatives from the two sides, and confirm and strengthen links of kinship (Carsten 2004). These "blood ties" are increasingly transgressing national borders because transnational migration disperses kin across the globe, whereas the global links created by children born by gamete donation and surrogacy are usually cut off, either by the agencies organizing the exchange or deliberately so by the new parents. Out of these exchanges arises a need for legal and social relationships that recognize new forms of biological citizenship (Rose and Novas 2005). This gives rise to paradoxical legal situations in which, out of tradition, genetic relations are still given priority but these are modified to make room for non-genetic relations. As already mentioned, Vora and Iyengar point out that a surrogate mother can give birth to a US citizen while herself remaining cut off from that same citizenship. A child can be conceived using gametes from providers of two different nationalities and be born into another, and the legal regulations pertaining to citizenship have not caught up with these developments in ways that take into account the donors, the intending parents, and the children. This may create new notions of "illicit" children, which Melhuus (this volume) points out as being a serious problem. Until now, questions of filiation and citizenship have been organized partly by interim and often conflicting regulations, partly by private initiatives challenging the legal regulations, and sometimes they are not really organized at all but fall into place via unruly trickster happenings that create enrollments and associations not actually planned for.

Chapter 6, "Governing New Reproductive Technologies across Western Europe: The Gender Dimension," by Isabelle Engeli, University of Ottawa,

Canada, and Christine Rothmayr Allison, University of Montreal, Canada, gives an overview of the legal frameworks regulating ARTs in a Western European context. The chapter builds on a comparative analysis of ART policies and regulations in 16 western European countries over time, highlighting three main issues: (1) the degree of autonomy granted to the medical community in terms of practicing ARTs, (2) the restrictions placed on access to ARTs, and (3) the availability of healthcare coverage. Against this background, Engeli and Rothmayr Allison demonstrate that the policies of these 16 countries can reasonably be sorted into three categories: "restrictive," "permissive," and "intermediate," the latter combining features of the first two. Through the chapter's comparative overview, it becomes possible to see how interactions between different key actors – the medical establishment, governments, and citizens in general, as well as queer groups and women's movements – and their relative strength vis-à-vis each other, play an important role in terms of setting national agendas and constructing legal frameworks for ARTs.

Chapter 7, "Norwegian Biopolitics in the First Decade of the 2000s: Family Politics and Assisted Reproduction Understood through the Concept of the Trickster," by Kristin Spilker, Norwegian University of Science and Technology/NTNU, Norway, focuses on a specific example: Norway. Spilker shows how the restrictive Norwegian legal framework is challenged, not only by the alternative family-building practices made possible by ARTs, but also by discursive contradictions and disruptions within the legal frameworks themselves. Spilker employs Donna Haraway's figuration of the trickster – a mythological figure embodying undecidability and in-betweenness – to theorize national-level tensions and paradoxes within ART policies and practices in Norway. With the trickster as theoretical tool, Spilker explores the disruptive effects of a clash between the different discursive regimes governing Norwegian biopolitics and family politics. She highlights the processes of discursive displacement, sliding, and disruption occurring within the legal frameworks, and the chapter spells out how tricksters seem to haunt Norway, an icon of a modern, semi-secular western welfare democracy with strong claims to equality.

Chapter 8, "Bringing it All Back Home: Cross-Border Procreative Practices. Examples from Norway," by Marit Melhuus, University of Oslo, Norway, continues to reflect on the Norwegian example. While the main focus of the previous chapter was clashes occurring within the framework of the legal discourses themselves, this chapter investigates the ways in which the reproductive practices of alternative families trouble and challenge the legal frameworks. Following up on the discussions of surrogacy in Part I of this volume, the chapter focuses on the ways in which transnational surrogacy arrangements initiated by Norwegian citizens who afterwards return with their babies expose gaps and inconsistencies in Norwegian legislation. Norwegian regulation of ARTs takes a restrictive approach, *inter alia* forbidding egg donation and surrogacy, although not making it illegal for Norwegian citizens to seek donors and surrogate arrangements in other countries. Melhuus discusses how the new reproductive practices clash with the national legal framework, disrupting and displacing conventional understandings of biogenetic filiation and definitions of children's rights to citizenship and legal parenthood.

Chapter 9, "Finland as a Late Regulator of Assisted Reproduction: A Permissive Policy under Debate," by Lise Eriksson, Åbo Academy University, Finland, reveals how Finland, a country that sits well within the framework of modern western semi-secular welfare democracies, is counted among the more permissive countries of Europe when it comes to ART legislation and practices. It is also a country that regulated ARTs very late compared to other Nordic countries with comparable welfare regimes. But, as Eriksson underlines, the Finnish situation is more complex than an analysis of the law as such and the liberal practices of clinics might suggest, particularly before the first Finnish Act on Assisted Reproduction was enacted in 2007. There is a significant difference between the wording of the actual act, and the heated debates that preceded its being approved by the Finnish Parliament. Eriksson shows how, to a large extent, the debates framed childlessness as a medical problem, excluding social aspects, making queer and other alternative families' use of ARTs dubious, and problematizing equality in terms of both eligibility and access. She also demonstrates how conservative religious views impacted on the debate.

Religious and Other Kinds of Fundamentalism

Part III, "Religious Fundamentalism, Humanist Values, and State Dilemmas in an Era of Technological Monsters," shifts the focus from national-level perplexities in more secular states to state contexts that are more strongly and explicitly embedded in different kinds of fundamentalism, primarily of a religious nature, but in some cases (e.g., Germany) also influenced by the value systems of classic humanist philosophy. In these contexts, ARTs are considered to be a kind of monster technology which threatens "natural" conception, heteronormative and patriarchal family-building, and notions of human life beginning at conception. As the contributions demonstrate, the perceived monstrous potentialities of ARTs seem to produce catch-22 situations for legislators. Difficulties with aligning the interests of creating "mother, father, child" families while preventing other kinds of family-building contribute to ambiguous legal constructions. Some countries with restrictive legislation based on religious values have some of the highest rates in the world of fertility travel to other countries – thus, paradoxically, they are not able to restrict the number of babies conceived by "artificial" means or within unconventional family structures by their citizens. The analyses in this section show that a shared feature is the ways in which state policies that are ideologically shaped by fundamentalist religiosities, whether Muslim or Christian, try to address the complex reproductive possibilities opened up by ARTs in a way that preserves rather than disrupts traditional family and kinship structures. But again, these efforts have generated contradictions and unintended side effects of trickster qualities, *inter alia* because of strong national interests in making progress within biotech science and medicine.

Chapter 10, "Reframing Conception, Reproducing Society: Italian Paradoxes," by Manuela Perrotta, Queen Mary University of London, UK, analyzes the blatant paradoxes that characterize the Italian situation regarding ARTs. In Italy, the Catholic Church has had a strong influence on the framing of ART regulations, and Perrotta notes that this has become even stronger over the past few decades, filling an ideological vacuum after the disappearance of the Italian Christian Democratic Party in 1994. Italy enacted its first law on ARTs in 2004. Before this, an image of Italy as a "test-tube Wild West" was created by incidents such as the media sensation of a 63-year-old woman who was impregnated using controversial ART practices. However, as Perrotta shows, there was a stark contrast between the media stories and the actual regulations and practices that existed in Italian infertility clinics. Even before the law, these regulations and practices were generally very conservative, strongly reinforcing traditional heteronormative family ideologies and sustaining "prolife" arguments prioritizing the rights of embryos over those of women. One of the paradoxes is that Italy also has a very high rate of fertility travel to other countries, so, as Perrotta argues, a large proportion of the population does not seem to let itself be controlled by the restrictive legislation and its moral underpinnings.

Chapter 11, "The Veto of Moral Politics: The Catholic Church and ARTs in Ireland," by Orla McDonnell, University of Limerick, Ireland, focuses on Ireland as another example of a national context in which the Catholic Church plays a major role. Although the influence of the Church has decreased, Catholic moral beliefs maintain a firm grip on state policies and national identities, profiling them along the lines of the "natural" family. For many years, this resulted in an impasse – what McDonnell describes as a situation of "moral veto" – which until very recently prevented anything from happening in the field of ARTs beyond maintaining a status quo which has served to underpin the image of Ireland as a nation committed to traditional heterosexual family values and a firm prolife ethics. McDonnell describes how, for a long time, a clash of values led successive governments to refrain from setting up an overall regulatory framework for ARTs, shying away from stirring up a confrontational public debate between Catholic defenders of a prolife stance and the "natural" family, and an opposing camp arguing for equality and the legitimacy of different family types (e.g., LGBTQ families). One result of this long-lived "passive" state policy, leaving the government prone to non-intervention, is that fertility clinics were left to self-regulate, and a new law enacted in 2015 which introduces legal regulation of the area only does so in a limited and partial way.

Chapter 12, "Desiring Bodies: Problematizing the Matter of ARTs in Poland," by Edyta Just, Linköping University, Sweden, discusses yet another case in which Catholic fundamentalism has had a major impact on the politics of ARTs. In parallel with Ireland, the situation in Poland was also characterized for a number of years by the lack of a legislative framework, and a political inertia generated by a very similar kind of moral veto and political reluctance to confront the issue as that described by McDonnell in the previous chapter. Still, in 2013, the Polish government launched an ART program intended as a possible pilot scheme for future legislation, and in the summer of 2015 a law on ARTs was passed addressing heterosexual couples with diagnosed medical infertility. As well as giving an overview of the Polish situation, Just's main focus is to confront one of the Vatican's key arguments against ARTs, namely that ART practices undermine the idea that conception is based on a loving, bodily-affective encounter. With a theoretical point of departure in the philosophy and ethics of Gilles Deleuze and Félix Guattari (1987), Just argues that affective and embodied processes of a shared becoming as parents can indeed take place for couples during ART procedures. She illustrates this through an example from her interview material of Polish heterosexual couples undergoing IVF treatment.

In Chapter 13, "Germany goes PGD: The Appeal to Women's and Human Rights Discourse in the Paradigmatic Amendment to the German Embryo Protection Act," Bettina Bock von Wülfingen, Humboldt University, Berlin, shifts the focus to Germany, which in terms of religious beliefs is split between a more Catholic south and a more Protestant north, with the former East Germany being influenced by a secular Marxist tradition. Of particular importance is the presence of strong Christian Democratic political parties and a humanist tradition that draws on Kantian notions of fundamental human exceptionalism, mobilized in postwar Germany against the dehumanization of the Nazi past. Against this background, ARTs have in general been handled very restrictively. But, in contrast to the kind of moral veto causing political inertia in other countries influenced by Catholicism, such as Italy, Ireland, and Poland, Germany regulated ARTs early, enacting a very strict Embryo Protection Act in 1990. This restrictive approach to ARTs should also be understood against the background of feminist movements and feminist researchers arguing strongly against ARTs. However, a paradigm shift took place during the late 2000s, leading to a radical revision of the Act in 2011, shifting from the prioritizing of the rights of the embryo (potentially in conflict with those of its mother) to those of the intending parents. Against a background of pressure from medical and pharmaceutical actors in favor of a more flexible way of treating the embryo, the chapter shows how earlier feminist discourses, related to abortion and anti-sterilization campaigns for women's basic rights to self-determination and reproductive choice, were used to accommodate arguments in favor of PGD (Preimplantation genetic diagnosis), and the rights of the intending parents.

In Chapter 14, "Matters of Donation and Preserved Relations: Co-Construction of Egg Donation and Family Structures in Iran", Tara Mehrabi, Linköping University, Sweden, takes us to Iran, another country where religion, in this case Shi'ite Islam, determines the politics and practices of ARTs. Iran is the first and, together with Lebanon, so far the only Islamic country to allow third-party gamete donation (since 2003), including medical practices that facilitate the use of ARTs, such as cryopreservation. However, Mehrabi also discusses how, in the absence of straightforward legislation on egg and sperm donation, clinics and infertile couples in Iran are relying mostly on the religious authorities and their fatwas, a majority of which sees sperm donation as incompatible with Islamic understandings of the key role of biological fatherhood, paternal genes, and blood-lines in the construction of kinship, while egg and embryo donation faces less restrictions from these religious authorities. Mehrabi combines multi-site fieldwork material with an analysis of the biopolitics of the Iranian theocracy, discussing dilemmas and paradoxes caused by ART practices both at the level of the state and from the perspective of women seeking infertility treatment. The chapter is based on fieldwork and interviews with religious Iranian women considering making use of egg donation at infertility clinics in Tehran. Mehrabi's main focus is how processes of Islamization and ARTs practices mutually co-construct each other.

Demographic Agendas and Biopolitics

Part IV, "ARTs as Eentangled in Demographic Agendas and Biopolitics," focuses on different kinds of biopolitical entanglements of ARTs, demographic policies, nationalisms, and normativities. Contributors explore how different aspects of biopolitics are being appropriated, resisted, or problematized within the framework of national projects. Warnings about a demographic crisis have been discussed in the countries of the European Union, based on a declining birthrate, a trend toward postponing the first pregnancy, and an increasing number of one-child families and singles who do not intend to procreate (Douglass 2005; Ellingsæter *et al.* 2013). These discussions have been even more outspoken in Russia and other states that formerly belonged to the Soviet Union, such as Ukraine. In Russia, the number of deaths started to drastically outpace the number of births in the early 1990s, attributed not only to a declining birth rate and the world's highest abortion rate, but also to increasing numbers of premature deaths due to poor health conditions and limited healthcare provision (DaVanzo and Adamson 1997). These discussions have paved the way for pronatalist policies and have also created tensions between restrictive views on ARTs and a strong impetus to encourage citizens to engage in (traditional) family-building. Ironically, social groups whose family-building has not traditionally been looked upon as socially acceptable, such as single people and same-sex couples, might contribute to more births through ART practices, but they are often excluded from these by national legislation. Current political negotiations in Russia about restrictions of access to ARTs, as illustrated in the last chapter of this part, are a case in point. The analysis of ARTs through the lens of biopolitics reveals how they are paradoxically being employed as technologies of gender and sexuality, reinforcing stereotypes and conservative and heteronormative family values (see Franklin 2013). However, as the first chapter of this part illustrates, demography is not only included in general national policies but is also involved in political struggles, such as that between Israel and Palestine.

Chapter 15, "Babies from Behind Bars: Stratified Assisted Reproduction in Palestine/Israel," by Sigrid Vertommen, Ghent University, Belgium, looks at how ARTs have become a tool in the conflict between Israel and Palestine. Vertommen focuses on the ways in which ARTs and the smuggling of sperm from

Palestinian political prisoners who are denied conjugal visits in Israeli prisons are used as an act of resistance on the part of the prisoners and their wives. She frames the discussion within an analysis of Israeli biopolitics and the regulation of ARTs, which she defines as grounded not only in a nationalist, but also in a Zionist, settler-colonial demographic logic. She shows how Israeli ART politics is extremely liberal, permitting the use of different ART practices and giving every Israeli citizen, irrespective of religion or marital status, full economic support for an unlimited number of IVF cycles until two live births have been achieved within the current relationship. Against this background, Israelis have become the biggest consumers of ARTs in the world. However, Vertommen argues that the apparent equality built into this regulatory framework should be seen as entangled with overall settler-colonial goals and a settler-colonial ideology bent on promoting Jewish-Israeli births, while preventing Palestinian ones.

Chapter 16, "From Precarity to Self-Governance: Performing Motherhood through IVF Treatment in Ukraine," by Polina Vlasenko, Indiana University, USA, discusses how the demographic crisis in Ukraine due to the decreasing birthrate has prompted successive governments to take a pronatalist stance, embedded in a strongly gender-conservative biopolitical rhetoric of promoting traditional family values, but also pinpointing the declining birthrate as a threat to national security. As far as ART policies are concerned, the situation has led to a liberal and permissive approach in the sense that ARTs are, to a large extent, unregulated. As the practice of ARTs is also predominantly left to private clinics, these practices have become commodified, which has led to them being too costly for most Ukrainian women, while, at the same time, the country has become a destination for fertility travel. Vlasenko discusses this rather messy situation, taking her point of departure in an understanding of the situation as framed by a biopolitical governmentality and notions of precarity. Pronatalist stances, combined with a gender-conservative rhetoric, make individual women responsible for remedying the demographic crisis through a self-styled urge to become mothers at any cost, including doing their utmost to conceive a child through ARTs, should they be diagnosed as infertile.

Chapter 17, "Russian Legislative Practices and Debates on the Restriction of Wide Access to ARTs," by Maria Kirpichenko, Norwegian University of Science and Technology/NTNU, Norway, scrutinizes another case of demographic crisis, prompting governmental pronatalism in combination with a gender-conservative and strongly homophobic focus on traditional family values in Russia. The chapter demonstrates how current Russian parliamentary debates on these issues are based on sharp demarcations between their own stance and "western" decadence, which is associated among other things with ART practices that make alternative family-building possible, while, paradoxically, western practices are also highlighted as a model to be followed when it comes to the restrictive regulation of surrogacy. Moreover, Kirpichenko explores the growing political influence of the Orthodox Church, which involves attempts to revitalize the cultural-national values of pre-Soviet Russia. In terms of ART policies, this means that the days of the current permissive and liberal state of the art, characterized by effectively no legal limits to access on either medical or social grounds, seem to be numbered.

"New Normals" and their Discontents

In Part V, "'New Normals' and their Discontents" – the last section of the volume – we take a look at some examples of normalization and discuss the kinds of "new normals" that can arise when ARTs become uncontroversial and accepted. A major concern throughout the volume so far has been the contradictions and clashes that occur between the wide range of reproductive possibilities opened up by ARTs and the ways in which they are being exploited in a context of neoliberal global consumerism and geopolitical inequalities. Contributors have amply demonstrated how ARTs are simultaneously being restricted in some countries by state regulations and cultural and religious belief systems, while being appropriated as technologies of settler-colonialism, nationhood, and traditional family values in others. We began this introduction by asking whether ARTs have become not only routinized as standard procedures, but also normalized. Seen against the background of the analyses of contradictions and clashes, normalization is not an apt term. ARTs have certainly become routinized as a standard medical practice, but in many countries and contexts they are definitely not normalized as uncontroversial and generally accepted procedures, smoothly made accessible to all citizens.

However, in some delimited cultural contexts, ARTs have, indeed, become normalized as an uncontroversial way to have children, and in the last part of this volume we will take a look at what happens in such contexts of normalization. Four case studies are discussed: the so-called "lesbian baby boom" as framed in popular culture in film and on TV; how IVF may be accepted to the extent that it is culturally included as a normal, even "natural" route to pregnancy; sperm banking as naturalizing or possibly de-naturalizing the link between sperm and paternity; and finally, how the recently introduced technology of Time-Lapse Embryo Imaging may challenge traditional human origin stories and pave the way for new ones. Each in their own way, these four case studies exemplify what normalization processes may imply, and how the "new normals" give rise to new constraints, troubles, and discontents.

Thus, it is *not* our conclusion that the normalization of ARTs is a general trend. We understand the "new normals" and the four chapters of Part V dealing with them to be articulations of specific and limited situations and locations where ARTs have become a normalized practice. However, it is still interesting to compare these final chapters with the previous ones and their discussions of strategies of resistance as well as restriction. We draw attention to these webs of forces and counter-forces in processes of normalization that take place over time, engendering "new normals," producing their own discontents and disruptions. It is the complex character of ARTs and the vital matters involved that over and over again invoke new tricksters.

Chapter 18, "Lesbian Kinship and ARTs in American Popular Culture: *The L Word* and *The Kids Are All Right*," by Julianne Pidduck, University of Montreal, Canada, discusses two popular fictional representations from the USA: the TV series *The L Word*, and the film *The Kids Are All Right*, both related to the "lesbian baby boom" – understood as a "new normal" which has characterized recent decades, beginning in the 1980s and increasingly facilitated by ARTs. Pidduck shows how the two productions, directed by established lesbian cultural producers, Ilene Chaikin and Lisa Cholodenko, respectively, portray lesbian uses of ARTs, queer female sexuality, and motherhood as normal and everyday phenomena. Both productions take for granted the access of their affluent middle-class lesbian protagonists to ARTs on a privately financed basis, and in this sense ARTs are normalized as an unproblematic precondition. Instead of taking ARTs as their focus, the plots of these productions revolve around other tensions that are related to ARTs as a normalized practice within lesbian family-building, such as the issue of finding a suitable sperm donor who does not want to claim fatherhood status. Another plot explores the problem of teenage children rebelling against their lesbian mothers by tracing and starting up a familial relationship with their sperm donor.

In Chapter 19, "Naturalization and Un-Naturalization: ARTs, Childlessness and Choice," Malin Noem Ravn, Norwegian University of Science and Technology/NTNU, Norway, looks at another "new normal" emerging as an outcome of the normalization and naturalization of ARTs. She uses an interview that was part of a broader project on gender, genes, and reproduction in Norway to discuss the ways in which the choice of IVF for an infertile heterosexual couple is considered normal and "conspicuously unprovocative." As Ravn points out, it is precisely this totally uncontroversial status which characterizes the case and makes it interesting. Using IVF is perceived by women such as this interviewee to be a self-evident and "naturalized" way to become pregnant and to experience pregnancy and motherhood – so self-evident and "naturalized" that the discourses the interviewee taps into when explaining her choices and desires unintentionally denaturalize other kinds of choices, in particular the choice to remain childless and *not* try the three IVF cycles that are offered free by the Norwegian public healthcare system.

In Chapter 20, "Sperm Stories: Sociotechnical Imaginaries of Sperm Donation and Sperm Banking in Denmark," Stine Willum Adrian, University of Aalborg, Denmark, continues the discussion of the ways in which the "new normals" may sustain stigmatizing and exclusionary discourses. Her analysis addresses the sperm donation business, taking as examples commercial Danish sperm banks operating on the global market, and an alternative, private, midwife-owned fertility clinic, originally set up to support queer family-building during the decade when Danish law prevented medical doctors from providing assisted reproduction to anyone except heterosexual couples. The focus of the analysis is sociotechnical imaginaries: how do the sperm bank and the alternative fertility clinic narrate and visualize stories of sperm donation? Adrian studies how narrations and visualizations reinforce or deconstruct stereotypes such as the hyper-masculine and hyper-fertile sperm donor, which collapse fertility, sexual potency, and fatherhood into one another, stigmatizing infertile men as well as lesbians and single women seeking to conceive via ARTs. Adrian demonstrates how "new normals" are being produced and challenged, but also how other stories of the making of kin are possible, for example stories that deconstruct the naturalized link between sperm and fatherhood, or query the image of the sperm donor as "invulnerable superman."

Finally, in Chapter 21, "Cellular Origins: A Visual Analysis of Time-Lapse Embryo Imaging," Lucy van de Wiel, University of Amsterdam, The Netherlands, takes the issue of the "new normal" to the embryonic level. She discusses a new technology for embryo selection which has recently been widely adopted in UK fertility clinics: time-lapse embryo imaging. This technique, which represents a non-invasive method of embryo selection, involves the close observation of early embryonic development in vitro, in order to select embryos for implantation in the womb. This is done on the basis of an evaluation of individual embryonic growth patterns against parameters based on the previous growth patterns of embryos that developed into healthy fetuses. Tentatively hailed by the scientific and clinical community as a paradigmatic shift in IVF, time-lapse imaging produces new visual mediations of extracorporeal embryos and foregrounds temporal parameters as key indicators in embryo selection. In her analysis of time-lapse embryo imaging, van de Wiel distinguishes three approaches to visualizing embryos: as individuals, collectives, and populations, and she considers what the implications may be if time-lapse imaging becomes the "new normal" in embryo selection. Van de Wiel suggests that such imaging is instrumental in a contemporary rewriting of human origin stories by shifting the value ascribed to early cell divisions and thus destabilizing fixed notions of what counts as life.

Notes

1 The alphabetical order of names of the two authors and editors means that we have contributed equally, and does not refer to a first or second author.

2 FINRRAGE – Feminist International Network of Resistance to Reproductive and Genetic Engineering. The network was started at a worldwide feminist conference in Groningen in 1984 as a protest against reproductive and genetic engineering, which were seen as instruments for exploitation of women's bodies, and reflected as harmful to women worldwide.

3 We could mention a range of studies from the USA and UK, such as Stanworth 1987, Strathern 1992, Ginsburg and Rapp 1995, Clarke 1998, Edwards 1999, Becker 2000, Franklin 2013.

4 We use the term "egg donation" in quotation marks to indicate that, on the one hand, this is the term generally used, while, on the other hand, it obscures the fact that money is often deeply involved, for example when it comes to international fertility travel and trafficking in gametes. In her doctoral dissertation on ARTs, our linguistic reviser, Liz Sourbut, has suggested the alternative term "egg provision," covering both donation proper and sale (Sourbut 2009, 83).

References

Almeling, Rene. 2011. *Sex Cells: The Medical Market for Eggs and Sperm.* Berkeley: University of California Press.

Becker, Gay. 2000. *The Elusive Embryo: How Women and Men Approach the New Reproductive Technologies.* Berkeley: University of California Press.

Birenbaum-Carmeli, Daphna, and Marcia Inhorn, eds. 2009. *Assisting Reproduction, Testing Genes: Global Encounters with New Biotechnologies.* New York, Oxford: Berghahn Books.

Carsten, Janet. 2004. *After Kinship.* Cambridge and New York: Cambridge University Press.

Clarke, Adele. 1998. *Disciplining Reproduction: Modernity, American Life Sciences, and the Problems of Sex.* Berkeley: University of California Press.

DaVanzo, Julie, and David Adamson. 1997. "Russia's Demographic 'Crisis': How Real Is It?" *Rand Issue Paper 162.* Santa Monica, California, USA: Rand Corporation. Accessed December 19, 2015. www.rand.org/pubs/issue_papers/IP162/index2.html.

Deleuze, Gilles, and Félix Guattari. 1987. *Thousands Plateaus, Capitalism and Schizophrenia.* London, New York: Continuum.

Douglass, Carrie B., ed. 2005. *Barren States: The Population "Implosion" in Europe.* Oxford, New York: Berg.

Edwards, Jeanette. 1999. *Technologies of Procreation: Kinship in the Age of Assisted Conception.* London: Routledge.

Ellingsæter, Anne L., An-Magritt Jensen, and Merete Lie, eds. 2013. *The Social Meaning of Children and Fertility Change in Europe.* London, New York: Routledge.

Firestone, Shulamith. 1971. *The Dialectic of Sex.* New York: Bantam.

Foucault, Michel. 1979. *The Will to Knowledge: The History of Sexuality.* London: Penguin.

Franklin, Sarah. 1997. *Embodied Progress: A Cultural Account of Assisted Conception.* New York and London: Routledge.

Franklin, Sarah. 2013. *Biological Relatives: IVF, Stem Cells, and the Future of Kinship.* Durham: Duke University Press.

Ginsburg, Faye D. and Rayna Rapp. 1995. *Conceiving the New World Order: The Global Politics of Reproduction.* Berkeley: University of California Press.

Haraway, Donna. 2004. *The Haraway Reader.* New York, London: Routledge.

Harris, Cheryl I. 1993. "Whiteness as Property." *Harvard Law Review* 106: 8.

Inhorn, Marcia. 2010. "'Assisted' Motherhood in Global Dubai: Reproductive Tourists and their Helpers." In *The Globalization of Motherhood: Deconstructions and Reconstructions of Biology and Care*, edited by Jane M. Maher and Wendy Chavkin, 180–202. New York: Routledge.

Inhorn, Marcia. 2012. *Islam and Assisted Reproductive Technologies: Sunni and Shia Perspectives.* New York, Oxford: Berghahn.

Inhorn, Marcia, and Frank van Balen, eds. 2002. *Infertility around the Globe: New Thinking on Childlessness, Gender, and Reproductive Technologies.* Oakland: California University Press.

Jasanoff, Sheila. 2005. *Designs on Nature: Science and Democracy in Europe and the United States.* Princeton: Princeton University Press.

de Jong, Willemijn, and Olga Tkach. 2009. *Making Bodies, Persons and Families: Normalising Reproductive Technologies in Russia, Switzerland and Germany.* Zürich, Berlin: LIT Verlag.

Lie, Merete, Malin N. Ravn, and Kristin H. Spilker. 2011. "Reproductive Imaginations: Stories of Egg and Sperm." *NORA: Nordic Journal of Feminist and Gender Research* 19 (4): 231–248.

Ong, Aihwa. 1999. *Flexible Citizenship: The Cultural Logics of Transnationality*. Durham: Duke Uniersity Press.

Petersen, Michael N., Lene Myong, and Charlotte Kroløkke. Forthcoming, 2017. "Dad & Daddy Assemblages: Re-suturing the Nation through Transnational Surrogacy, Homosexuality, and Norwegian Exceptionalism." *GLQ: A Journal of Lesbian and Gay Studies*.

Puar, Jasbir. 2007. *Terrorist Assemblages: Homonationalism in Queer Times*. Durham, London: Duke University Press.

Rose, Nikolas. 2001. "The Politics of Life Itself." *Theory, Culture & Society* 18(6): 1–30.

Rose, Nikolas, and Carlos Novas. 2005. "Biological Citizenship." In *Global Assemblages: Technology, Politics and Ethics as Anthropological Problems*, edited by Aihwa Ong and Stephen J. Collier, 439–463. Oxford: Blackwell.

Sourbut, Elizabeth M. 2009. "Property in Reproductive Body Parts." PhD diss., University of York.

Squier, Susan M. 1994. *Babies in Bottles: Twentieth-Century Visions of Reproductive Technology*. New Brunswick: Rutgers University Press.

Stanworth, Michelle, ed. 1987. *Reproductive Technologies: Gender, Motherhood and Medicine*. Cambridge: Polity Press.

Strathern, Marilyn. 1992. Reproducing the Future: Anthropology, Kinship and the New Reproductive Technologies. Manchester: Manchester University Press.

Thompson, Charis. 2005. *Making Parents: The Ontological Choreography of Reproductive Technologies*. Cambridge: MIT Press.

Waldby, Catherine, and Robert Mitchell. 2006. *Tissue Economies: Blood, Organs, and Cell Lines in Late Capitalism*. Durham: Duke University Press.

Part I

ARTs in a Neoliberal World of Transnational Reproflows

1 Citizen, Subject, Property

Indian Surrogacy and the Global Fertility Market

Kalindi Vora and Malathi Michelle Iyengar

International fertility travel engages structural inequalities arising from histories of conquest, capture and colonialism, and is entwined with the landscape of mobility, migration and rights. To better understand these relationships and their effects on participants in transnational fertility markets, this chapter explores how transnational surrogacy arrangements in India raise new issues around the legal and social construction of citizenship as a technology of mobility and of marking rights-bearing subjects. Locating foreign-born offspring, who are born to Indian surrogates but have the citizenship of their parents, within the history of birth and citizenship in the USA, we raise the question of how histories of labor, mobility, and citizenship influence the market for surrogacy. By bringing recent research on surrogacy together with critical theoretical work on the construction of citizenship, we highlight the ways in which the practice of transnational commercial surrogacy both grows out of and reinforces structures of inequality produced and controlled through apparatuses of the state.

We use theories of citizenship and the nation-state to analyze the practice of US commissioning parents who contract commercial surrogacy in India, focusing in particular on US citizenship and its racial underpinnings, and suggest lines of inquiry for the ongoing scholarly examination of transnational surrogacy. Using the concepts of differential and flexible citizenship, we think through the consequences of the relatively weak citizenship of low-earning subjects like those who become surrogates in India by relating this to scholarship on women of color who are mothers in the USA. We also compare the context of citizenship issues raised by Indian surrogacy to historical instances where infants have been regarded as property, aliens, or citizens in the USA and India. We focus specifically on how foreign-born offspring complicate the history of citizenship through *jus sanguinis* in the USA. Through these relational and comparative analyses, this chapter brings a new analytics to scholarship on the exposure to risk of actors in surrogacy arrangements in terms of long-term health and social consequences, precarity and potential rightlessness.

Background to Commercial Surrogacy in India

Commercial gestational surrogacy in India, which arose out of historical, social and market inequities, is already a sociologically complex phenomenon that is increasing in volume and scope. Rapid growth in the surrogacy market is occurring without the resolution of legal inequalities and medical risks that are likely, in different ways, to affect surrogates, commissioning parents, and the children born from these arrangements. ART clinics in India are currently encouraged to adhere to national "guidelines," but are not actually bound by any enforceable legislation, a situation similar to that of South Africa (see Namberger, this volume). There is also no mandatory reporting by clinics, so the full scope of clinics and their practices can only be estimated. Research suggests that around 2000 babies were born to gestational surrogates in India in 2011. For example, as many as 1000 are thought to have been commissioned by British client-parents, although figures involving British citizens may be underreported because commercial surrogacy is illegal in the UK (Knoch 2014). The number of clinics offering surrogacy services in India is roughly estimated to be in the 600s, and the Indian Council for Medical Research predicts that fertility travel to India will soon be a six-billion-dollar industry (Rudrappa 2012).

The global geography of commercial surrogacy arrangements, like that of reproductive tourism in general (Deomampo 2013), is racialized and gendered in complex ways. The first surrogacy clinics established in India catered primarily to North American, Israeli, Australian, and European clients, with additional clients from Taiwan, Japan, and Gulf nations. Newer clinics serve populations from Pakistan and Bangladesh, where ART technology and practice is less available (Kashyap 2011), with a similarly motivated growth in clients from Tanzania, Nigeria, and Ethiopia (Deomampo 2013). Marcia Inhorn has argued that, in nations where lack of preventative medicine is the primary cause of infertility, earlier intervention is more important than ART treatments for fertility issues in local populations (Inhorn 2003), and so ARTs are not a demographic necessity for the local population. India is one such country, and despite the rapid development of fertility services, this growth is not in areas of necessity for local residents. For these reasons, ART clinics offering surrogacy arrangements usually do not serve the needs of their local communities, nor the communities of the women who are recruited to become surrogates.

The long-term health impacts of gestational surrogacy are understudied, particularly in light of how rapidly the number of clinics offering this service is multiplying (Knoch 2014). Obstetrics research has shown that conception through IVF increases the risk of gestational hypertension, pre-eclampsia, placenta previa, hyperemesis gravidarum, venous thromboembolism, and cholestasis (Knoch 2014), and the low-resource context of women who become surrogates in India is likely to increase the chances of these complications, many of which can have long-term health consequences. Despite the fact that surrogates are at risk of serious adverse health effects, permanent injury, and death, ethnographic accounts make it clear that the surrogate is not seen as a patient in

ARTs, but as a tool for commissioning parents who are the patients (Vora 2009, 2012; Riggs and Due 2010; Sama 2012; Saravanan 2013).

Surrogates are provided with little information about the process of IVF and, although clinics may obtain formal consent through a signed form, in general surrogates are not treated as clinical subjects and therefore informed consent is not sought. Surrogacy contracts offer little protection for women in cases where long-term care becomes necessary. The Draft ART Bill (2012),[1] if passed, will require that commissioning parents pay for one year of medical insurance for the surrogate following delivery of the infant, but the Bill provides no rights, compensation, or care for the surrogate and/or her family in cases of longer-term illness or permanent injury. This lack of long-term protection means that the surrogacy arrangement has the potential to pose substantial financial risk for the surrogate's family, as well as medical risk for the surrogate herself.

While commissioning parents are conscious of the economic disparity between themselves and surrogates (Førde this volume; Vora 2014), they are less likely to be aware of the health risks to surrogates. Not only is a woman's regular income lost to her family if she is unable to return to her usual work due to a pregnancy-related injury; the family is also burdened with the financial costs of the woman's lifelong care. Adverse outcomes of pregnancy and delivery can include paralysis, blindness, the need for repeated surgeries, and lifelong dependence upon medications to compensate for damaged organs. The single year of medical care proposed in the Draft ART Bill 2012 does not protect surrogates and their families from medical and financial devastation in such cases.

Most Indian surrogates are recruited from the informal economic sector, and therefore they and their families receive low wages for unstable employment with few if any benefits, despite sometimes unsafe working conditions that can endanger their health (Sama 2012, 58). Ethnographic research shows that surrogates and their families:

> often do without many necessities that commissioning parents would not do without, including basic health insurance, medical privacy, reliable electricity, clean and reliable water, a permanent home/residence, the ability to seek and find another job when one is lost, access to a variety of foods or the ability to grow them (requiring land and water), and so on.
>
> (Vora 2012, 687)

Many are in situations of "acute financial desperation" (Pande 2014, 49). This type of financial desperation on the part of potential surrogates, alongside India's technological, medical and economic infrastructure, makes it possible for commissioning parents from the global North to avail themselves of surrogacy services in India much more cheaply than they could in their home countries.

The nature of transnational surrogacy in India is further obscured by less-than-accurate assumptions about who the participants are – i.e., whose labor is making the surrogacy process possible. While only the clients, the medical staff and surrogacy brokers, and the surrogate herself are named in the contract, the entire arrangement is also underpinned by the labor of the surrogate's family. Surrogacy clinics often require surrogates to live away from their families, in clinic-run hostels, throughout their pregnancies (Vora 2009). The family – notably the surrogate's own children – thus bear the affective burden of making the surrogacy possible via this prolonged familial separation. The labor normally performed by the woman within her household must be taken on by others during her absence. The mandate that surrogates reside in hostels also speaks to the artificially low cost of transnational surrogacy in India: when clinics require surrogates to live in hostels to make sure they are getting nutritious food, clean water, and medical services during pregnancy, it suggests that the surrogates' usual family lives do not include such benefits. Rather than paying enough for a surrogate's family to eat a variety of healthy foods, drink consistently safe water, and access professional medical care, the clinic can simply require the surrogate to leave her family and stay in a hostel. The bulk of the surrogacy fee is generally paid upon successful delivery of the infant to the commissioning parents but, given the uncertainty of this outcome, a woman could theoretically undergo six or seven months of pregnancy (with all of its accompanying dangers and discomforts), separation from her family, and absence from her normal paid employment, only to have a miscarriage which (in addition to potentially endangering her own life) means that the whole process has resulted in a net financial loss for her family.

The exponential growth of the transnational surrogacy market in India demonstrates the satisfaction of international clients, who see in India an amenable and affordable location for the outsourcing of gestation and reproduction. At the same time, the low cost of surrogacy arrangements in India is actually enabled through the enforcement of a de facto lower standard of living and more limited understanding of rights for the Indian classes from which surrogates are drawn. While the fees promised upon successful completion of the pregnancy are many times what the woman would make through her regular work, the exposure of the surrogate's body and family to long-term risk and potential rightlessness is elided in the limited understanding of surrogacy as a nine-month labor contract.

Race and Reproduction in the Construction of Citizenship and Property

The conditions of possibility for transnational surrogacy in India, in addition to involving new developments in biotechnology, arise from very old structures of imperialism and race. In this regard, the different types of human commodification involved in nineteenth-century racial slavery and twenty-first-century Indian gestational surrogacy, while clearly distinct and incommensurable, are not structurally unrelated. Thinking about the economies of slavery, particularly in terms of United States history, both provides historical context for the current position of middle-class US clients (as having the means to outsource the bodily labor of biological reproduction) and helps to set up an analytical lens for an examination of the relationships between citizenship, non-citizenship, and the commodification of reproduction.

During the seventeenth and eighteenth centuries, evolving structures of race and empire gave rise to an international economic order founded upon the circulation of captive humans as commodities. The commoditized human body played a foundational role in the political and economic development of the US settler state (Takaki 2000). Even before the US separation from Great Britain, white settlers in what would eventually become "the United States" had developed a profitable economy built upon the labor of enslaved Black and Native peoples. By the nineteenth century, the profitability of the enslaved Black body for the white owner (or potential owner) was understood to be divisible into a number of constituent components: slaves too old or sick to work might be sold to medical colleges or to individual scientists for experimentation and dissection, and the reproductive capacity of the enslaved Black woman was regarded as possessing a financial value separate from and in addition to her capacity for field labor or domestic work (Morgan 2004). The enslaved Black woman had the potential to give birth to children who would inherit their mother's slave status; hence, to purchase a female slave was to invest in a self-multiplying commodity (ibid.). In this sense, to pay a higher price for an enslaved female regarded as a "breeder," or for a visibly pregnant enslaved woman, was to make an investment in the predicted financial value of lives yet to exist. After the formal banning of the transatlantic slave trade in 1808, the still rapidly expanding domestic slave trade relied entirely upon the reproductive capacities of enslaved Black women (Harrison 2009). In other words, economies depending on human reproduction are not a *new* phenomenon. Rather, the accumulated resources allowing some people to access transnational surrogacy arrangements emerge from generations of commodified human reproduction.[2] In the USA, this process also recapitulates racialized constructions of citizenship and non-citizenship, as we will now discuss.

Racialized Constructions of Citizenship and Non-Citizenship

Gestational surrogates in India lack full protection as Indian citizens as a result of their low-earning status and as contracted workers in a transnational agreement. "Citizenship," notes Lynn Fujiwara, "is a multilayered construct at constant play on the local, national, and international political terrain" (Fujiwara 2008, 24). The notion of citizenship serves as an instrument for sorting and classifying bodies and subjects. The hegemonic status of the concept of citizenship naturalizes the ability of the nation-state to prescribe and enforce notions of who belongs where, of which bodies are allowed to move into and out of which geopolitical spaces, and when, and under what circumstances. Within the US context, citizenship, like property, has always been constructed through the technology of race. In this regard, Cheryl Harris's analysis of "whiteness as property" (Harris 1993) provides a generative model for the analysis of US citizenship.

Harris outlines the ways in which the legal construction of property in the US settler state has been co-constituted with the social construction of race. The development of the US economy, and of the US state itself, has been predicated upon a racialized system of property, a system based on "the valorization of whiteness as treasured property in a society structured on racial caste" (1713). The nineteenth-century Market Revolution, the formative historical "moment" for the US settler state as a political and economic entity, hinged upon a particular set of articulations between racial identity and property: Indigenous people were displaced and killed in order to free up land which could then become the basis of white property; whites had the potential to *own* this property, while Blacks were enslaved and therefore could not own property because they were legally figured as property. Later in the nineteenth century, the construction of "Asian" as a racial identity became linked to an ambivalent set of relationships to property: Asians could sometimes hold property, but could also have their property – including citizenship-as-property – revoked on the basis of their nonwhite status (Ngai 2004). The value of whiteness-as-property has always been generated through the labor of people excluded from the category of whiteness.

The material benefits of US citizenship, like the material benefits of whiteness, depend on the structural relationship between a designated privileged group (US citizens) and its various non-privileged others (people of the Third World, particularly in geopolitical areas that have a distinct neocolonial relationship with the USA). We can also note that the social constructions of whiteness and US citizenship are articulated together in the sense that federal law and policy around who is and is not eligible to become (and remain) a US citizen have historically been inseparable from notions of race and whiteness (Lopez 1996). Of course, the differential nature of US citizenship means that not all US citizens are able to equally access their citizenship-as-property. The same can be said about whiteness-as-property: as race is inflected by other social constructions such as gender, sexual identity, and socio-economic class, the fact that all whites possess whiteness-as-property does not mean that all whites can leverage this property to the same degree. Whiteness and US citizenship are thus similar to other forms of property in that they do not possess the same use-value for all who hold them, although they do consistently possess value in the abstract, and hence do constitute property for all who possess them.

During the nineteenth-century Market Revolution, the alienated labor of enslaved people became congealed not only in the form of white property and whiteness-as-property, but also in the form of US citizenship-as-property. US citizenship today, in addition to containing the alienated and congealed labor of generations of enslaved people, also increases its value by absorbing the alienated and congealed labor of subjects who produce value for the US nation-state but are not permitted to enter or legally inhabit the geopolitical space for which the fruits of their labor are destined. Indian gestational surrogates fall within the category of Third World workers who produce value for the US state and who labor toward the increase of US citizenship-as-property, but who are not allowed to legally inhabit the US state and hence do not have access to this type of valued property themselves.

Indian gestational surrogates produce commodities for the United States, for artificially depressed compensation, that reflect a global economic order featuring unequal exchange between the global North and South. On this very basic level, gestational surrogates occupy a structural position akin to Third World garment workers, or like the undocumented immigrants who labor in fields producing American food, or in cleanrooms producing American digital equipment. But gestational surrogacy centrally involves affective and biological labor, involving the commodification of unquantifiable life energy extracted from Indian workers and re-invested in US families, US communities, and US society-at-large (Vora 2015). As several chapters in this book explain, the nature of this labor means that its impact, and the social relations surrounding it, are highly mediated by the cultural investments in, and negotiation of, the meaning of gametes, gestation, and childbirth (Lykke and Lie, Kroløkke, Førde, Namberger, Smietana in this volume).

Positioning transnational Indian surrogacy arrangements within the history of US citizenship laws, we observe that, first, they offer commissioning parents bearing US citizenship an opportunity to utilize services provided by low-earning Indian citizens with limited mobility and relatively weak citizenship in India. Second, they convey the commissioning parents' citizenship status, with its historical accretion of value, to a child birthed by a woman who does not have legal access to that status. Indian surrogates become a new point in a spectrum of exclusion, most recently Asian immigrants to the USA. Lisa Lowe notes that, "In the last century and a half, the American *citizen* has been defined over against the Asian *immigrant*, legally, economically, and culturally" (1996, 4; emphasis in original). Transnational surrogacy arrangements preserve the privilege/property of commissioning parents that resides in their citizenship and depends on the exclusion of undesirable subjects, "reproducing the capitalist relations of production as *racialized gendered relations* and are therefore symptomatic *and* determining of the relations of production themselves" (Lowe 1996, 22; emphasis in original) in a way that complements and extends the history of immigration law in the USA.

Inside the State, Outside the Protections of Citizenship

Recent theories of citizenship highlight the politics of closure whereby some citizens are in fact excluded from full participation, resulting in a de facto structure of differential citizenship (Fujiwara 2008). Citing T. H. Marshall's classic concept of "social citizenship," Glenn points out that "the right to a modicum of economic security, education, and other resources" (2004, 53) is obviously "necessary to realize one's civil and political rights" (ibid.). Fujiwara suggests that scholars have tended to focus either on the study of legal citizenship or on issues of social citizenship, leading to the sense that "a tendency has emerged to examine citizenship at two disconnected levels" (Fujiwara 2008, 24). In reality, these different valences of citizenship are inextricably entangled – and are caught up together in a vicious circle: Just as factors such as access to education and "a modicum of economic security" are necessary to an individual's or community's realization of civil and political rights, citizenship as legal status is necessary to the individual's or community's effective pursuit of things like meaningful education and fair employment.

Over the past few decades, developments in technology and finance have become incorporated into the structuring of differential citizenship, thereby modifying it. Aihwa Ong (1999) uses the term *flexible citizenship* to denote the ways in which both nation-states and individual citizens (as individuals per se and as members of families and communities) bend the citizenship binary, in which subjects are understood to simply either have national citizenship or to be without it, and take advantage of this flexibility in order to pursue a range of goals – from national prestige and the growth of national economies, to individual and familial financial profits, to social mobility and a sense of economic security. Citizenship is "flexibilized" when the law and public policy position particular regions, populations, activities, and individual bodies as simultaneously within and outside of the nation-state. Ong points to the suspension of national labor laws and other protections in "export processing zones" (also known as "special economic zones," "free trade zones," etc.); workers entering these zones lose many of the rights and protections they would otherwise possess as citizens of the nation-state. They are "inside" the state, but "outside" the protections normally afforded to citizens of the state.

Flexible citizenship is not only a nation-state strategy; it also refers to the ways in which individuals and kinship groups utilize their own citizenship in "flexible" ways, and take advantage of the "flexibility" of the nation-state system in order to promote their own interests. Ong writes: "In this sense 'flexible citizenship' also denotes the localizing strategies of subjects who, through a variety of familial and economic practices, seek to evade, deflect, and take advantage of political and economic conditions in different parts of the world" (1999, 113). Such strategies include collecting multiple passports, sending offspring to study in particular nation-states in order to establish business and social connections in those areas, etc. State regimes "are constantly adjusting" to fluctuating trends in the global circulation of both money and bodies (ibid., 112).

Flexible and differential citizenship come into play on both sides of the transnational surrogacy contract between US and Indian citizens. Potential surrogates, although they hold formal citizenship in the Indian state, do not have social citizenship in Marshall's sense; their families do not always have access to things like education or "a modicum of economic security"; indeed, it is often these things that they are attempting to access through participation in the surrogacy process. Furthermore, the ART clinic – indeed, the surrogate's body itself – becomes analogous to an "export processing zone," in which the rights of the subaltern Indian citizen (i.e., the surrogate) are suspended in the interest of cheap, efficient production for the transnational client. The woman who becomes pregnant through ARTs under a surrogacy contract, although she remains inside the geographic borders of the Indian state, is outside of the protections normally afforded to Indian citizens: since the ART clinic is not legally bound to follow the national "guidelines" regarding surrogacy, the woman is not protected by the nation-state and is instead essentially "governed" by the clinic, an institution which – as stated earlier – regards her less as a patient than as a means of production.

Meanwhile, the commissioning parents in transnational Indian surrogacy arrangements benefit from the surrogate's lack of social citizenship in her home country and the flexibilization of her citizenship status once she enters the surrogacy clinic. Simultaneously, they benefit from their own "strong" US citizenship to exercise forms of cross-border mobility and rule-bending. For example, Deomampo's ethnographic research shows how US clients argue with US and Indian officials and insist that rules and procedures be changed in order to accommodate their preferred timelines for leaving India with their surrogate-born infants. Flexible citizenship thus facilitates the transnational surrogacy process: for the surrogate, the *rights* of citizenship are flexibilized; for the clients, the *rules* of citizenship (and borders) are flexibilized. The infant produced by the surrogate's body, labor, and vitality ceases to be a commodity as soon as it is delivered to the intended recipients, the commissioning parents. Thereafter, the infant is no longer a commodity, but a self-authenticating subject of rights: a citizen. Under the current US legal system, the infant produced through surrogate gestational labor inherits, not the non-citizen status of the mother who gives birth to it, but the citizen status of the commissioning parents whose gametes have been used to produce the embryo gestated by the surrogate.

Under US law, birthright citizenship is conferred according to two principles: *jus soli*, or the "right of the soil," and *jus sanguinis*, the "right of the blood." Prior to 1868, birthright citizenship was the exclusive provenance of whites – a long-standing fact that was reconfirmed with the 1857 Dred Scott case, in which the Supreme Court declared that persons of African descent could not be regarded as citizens of the United States. With the 1868 passage of the Fourteenth Amendment, birthright citizenship was conferred upon the descendants of slaves, along with all other "persons born or naturalized in the United States, and subject to the jurisdiction thereof" (U.S. Const. amend. XIV sec. 1). The phrase "subject to the jurisdiction thereof" was used to exclude Native Americans born within reservations or tribes, although these individuals clearly were subject to US jurisdiction in practice. Birthright citizenship was granted to Native Americans as a group in 1924, with the passage of the "Indian Citizenship Act" (Indian Citizenship Act, Public Law 68–175, U.S. Statues at Large 43 (1924): 253).

As compared with *jus soli*, the legal adjudication of *jus sanguinis* is currently much less clear-cut. The mythical notion of American "blood" suggests that anyone who has such "blood" should naturally have US citizenship. While the foreign-born offspring of US citizens are generally granted US citizenship on the principle of *jus sanguinis*, this is by no means always the case. The granting of US citizenship to a child born outside the USA is contingent upon a number of factors, including whether or not the parents are married, whether or not *both* parents are US citizens, whether or not the father acknowledges the child, and whether or not the US citizen parent (if only one parent is a US citizen) has resided within the USA for a total of at least five years, at least two years of which must have been after that individual's fourteenth birthday.

Not being eligible for *jus soli*, the children gestated by Indian surrogates on behalf of US commissioning parents are considered US citizens on the basis of *jus sanguinis*. Of course, the actual "blood" that produces the child is not "American," nor does the subject-body that produces this blood have the opportunity to gain the status of US citizen.[3] Nevertheless, the child is considered to be a US citizen on the basis of *jus sanguinis*. The surrogate mother whose *blood* has produced the child, by contrast, remains a subaltern citizen of the Indian state.

The Latin term *jus sanguinis* becomes confusing and contradictory in the context of granting birthright citizenship to an infant generated and birthed through the blood of an Indian surrogate mother nine months after implantation of an embryo produced in an Indian lab using gametes from a US couple. Under these conditions, a different term is perhaps needed in order to more accurately reflect the basis upon which the infant is considered a US citizen. *Jus gametas*? In cases where a commissioning pair or individual cannot produce a viable egg, eggs from an Indian donor, or frozen eggs from a donor outside India, may be used (Vora 2013, 98). In such cases of *jus gametas*, when the child is generated through the blood of an Indian birth mother nine months after implantation of an embryo created in an Indian lab from an egg donated by an Indian or other national and a US citizen's sperm, we might conjecture about the connection between citizenship and national origin. For example, is the source of sperm required to prove that he has met the five-year US residency requirement, with at least two of those years of residency having taken place after his fourteenth birthday?[4] Or is the infant granted US citizenship on the basis of *jus spermae*?

It is interesting to note that the connection between kinship and citizenship implied by the principle of *jus sanguinis* has traditionally functioned in multiple directions: not only can foreign-born offspring of US citizen parents gain US citizenship through this principle, but (naturalized or *jus soli* birthright) US citizens over the age of 21 can petition for permanent US residency status for their foreign-born parents and siblings, who can then become naturalized US citizens on this basis. Indian (and other) surrogate mothers who give birth to US citizen children are unique in this regard: they produce US citizens, but are granted no corresponding ability to become US citizens themselves.

The point is not to suggest that Indian mothers who give birth to US citizen children via transnational surrogacy arrangements are seeking US citizenship as a part of their compensation, because to our knowledge this issue has not been raised. Our point, rather, is twofold: First, the racialized structures of US citizenship and property rights that have created the conditions enabling transnational surrogacy arrangements are then reproduced when Third World women who give birth to US citizens are permanently denied US citizenship themselves. Second, the traditional rubrics of *jus soli* and *jus sanguinis* as determinants of US citizenship are displaced by the transnational surrogacy process. The citizenship traditions that endure within this process are not those of *soli* or *sanguinis*, but of property and race.

By producing value for US society while being forced to remain outside of that society themselves, Indian surrogates contribute value to US citizenship. In this regard they are structurally similar to Third World sweatshop workers, and to various (historical and contemporary) non-citizen laboring populations within the US. But Indian surrogates are unique in that the extraction of their vital energy not only enhances the property value of US citizenship, but also biologically reproduces the citizenry itself. In this sense, transnational gestational surrogacy in fact represents an entirely new phenomenon. While the labor of producing the property value of US citizenship has always been "outsourced," so to speak, the rise of transnational surrogacy represents the outsourcing of the cellular-biological reproduction of the US citizenry. In these ways, we have argued that different valences of citizenship are inextricably entangled in transnational Indian surrogacy, and need to be considered when assessing access to rights and entitlements by and for subjects of surrogacy arrangements.

Notes

1 The 2012 Draft remains the most recent revision to date, and the Bill has not been passed into law as of 2015.

2 In fact, the practices of colonial labor allocation following the abolition of slavery in the British Empire preserved the centrality of human reproduction when it instituted indentured labor to supplement enslaved labor (Vora 2015).

3 For a discussion of how surrogates in India view the importance of their own blood in gestation, see Pande 2009.

4 When a child is conceived by a couple without the aid of technology, and is not born in the US, and only one parent is a US citizen, then there are a number of conditions that have to be met in order for that child to have US citizenship. But when a child is conceived via IVF, using a non-U.S. egg and a non-US gestational mother, and only one parent (the commissioning father) is a US citizen, and the child is not born in the US, do the same restrictions apply? Or is the child automatically given US citizenship on the basis of *jus spermae*?"

References

Deomampo, Daisy. 2013. "Gendered Geographies of Reproductive Tourism." *Gender & Society* 27 (4): 514–527.

Fujiwara, Lynn. 2008. *Mothers without Citizenship: Asian Immigrant Families and the Consequences of Welfare Reform*. Minneapolis: University of Minnesota Press.

Glenn, Evelyn N. 2004. *Unequal Freedom: How Race and Gender Shaped American Citizenship and Labor*. Cambridge, London: Harvard University Press.

Harris, Cheryl I. 1993. "Whiteness as Property." *Harvard Law Review* 106 (8): 1707–1791.

Harrison, Renee K. 2009. *Enslaved Women and the Art of Resistance in Antebellum America*. New York: Palgrave Macmillan.

Inhorn, Marcia C. 2003. "Global Infertility and the Globalization of New Reproductive Technologies: Illustrations from Egypt." *Social Science & Medicine* 56 (9): 1837–1851.

Kashyap, Pooja. 2011. "Test-Tube Babies No Real Option in Patna." *Times of India*, 20 October.

Knoch, Jonathan K. 2014. "Health Concerns and Ethical Considerations Regarding International Surrogacy." *International Journal of Gynecology & Obstetrics* 126 (2): 183–186. April 27.

Lopez, Ian H. 1996. *White by Law: The Legal Construction of Race*. New York: NYU Press.

Lowe, Lisa. 1996. *Immigrant Acts: On Asian American Cultural Politics*. Durham: Duke University Press.

Morgan, Jennifer. 2004. *Laboring Women: Reproduction and Gender in New World Slavery*. Philadelphia: University of Pennsylvania Press.

Ngai, Mai. 2004. *Impossible Subjects: Illegal Aliens and the Making of Modern America*. Princeton: Princeton University Press.

Ong, Aihwa. 1999. *Flexible Citizenship: The Cultural Logics of Transnationality*. Durham: Duke University Press.

Pande, Amrita. 2009. "It May Be Her Eggs but It's My Blood: Surrogates and Everyday Forms of Kinship in India." *Qualitative Sociology* 32 (4): 379–397.

Pande, Amrita. 2014. *Wombs in Labor: Transnational Commercial Surrogacy in India*. New York: Columbia University Press.

Riggs, Damien W, and Clemence Due. 2010. "Gay Men, Race Privilege and Surrogacy in India." *Outskirts: Feminisms along the Edge* 22. www.outskirts.arts.uwa.edu.au/1179040.

Rudrappa, Sharmila. 2012. "Working India's Reproduction Assembly Line: Surrogacy and Reproductive Rights?" *Western Humanities Review* 66 (3): 77–96.

Sama: Resource Group for Women's Health. 2012. *Birthing a Market: A Study on Commercial Surrogacy*. New Delhi: Sama.

Saravanan, Sheela. 2013. "An Ethnomethodological Approach to Examine Exploitation in the Context of Capacity, Trust and Experience of Commercial Surrogacy in India." *Philosophy, Ethics, and Humanities in Medicine* 8 (10): 1–12.

Takaki, Ronald. 2000. *Iron Cages: Race and Culture in 19th-Century America*. New York: Oxford University Press.

Vora, Kalindi. 2009. "Indian Transnational Surrogacy and the Commodification of Vital Energy." *Subjectivity* 28: 266–278.

Vora, Kalindi. 2012. "Limits of Labor." *South Atlantic Quarterly* 201 (111): 681–700.

Vora, Kalindi. 2013. "Potential, Risk and Return in Transnational Indian Gestational Surrogacy." *Current Anthropology* 54 (S7): S97–S105.

Vora, Kalindi. 2014. "Experimental Socialities and Gestational Surrogacy in the Indian ART Clinic." *Ethnos: Journal of Anthropology* 79 (1): 63–83.

Vora, Kalindi. 2015. *Life Support: Biocapital and the New History of Outsourced Labor*. Minneapolis: University of Minnesota Press.

2 Fair Play in a Dirty Field?

The Ethical Work of Commissioning Surrogacy in India

Kristin Engh Førde

Introduction

> You want to do good, so [the surrogates] are treated well. But sometimes it feels as if it's impossible. It feels as if it's not possible to do this in a good way in India. That's what a lot of our ambivalence is about, can we really do this and own up to it? Can we defend it?
>
> (Emma[1])

This chapter explores the experiences of Western so-called Indented Parents (IPs) i.e., couples or individuals who commission a commercial gestational surrogacy arrangement in India in order to have a child. As indicated by the quote above, these experiences were usually characterized by ambivalence and a sense of moral risk associated with the practice. In the following, I will discuss how the IPs deal with their ambivalence through what I analyze as *ethical work*.

The analysis is based on data from long-term ethnographic fieldwork on commercial gestational surrogacy in Mumbai, India. Seven heterosexual couples, seven homosexual couples and four single men participated in the study. The ages of the participants ranged from 25 to 51. They all came from Western countries, all but four individuals from Scandinavia. Interviews and participant observation were conducted both in Mumbai and Scandinavia during the period from August 2012 to May 2014.

The ethics and feminist politics of commercial surrogacy in India have been discussed in several studies (Smerdon 2008; Qadeer 2010; Kroløkke 2012). The imbalanced power relations between the parties, relating to global inequality, gender, and race, have been explored and problematized (Pande 2009, 2010; Vora 2009, 2014; Vora and Iyengar, this volume). By making the IPs' experiences and reflections my starting point, I wish to contribute to the on-going discussion with an analysis of these power relations and the ethical dilemmas they entail, as experienced and handled by the dominant party.

In her discussion of the Norwegian public debate on transnational surrogacy, Andersen (2013) notes that media discourses position Norwegian commissioning parents as victims in relation to the state, in terms of their lack of reproductive rights, and as a result exclude surrogates from such a position, reversing the roles of dominant versus dominated within the North–South divide. The IPs in my study did to some extent refer to what they saw as reproductive disempowerment by their home countries to legitimize choosing surrogacy in India, referring to it as the "only possibility" or "last resort," in the sense that health issues, gender/sexual orientation, age and/or economic situation had made "natural" procreation unavailable to them. More common methods of "unnatural procreation" (Melhuus and Howell 2009), adoption and various forms of ARTs were also unavailable to most, due to legislation, health service regulations, and the international adoption system.

However, their concrete experiences, actions, and relationships in India were mostly not presented within this discourse of victimization. Rather, the IPs' feelings of ambivalence and moral risk related to the experience of being in a position of power that they themselves did not consider fully legitimized. The means of having a child were there for them to purchase in India. Still, the IPs did not see themselves as mere consumers in a liberal market. Most of the actions they took during the surrogacy process were preceded by ethical work; i.e., active intellectual involvement with what they perceived as moral dilemmas entailed by their alternatives. Although taking part in "exploitation" of the surrogate was perceived as the main moral risk, the IPs only involved the surrogate herself in their ethical work to a very limited extent, due to the constitutive and multidimensional distance between the parties – made up of social inequality, cultural difference (including an almost complete language barrier), and very limited direct contact. Instead, they focused their ethical work on *being accountable* for their surrogacy experience in the face of their own communities, to which they would return with their children.

Culture and Morality – When Do Our Actions Have Moral Weight?

In order to analyze how the IPs attempted to solve their dilemmas, I turn to recent anthropological theories of ethics. Criticizing the Durkhemian tradition, in which all culture is understood as morally charged, leaving the meaning of morality to be "everything and nothing" (Laidlaw 2002), a common ambition among these anthropology scholars has been to theorize how some actions and relations come to be understood as morally loaded while others do not. The answer seems to lie in a disruption of ordinary normative structures (Robbins 2012). Such disruption could be caused by social and cultural change creating a need to reconsider values and their application (Robbins 2007; Zigon 2007; Faubion 2011). I argue that the change from a position in which they felt marginalized to one of power and agency implied such a disruption for the IPs, and that the shift of position created the need to reflect on their central values and the relation between them in order to make choices.

The displacement of procreation from the domain of intimacy into the marketplace constituted another such disruption. Lambek (2008) suggests thinking about the distinction between economic and ethical value in terms of *incommensurability*, a concept that sheds useful light on the IPs' experiences. Lambek argues that ethical value and market value are incommensurable to one another – at least under capitalism. The reason for this, according to Lambek, is their respective methods of dealing with commensurability. To put it very bluntly: Market value reduces everything to the same, whereas ethical value strives to keep things apart. A changed context forced the IPs to establish new criteria that would enable them to engage in commercial surrogacy without feeling that they had become exploiters. In practice there were potential value conflicts on several levels: between their goal and the means employed to achieve it, between market values and ethical values, and between their own Western values and those of Indian culture and society.

Inequality held a particularly central place here. While *hierarchy* has been seen as the key concept characterizing social life in India, the corresponding key value in the West is *individualism*, according to Dumont's very influential comparative study of the Indian caste system (1998 [1966]). Dumont stresses that hierarchy in the Indian context, or more specifically the caste system, should not be understood as an "extreme form of social stratification." Dumont argues that stratification is a Western concept, in which the idea of equality as the "natural" condition is already implied (Dumont 1986). Although equality is said to be an all-encompassing value for Western cultures, it has a special content in Scandinavia, home to the majority of the participating IPs. It has been argued that the Scandinavian concept of equality, unlike that of the rest of the West in general, contains an implied *sameness* (Gullestad 1992, 1984). Gullestad argues that difference is usually dealt with through avoidance, creating an inclination to surround oneself with equals in the sense of sameness, and correspondingly to avoid close relations with people who are thought of as different and thus unequal. Engaging in surrogacy in India – a practice that in many ways depends on inequality – implied having the value of equality challenged, and handling these challenges was another key element of the ethical project.

"Buying Oneself a Pregnancy?" The Incommensurability of Commercial Surrogacy

So what exactly are the moral values that become so challenged by transnational commercial surrogacy in India? Why is it such a dirty field? Among the participating IPs, the ethical risks were usually conceptualized as "exploitation." "Explotiation" I argue, related to the key values of commensurability and human equality. A crucial part of the ethical project would hence be creating and enhancing these values through speech and action.

> [Critics of surrogacy] find it awful that women are being "exploited" ... at the same time they wear €5.9 t-shirts and buy themselves a new mobile phone every six months. Without knowing which minerals and metals are in

> them, or how they are made. It's like vegetarians wearing leather ... I mean, it's ok to be principled and have an opinion, but you have to be consistent, it must be a committed choice. There was this recurring double standard in the debate, which annoyed me. It didn't hurt me, but it did annoy me.
>
> (Carl)

Carl's question is: Why is the commissioning of commercial surrogacy in India not morally evaluated like any other transnational market transaction that happens within the same frames of extreme global inequality? Dismissing the differentiated evaluation, Carl termed it a "double standard." Another way of understanding it would be as *incommensurability* in Lambek's (2008) sense. The exchange of bodies, reproductive functions or – worse – babies, for money, negates the distinction between ethical value and market value. Carl's ethical response was to create commensurability by equating surrogacy with any other exchange of services for money. Surrogacy was a business like any other, and he argued that to oppose surrogacy in India and accept exploitation of other labor was simply hypocritical (a "double standard").

Most of the IPs, however, expressed varying degrees of discomfort about the incommensurability inherent in commercial surrogacy, for example Mark:

> ...I must admit I do feel a little uncomfortable, coming from Western Europe, going down there, spending several Indian annual salaries on buying ourselves a pregnancy.

Here, Mark took a somewhat self-conscious view of himself from the outside. In the phrase "buying ourselves a pregnancy" he deliberately juxtaposed elements usually kept apart to illustrate a point. Unsurprisingly, he did not say "buying a baby" or "buying a woman's body." In theory, or rather at the rhetorical level, distinguishing surrogacy from "human trafficking" in this sense was quite simple for most of the IPs; they certainly did not pay for the baby, nor were they buying the surrogate's body. Rather, they were paying for a service i.e., the pregnancy. However, some sense of incommensurability remained: buying the "service" of a pregnancy was perceived by most as very different from buying a t-shirt or even the tailoring of a t-shirt.

On Unequal Terms – The Value of Equality at Risk

The second key value that I will discuss as being at stake here is that of *equality*. The risk of being guilty of "exploitation" was often – although not always explicitly – related to the power imbalance, or inequality, between the IPs themselves and the surrogate. Most of the IPs were well aware of the fact that a precarious socioeconomic position was the main factor motivating the surrogates. Nonetheless, social inequality between themselves and the surrogates was often portrayed as a form of undesired by-product. Christopher and Benjamin, a young couple, also from a Scandinavian country, said:

CHRISTOPHER: Here we come, being relatively rich. And we do come to rent her womb. And … that means we are not equal, we are not on equal terms. She is in a way a servant from whom we buy a service. And although it is by her own choice.... Oh, this is really difficult … to know.

BENJAMIN: It's also about how Indians.... Take when we Skype, the way she behaves. She acts a bit suppressed.... Or maybe it's more that she lets herself be suppressed, resulting in this difference in who takes the initiative and everything.

CHRISTOPHER: I think it would all be very simple if Poonam were as rich as us. And said "Yeah, sure I do it for the money, but I would be fine without this money, too. It's just a nice bonus, because now I can build a cabin in the mountains." That would make us much more on equal terms. I am sure she would have survived even without this money, they said they would themselves. But when you see how much difference the money makes, you realize that…

First, this quote clearly illustrates that the IPs saw the IP–surrogate relationship as ambiguous. Christopher and Benjamin came to "rent her womb" and "buy a service," and Poonam was "a servant," hence the nature of the relationship is economic. Yet, the Scandinavians were uncomfortable with the fact that they were not "on equal terms," suggesting that the relationship is not in fact merely one between buyer and seller in a market, or between employer and employee. As argued in the previous section, this ambiguity related to the fact that the nature and moral value of Poonam's contribution did not unequivocally belong in the marketplace.

However, the poverty and hence genuine need for money of Indian surrogates did play various roles in the moral discourse of the IPs. Framing surrogacy as a form of international aid was a way of recasting the role of inequality, handling the peril of incommensurability, and turning the choice of India into a morally good one.

> When we decided to go with India, we were very happy to go with India, because in our heads we knew that the surrogate needed the money and that it could help her as well as helping us. So it would be like a win-win situation for both of us too, that surrogacy agreement.
>
> (Nina)

From this perspective, rather than being a problem, inequality added to the ethical value: As huge amounts of money would be spent anyway, it was better to share it with a genuinely needy Indian woman and her kids. Surrogacy in India – as opposed to in the West – was interpreted as a kind of international aid more than a mere market transaction.

Although the IPs to some extent negotiated all the varieties of inequality implied in their relationship with the surrogate, they differentiated between morally legitimate and morally illegitimate inequality, a distinction that to a very large degree corresponded with the categories "Western" and "Indian." Even Carl, who was unusually relaxed with the process as a whole and had a strong faith in the ability of the market to maximize benefit for all parties, perceived a certain risk related to the "Indian" brand of inequality:

KRISTIN: Do you trust the clinic?
CARL: Not a hundred per cent.
KRISTIN: Could you say something about…
CARL: What the distrust is about? There is 10 to 20 per cent distrust. Maybe 10. That they will pretend everything is ok no matter what. I wish there was more certainty concerning that. But I have the feeling – it might be a little cynical – that this is one of those Indian things. "Don't mind them," sort of.
KRISTIN: By "them," you mean the surrogates?
CARL: Well, yeah. Or those who are poorly paid, and can't … those who are poorly paid and have bad jobs, how they feel is not considered to be that important.

Inequality relating to differences in wealth were perceived as being a result of global structures for which the IPs took limited – if any – moral responsibility, or it was considered to be the result of processes of distribution (markets) that were portrayed as morally good, or at least morally neutral, in this context. I argue that the "Indian" brand of inequality was the one that was experienced as the real threat to their moral subjectivities. This notion of inequality, which differed from financial inequality that was perceived as less morally defiling, does not stratify people solely in social terms, i.e., wealth and power, but also in terms of moral value, ascribing some humans less value.

The Practice of "Good Surrogacy"

At the heart of the IP's ethical work lay the making of choices that minimized the risk of engaging in "exploitation" and created and/or enhanced commensurability and equality. Picking the right Indian ART clinic was perceived as the most crucial choice in this regard.

Simon and Phillip, a couple in their early forties, had spent months researching surrogacy in India and were about to launch a surrogacy contract arranged by a fertility clinic in Mumbai when a series of events made them rethink their decision. First, they got some very bad news from another couple who were expecting a child through an Indian surrogate: Intrauterine death of the fetus in the eighth month. Around the same time as this incident, which the couple referred to as "a traumatic shock," they saw a TV documentary about surrogacy in Anand, India, which they found disturbing.

PHILLIP: It gave me nightmares.
SIMON: It gave him nightmares! How they treat the women and how they sort of … a very different attitude towards the women.

PHILLIP: The language.... Everything was bad.
SIMON: Evil people!
PHILLIP: Yeah. So we said "No, for fuck's sake, no, no!"
SIMON: So we pulled the plug and shelved it and said: "No, this is not for us."

After a year had passed, Simon and Phillip realized they were having difficulty "letting go" of the idea of having a child. So they looked into the available options again. Adoption was still out of the question; no donor countries accepted gay couples. It would have to be surrogacy, preferably in India where they could afford it. Simon and Phillip decided to go over their decision anew.

> And we did some more research and realized that there are clinics and there are places where it's all humane, where they have a humane attitude and a Western way of thinking. Where they don't ... we've realized now that Indians can treat Indians in a horrible way. They treat them like rats sometimes.... It's quite shocking, you get all: "How can you say something like that to a fellow human being?" But thanks to this clinic, [chosen clinic], we learned that there is a clinic that takes good care of the surrogates.

Simon and Phillip felt they had solved their dilemma between desiring a child and fearing the potential "evil" of surrogacy in India when they selected a specific clinic recommended by other IPs, a clinic which was "humane" and had a "Western way of thinking". Choosing the right clinic was thus above all about finding – or perhaps constructing – a morally clean enclave in a dirty field. The perceived source of immorality was not so much surrogacy itself or a crude global capitalist market for reproductive services. Rather, the IPs to a large extent related the moral risks to the internal qualities of Indian culture and society. The vast majority of IPs shared the view that, although social inequality and a hierarchal culture made India a "dirty" place, morally good enclaves in which they could practice non-exploitative surrogacy could be found.

The clinic was crucial because it was the IPs' proxy in their relation to the surrogate. Legally, the parties to the surrogacy contract were the IPs and the surrogate, the clinic only playing the part of facilitator. In practice, however, due to the distance between the IPs and the surrogates – geographically, obviously, but also socioeconomically, culturally, and linguistically – the clinics managed the morally loaded relation between the IPs and the surrogate throughout the process. Unlike in the case of Western surrogacy arrangements, very little – if any – interaction took place between the parties directly.

Another couple Emma and Sebastian, had multiple doubts about the conditions provided for surrogates by the clinics in India; they did not feel they could come to terms with the ethical dilemmas, and in the end they withdrew from their contract with the Indian fertility clinic. The issue that destroyed their ethical project was the clinic's regime for surrogates: the accommodation and the fact that the surrogates were separated from their families. These were practices that did not correspond with the couple's idea of "good care." Emma and Sebastian's case also illustrates the dilemma of reinterpretation and judgment. The Scandinavian couple did not wish to be responsible for the separation of small children from their mother; neither did they feel comfortable about letting the surrogate live in what they perceived as unhygienic and impoverished conditions.[2] The doctors at the clinic had justifications for most of the objections raised by the Scandinavians, often appealing to their understanding of cultural and social difference between Scandinavia and India. When I met them in Mumbai, Sebastian expressed sympathy with this dilemma:

> It feels like they're trying, but it still.... That it's like that ... like there are these gaps in India which ... which make the surrogates risk both the child's health and that of their own with their behavior.... These enormous gaps make them choose not to use the money on what it's meant for.

Can a severe restriction on the autonomy of an adult – the surrogate – be made ethical via the encompassing value of "good care"? Emma and Sebastian could not come to terms with their concerns. This made them an exception, however. The other IPs ended up trusting the clinic, usually after an only partially successful process of establishing the truth about their practice. A certain degree of doubt and ambivalence thus remained with the majority of IPs throughout the surrogacy process.

The Good Surrogate

A good surrogate, apart from being healthy and fertile, was primarily defined in negative terms, in the sense that it was *what she was not* that qualified her. Most importantly, a good surrogate was not "exploited." This term, however, was given a complex range of meanings, from "victim of trafficking" to simply "unhappy," involving practically any quality, motive, or experience that could impact negatively upon the IPs as ethical subjects.

Being "exploited" was often seen as an individual trait, or at least related to the individual surrogate's specific relations and conditions, as opposed to something systemic. Thus some surrogates could be "exploited" while others were not, and to some extent the IPs felt responsible for ensuring that the woman carrying their child was among the latter. Many of the IPs put great effort into assessing this question, and not all trusted the clinic's recruitment procedures. Some requested a meeting with the surrogate around the time the contract was signed to get an impression of her motivation and willingness (whether she was "exploited" or not), to reduce the risk of engaging in a morally illegitimate relation. "Gut feeling" was the primary tool of assessment available, as direct communication with the surrogate was complicated by the interference of clinics, language barriers, and shyness, especially on the part of the surrogate.

The morally important quality "not exploited" was strongly associated with the surrogate's motivation, meaning that she was willing and "not forced."

However, *why* the surrogate was willing was also morally significant. This was the case despite the fact that "they do it for the money" was repeatedly mentioned as an indisputable truth about surrogate motivation, often accompanied by phrases like "let's be honest," suggesting that denying this fact would be naive or unrealistic. However, the surrogate's need for money could, as already noted, play multiple parts in the IPs' ethical judgment. It was very common for IPs to construct the surrogate's fee as a kind of "special money" (Zelizer 1989), having different moral qualities from money in other contexts.

ALEXANDER: In [Scandinavian home country] the issue of money is often linked to prostitution and human trafficking. There has been some speculative linking so that people associate it with prostitution. So what I'm saying is that money is not a bad thing.... In [home country] it sounds somewhat dirty, but here [in India] it can be a future, for a family.

ELIAS: It creates opportunities.

ALEXANDER: It creates opportunities. I had to come here to realize that. I too was influenced by the view in [home country].

Framed in this way, the poverty and inequality in India transformed the meaning of money, giving it the power to alter the lives of a woman and her family. Thus the money is given higher moral value, as it adds to the encompassing values of "the good life" and "good parenthood." Money – the ultimate expression of market value – is thus converted into ethical value, making the transaction one of life-transforming values: the IPs get a child, the surrogate gets a better life and/or the opportunity to be a better mother. The surrogate's poverty, and hence the huge socioeconomic inequality between the parties, could thus not just play a neutral role in the moral evaluation, but even add moral value to it:

> It's a transaction of mutual benefit. Some describe it as an exchange of favors, giving one another a gift. And it is a sort of gift that we get. It is perhaps more of a gift to us than it is to her, but the gift she and her family get in return is the opportunity for her to give herself a better life, and give her own children a better life. That too, is a valuable gift.
>
> (Susanne)

Also note the role of motherhood in this framing. The fact that being a surrogate can turn an assumed "bad mother" (inadequate due to poverty and powerlessness) into a "good mother" transforms morally problematic money into a means to enable the most moral relation of all: that of a mother to her children. In his thorough discussion of values and meta-values, Lambek (2008) suggests (self-) sacrifice as an ultimate meta-value. The fact that the surrogate sacrifices herself for her children thus becomes a powerful agent of moral transvaluation.

On the other hand, the need for money could also be understood as "exploitedness" in the sense that the surrogate did not have any other choice (she was "forced"). Hence, a good surrogate was not *too poor*:

> In India.... It has been said a lot that they use destitute women who are forced to do it, that this is the rule rather than the exception.... But it's.... You are in fact not allowed to be a surrogate mother in India unless you could do without the money. That's how I understand it anyway.[3]
>
> (Mark)

Other IPs stressed that Indian surrogates were not "picked up off the streets," that they were far from being the "worst off." Again, economic inequality as a global relation, between Westerners and Indians, was considered morally neutral, whereas inequality between Indians was seen as more problematic.

Although financial motivations were seen as prevailing, for many of the IPs an additional element of non-monetary motivation was desirable in a good surrogate. More often than not, the IPs would state that, although Indian surrogates in general "did it for the money," they had a strong impression that "their" surrogate was somewhat different. Marta's emotionally loaded account of her first meeting with her surrogate clearly illustrates the moral value attributed to motivations.

> It was a very moving meeting. She didn't speak English, so we needed a translator.... But, it was a very moving meeting. Because I tried to explain to her that it was important to me that she realized that this ... This was not about me not wanting to get pregnant, it was not that I worried about stretch marks or refused to give birth, nothing like that. So I started crying, of course. And then she said: "I will take good care of your child." And that was very moving in a way. She was sitting there and ... was sort of willing to lend her body, you know. And people see it as an ugly thing, I find that really sad. That they only talk about exploitation, not about all the really beautiful things.

To Marta, the surrogacy transaction became "really beautiful" after a mutual acknowledgment of morally good motivations. Martha experienced that the surrogate saw her suffering and expressed her willingness to help put an end to it. She was "willing to lend her body," a priceless gift, even a brand of self-sacrifice, distinct from "exploitation" and far from morally bad ("ugly"). I interpret the appreciation of altruistic motives, or maybe more precisely motivation through a desire for rewards of ethical value, as another way of creating commensurability. The ambiguous – and dynamic – understanding of the surrogate's motives that I found amongst a majority of IPs, reflected their equally fluctuating and dynamic understanding of the nature of the transaction, between a pure market transaction and an exchange of ethical values (gifts).

Conclusion

Generally, the IPs claimed that they could indeed defend their choices in the face of their communities back home, and as such had succeeded with their ethical project. However, a great deal of ambivalence remained for most, demonstrated for instance in the degree of unease that could be evoked by criticism or access to new information that might alter their perception of their experience, especially concerning the surrogate. Moreover, my own study, as well as others (Sarojini, Marwah, and Shenoi 2011; Saravanan 2013), document the prevalence of practices and relations that would very likely be deemed unethical ("exploitation") according to the IPs' standards, indicating a high risk that many of them have participated in "exploitation" despite their best efforts. At one level, this illustrates how the efficacy of the ethical work in this particular context was severely constrained by the IPs having only partial access to relevant information, caused by both cultural and linguistic barriers and the clinics' more or less intentional lack of transparency. At a more general level, the experiences of the IPs illustrate the limited ability of individualized ethical projects to deal with inequalities and power imbalances that are ultimately caused by structures and processes beyond the scope of individual choices: the global, racialized, and gendered power relations of capitalism, neoliberal politics, and patriarchal societies.

Notes

1 All names have been changed and references to nationality removed to avoid identification of the participants.
2 This concern was not only about the surrogate's wellbeing, but also about pregnancy risk management and hence the wellbeing of the fetus.
3 I believe that Mark has been misinformed here. To my knowledge a stable financial situation is not a common criterion when Indian surrogates are recruited.

References

Andersen, Unn C. 2013. "The Paradox of the Victim Position – Public Debate on Surrogacy." [Offerposisjonens paradoks – Offentlig debatt om surrogati]. *Tidsskrift for samfunnsforskning* 54 (01): 31–62.

Deomampo, Daisy. 2013. "Gendered Geographies of Reproductive Tourism." *Gender & Society* 27 (4): 514–37.

Dumont, Louis. 1986. *Essays on Individualism: Modern Ideology in Anthropological Perspective*. Chicago: University of Chicago Press.

Dumont, Louis. 1998 [1966]. *Homo Hierarchicus: The Caste System and Its Implications*. Complete Revised English Edition. Delhi: Oxford University Press.

Faubion, James D. 2011. *An Anthropology of Ethics, New Departures in Anthropology*. Cambridge: Cambridge University Press.

Gullestad, Marianne. 1984. *Kitchen-Table Society: A Case Study of the Family Life and Friendships of Young Working-Class Mothers in Urban Norway*. Oslo: Universitetsforlaget.

Gullestad, Marianne. 1992. *The Art of Social Relations: Essays on Culture, Social Action and Everyday Life in Modern Norway, Scandinavian Library*. Oslo: Scandinavian University Press.

Kroløkke, Charlotte. 2012. "From India with Love: Troublesome Citizens of Fertility Travel." *Cultural Politics* 8 (2): 307–325.

Laidlaw, James. 2002. "For an Anthropology of Ethics and Freedom." *The Journal of the Royal Anthropological Institute* 8 (2): 311–332.

Lambek, Michael. 2008. "Value and Virtue." *Anthropological Theory* 8 (2): 133–157.

Melhuus, Marit, and Signe Howell. 2009. "Adoption and Assisted Conception: One Universe of Unnatural Procreation: An Examination of Norwegian Legislation." In *European Kinship in the Age of Biotechnology*, edited by Jeanette Edwards and Carles Salazar, 144–161. New York: Berghahn Books.

Pande, Amrita. 2009. "Not an 'Angel', Not a 'Whore.' Surrogates as 'Dirty' Workers in India." *Indian Journal of Gender Studies* 16 (2): 141–173.

Pande, Amrita. 2010. " 'At Least I Am Not Sleeping with Anyone': Resisting the Stigma of Commercial Surrogacy in India." *Feminist Studies* 36 (2): 292–329.

Qadeer, Imrana. 2010. *New Reproctive Technologies and Health Care in Neo-Liberal India: Essays.* New Delhi: Centre for Women's Development Studies.

Robbins, Joel. 2007. "Between Reproduction and Freedom: Morality, Value, and Radical Cultural Change." *Ethnos* 72 (3): 293–314.

Robbins, Joel. 2012. "On Becoming Ethical Subjects: Freedom, Constraint and the Anthropology of Morality." *Anthropology of this Century* (5). Accessed October 31, 2014. http://aotcpress.com/articles/ethical-subjects-freedom-constraint-anthropology-morality/#sthash.KE1yZOsu.dpuf.

Saravanan, Sheela. 2013. "An Ethnomethodological Approach to Examine Exploitation in the Context of Capacity, Trust and Experience of Commercial Surrogacy in India." *Philosophy, Ethics, and Humanities in Medicine* 8 (1). doi: 10.1186/1747-5341-8-10.

Sarojini, Nadimpally, Vrinda Marwah, and Anjali Shenoi. 2011. "Globalisation of Birth Markets: A Case Study of Assisted Reproductive Technologies in India." *Globalization and Health* 7: 27. doi: 10.1186/1744-8603-7-27.

Smerdon, Usha Rengachary. 2008. "Crossing Bodies, Crossing Borders: International Surrogacy between the United States and India." *Cumberland Law Review* 39 (1): 15–86.

Vora, Kalindi. 2009. "Indian Transnational Surrogacy and the Commodification of Vital Energy." *Subjectivity* (28): 266–278.

Vora, Kalindi. 2014. "Experimental Sociality and Gestational Surrogacy in the Indian ART Clinic." *Ethnos* 79 (1): 63–83.

Zelizer, Viviana A. 1989. "The Social Meaning of Money: 'Special Monies.' " *American Journal of Sociology* 95 (2): 342–377.

Zigon, Jarrett. 2007. "Moral Breakdown and the Ethical Demand: A Theoretical Framework for an Anthropology of Moralities." *Anthropological Theory* 7 (2): 131–150.

3 "Families Like We'd Always Known"?

Spanish Gay Fathers' Normalization Narratives in Transnational Surrogacy

Marcin Smietana

In this chapter, I examine how Spanish gay men who became fathers through transnational gestational surrogacy normalize their path to this ART method. I ask how far they draw upon normative family models during this process, and to what extent they transform them. I pursue these questions because, as relatively new reproductive subjects using ARTs, these fathers face a double dilemma in deciding how to account for their new methods of family formation in the face of conventional paths to parenthood. Through their use of surrogacy, Spanish gay fathers must normalize both surrogacy and gay parenting. I argue that they do this by equating their families to previously existing family formation practices. Even though their identity politics is innovative in certain respects, they distance themselves from unconventional family models, to bring themselves more into alignment with dominant social expectations.

Normalizing Families of Choice?

My analysis resonates with Charis Thompson's (2005) study of assisted reproduction, which demonstrated how ARTs were normalized and naturalized by their users as "new examples of old things" (ibid.: 80, 141). In the ART clinics she studied, heterosexual patients' gender and kinship identities were disrupted due to their infertility, and in order to repair them they strategically resorted to scripted gender and kinship roles that might not have been particularly salient in other aspects of their lives. Similarly, in my study, gay men's identities were disruptive of the normative gender and kinship scripts of heterosexual fathers in Spain (Pichardo Galán 2009), posing the question of how to address this situation.

Following queer theory (Kean 2015; Wiegman and Wilson 2015), as well as early lesbian and gay family studies (Weston 1991; Weeks, Heaphy, and Donovan 2001), one option these fathers have would be to challenge the normative scripts and create their own families of choice in novel ways. However, the biological and social barriers these men face on their way to parenthood may have led them to opt for more pragmatic normalization strategies. Such a course of action would also be in agreement with Thompson's argument, as well as with a recently growing body of studies on gay and lesbian parents and the social constraints they face in the UK, the USA (e.g., Stacey 2004; Jennings *et al.* 2014), and Spain (Pichardo Galán 2009). Psychological research on the development of children and the well-being of heterosexual intended parents and surrogates over time (e.g., Jadva and Imrie 2014) has shown that parties involved in domestic altruistic surrogacy in the UK followed normative family structures and relationships. These studies have been focused on the USA and the UK, and have not included gay fathers employing surrogacy. In this chapter, I aim to see whether and how Spanish gay men who become fathers through transnational surrogacy deal with the normative scripts of family formation in order to access reproduction and benefit from the social protections and privileges of sex, gender, kinship, and nation.

Europe, Spain, and Reproductive Travel

Surrogacy is prohibited or unrecognized by law in almost all Western European countries. Only Greece, the Netherlands, and the UK allow so-called altruistic surrogacy, whereby the surrogate can receive compensation for costs incurred during her pregnancy from the intended parents, but she cannot earn income or advertise her services (Brunet *et al.* 2013). Therefore, many Europeans seeking surrogacy commission it in other countries, where commercial surrogacy is legal and available to foreigners, particularly in the United States, Ukraine, Russia, or until recently India (Twine 2015). The resulting transnational movement of babies is creating legal issues for intended parents who seek recognition of their parenting rights and their children's citizenship in their home countries, and adding fuel to a global debate about transnational surrogacy and the rights of surrogates and egg donors (for a detailed discussion of global inequalities, see Vora and Iyengar, this volume).

The Spanish context is conducive to exploring the dynamics of innovation and normalization. Until 1979, homosexuality was criminalized and conservative social mores were promoted by General Franco's regime and the allied Catholic Church; however, with the onset of democracy a major social shift took place toward a greater acceptance of non-traditional values (Pichardo Galán 2009). This culminated in the recognition of same-sex marriage with the right to adopt and raise children in 2005 (Ley 13/2005) and the relatively progressive Assisted Reproduction Act in 2006 (Ley 14/2006), which gave all women access to ARTs regardless of their sexual orientation or civil status. Nevertheless, men as primary caregivers continue to be a rare minority; opportunities to adopt children are very limited (as discussed below), and surrogacy arrangements are not legally recognized (Ley 14/2006: Art. 10). Not surprisingly, then, in the international context of the rise in gay and lesbian procreative consciousness over the last decade (Berkowitz 2007), Spanish gay men have started to seek surrogacy abroad.

Surrogates working with them often continue to be the babies' legal mothers even after the intended father(s) and baby/ies return to Spain. A lengthy judicial process is usually required for parental rights and citizenship to be transferred, and for the genetic father's spouse to be able to co-adopt the child. In 2010, the Spanish Ministry of Justice issued a directive facilitating the recognition of transnational surrogacy (Ministerio de Justicia 2010), however, in 2015, the Spanish Supreme Tribunal vetoed it (Tribunal Supremo 2015). In this uncertain legal context, Spanish gay fathers through surrogacy may find the social normalization of their families even more important.

Methodology

I carried out a qualitative study in Spain, including in-depth semi-structured interviews with 23 gay fathers in 12 families created through transnational gestational surrogacy. Ten of these families contracted the surrogacy arrangement in the USA and two in India. The findings thus give more insight into the US situation than that in India. The families were recruited from gay family associations, community announcements, and personal networks. Their children were aged between one and six years at the time of the interviews. All of the fathers I encountered during this research were white and middle to upper class.[1] Parents with this profile have more access to intentional gay family formation (Jennings *et al.* 2014), and even more to costly transnational surrogacy. Apart from one single father, all the parents were couples of two fathers, married or not.

My analytical strategy is indebted to the narrative tradition of qualitative sociology, which asks why speakers tell certain stories. Inspired by Erving Goffman (1963), I assume that speakers who face stigma, such as my interviewees, may feel coerced into constructing their public identities in a way that will protect them from the negative effects of the stigma.

Spanish Recognition by Global Means

Among the men I interviewed, two main reasons for the choice of a surrogacy destination country were dominant: first, mundane circumstances such as legal recognition or prices and, second, their perceptions of the cultural closeness or distance of the country and people involved in surrogacy arrangements, including the ethical side of the process.

The families who had completed surrogacy in the United States depicted it as the most common and least controversial surrogacy destination, despite its high financial cost (approximately US$100,000[2]). Their major practical motivation was surrogacy laws that in some parts of the USA give intended fathers explicit parenting rights, which were also recognized with greater ease by the Spanish administration; including attaining Spanish citizenship for the children since the 2010 directive from the Spanish Ministry of Justice (Ministerio de Justicia).

These fathers reported feeling culturally closer to the part of the USA to which they traveled than to other surrogacy destinations. They felt that they shared a Western culture they considered "normal" with the surrogates, egg donors, and agency or clinic practitioners in the USA, as well as English or Spanish as languages (some of the US surrogates being of Mexican origin). This, enhanced by the legal freedom to choose and contact the surrogate and egg donor, gave the fathers a feeling of control over the process, as well as the feasibility of contacting the involved women in the future.

> We preferred a person who had a normal life, in a normal family. So India was much cheaper, but the United States gave us much more security and tranquility. And the language too, the surrogates in India don't speak English either, most only speak Hindi. And then, when our daughter is older, we're going to explain to her what we have done and who her surrogate is, and that we have a relationship with her, and of course, with India it's a bit more difficult. The issues of paperwork and documentation are also much more difficult.[3]

Furthermore, certain common practices at US surrogacy agencies and clinics gave these men a perception of the process as ethically trustworthy. They praised the mutual choice taking place between surrogacy parties through internet profiles, which bore some resemblance to dating, and stressed the self-determination and agency exercised by the egg donors and surrogates.[4] In the same vein, many of these men highlighted what they perceived as the women's pro-social and altruistic motivations, their socially inclined professions or interests, as well as the friendship and exchange of life favors they established with their surrogates throughout the process.

> Some people think that surrogacy is a pure and tough economic transaction. But we were very lucky in the relationship we are maintaining with the woman who had them in her belly; we called her the godmother, because we thought it was someone closer and we wanted to give her a more important place in our family. And for the girls the godmother is very important. From time to time we talk on the phone to her and her family; we know her husband, her children, her mother.

On the other hand, the men who had completed surrogacy in India justified it by its lower cost (approximately US$50,000), as well as their understanding of global justice, in terms of which they preferred to help a poor Indian family rather than contribute to wealthier American agencies, clinics, and women (see the discussion of ethical dilemmas in Førde, this volume). These fathers also rejected what they called the US "dating" style of relationships with surrogates and donors, which, in their view, was exaggerated given that surrogacy is in fact an exchange of services. Nevertheless, these men had to contend with social criticisms of Indian surrogacy as ethically problematic toward the involved women.[5] They reported that Spanish gay fathers who conducted surrogacy in the USA, as well as major associations of parents through surrogacy in Spain, distanced themselves from Indian surrogacy due to the global inequalities upon which it was based and its unregulated nature. These fathers exchanged information within an online group of Spanish parents through surrogacy in India.

> Obviously, I'm doing it to help myself. But I prefer this money to serve an Indian family, because it will change their lives; rather than an American family whose lives it won't change, and where most of the money you spend (and you spend a lot) is due to the type of health care they have in the USA.... What I can assure you is that in the clinic where I went and where the other people I know went, there is no exploitation. I met the surrogate, and my eldest son met her, we stayed with her, and there's nothing like that.

All of the interviewed men insisted on the human values that are present in surrogacy alongside the economic, an example of which was their rejection of the common Spanish term "belly for rent" (*vientre de alquiler*), which they considered reductionist and inadequately implying an impersonal and purely commercial exchange. At the same time, they did not deny the economic nature of the process, but rather normalized it by comparing surrogacy to different aspects of raising children nowadays, in which economic exchanges are also present, such as education and health care.

In navigating among these arguments, most of these fathers claimed they had chosen surrogacy because for them it was the most accessible path to parenthood. Almost all of them reported that before completing surrogacy they had first contemplated or attempted adoption, but that it had not worked for numerous reasons (the long process of obtaining a parental suitability certificate, subjective or homophobic decisions made by some psychologists or officials, age limits for intended parents, legal homophobia in international adoption toward gay couples or single men). Apart from these practical difficulties in the adoption process, some of the men also opted for surrogacy because they felt incapable of bringing up adopted children whom they would only receive at an older age, when they would face more issues of re-enculturation and less "normal" parenting from infancy.

> When I started having all this desire for fatherhood, it was not about having my own biological offspring [*de mi sangre*], so if it had been easier to adopt, I would have gone for adoption, but when I inquired a little I saw it was virtually impossible, unless I wanted to get a child after a long fight of six or seven years. And I sincerely wanted to be a father from the beginning or for as young a child as possible, because I honestly do not see myself prepared for all the problematics related to adopting a five- or six-year-old, who would surely come from another culture, speak another language...

Normal Families by Novel Means

Even though these men eventually managed to create the families they desired, during the process they struggled with what they experienced as priority being given to women as parents by biology, society, and Spanish law. One example of this, according to the interviewees, was the 2006 Assisted Reproduction Act, which many of them criticized for granting access to assisted reproduction to all women whilst denying it to men. In this context, given the high cost of transnational surrogacy, accessible only to intended parents of higher social class backgrounds, the terms under which assisted reproduction was incorporated into the available options of family formation in Spain were classed and gendered.

> The law allows lesbians to register the child of one under the names of both, it is allowed for two women, and the Constitution says you cannot discriminate by gender, but it is not allowed for two men.

Similar patterns could be seen in the fathers' social experiences, suggesting an ongoing but as yet incomplete change in social perceptions of surrogacy. Many of the interviewed men reported that, before embarking on their surrogacy arrangements, they had to contend with their own doubts, lack of knowledge, or even prejudice with regard to the process. Some also mentioned the mixed feelings or reservations with which their decision to pursue surrogacy was received by some of their extended family members or friends, not only because they were a family of two men, but also specifically because of the perception of surrogacy as a controversial technique. Nevertheless, despite these initial reservations, in the end all of the interviewed fathers and their children reported being warmly welcomed by their local communities, schools, friends, and families.

> When we decided to do surrogacy, my sister and my husband's sister initially had some reservations, I think due to the lack of knowledge, because they thought it was like an exploitation of the female body and all that.

From the very beginning, all the interviewees were open in all their social milieus about being gay father families created through surrogacy, non-disclosure not being an option due to their social visibility. Apart from some initial reactions of surprise or disbelief on the part of their school mates, the interviewed families' children claimed not to have experienced bullying or exclusion in their schools (for interviews with the children see also: Smietana 2011). As I argue throughout this chapter, this inclusive situation seems to have been possible in the Spanish context thanks to the fathers' framing of their families as "normal" and "conventional." Indeed, such identity politics appeared to be expected from these gay father families by many of the social actors they addressed in their narratives, such as legislators or psychologists, who could impact on their custody rights. At the same time, however, the "normalcy" narrative could also be said to accurately describe the families' everyday lives, which revolved around home, childcare, school, and work.

> In reality we are a conventional family, and every day, when you see other families, you see we're exactly like the rest. We have a life of school, buying food, we really have the life of a conventional family, even though we may have found it hard to admit.

Consistently, the men also held rather conventional beliefs about family structures in the context of interviews about surrogacy. Despite the participation of surrogates and egg donors in their family formation projects, all of the interviewed fathers retained exclusive parenting rights, and the children lived with them permanently. At the same time, the families created through surrogacy in the USA did maintain contact with the surrogates, even though these women were not considered mothers but rather family friends, aunts, or godmothers. Contact with egg donors was much more limited by the agencies, clinics, and the women themselves, who usually preferred not to be contacted before the child was adult. Given the nature of gestational surrogacy, the egg donors were not involved during the pregnancy, unlike the surrogates. Alongside their relationships with the involved women, however, the interviewed men aimed to form nuclear two-father families.

> We wanted to raise her ourselves, we did not want her to spend a weekend with us and a weekend with others.... We had an idea of a family like we'd always known, but with two men, that was the idea we had. But, well, perhaps because that's what we had access to.

This rather conventional family structure corresponded to the biopolitics of race and class pursued by the fathers during the family formation process in the USA. In their choice of egg donors, the men usually opted for educated women with Mediterranean white skin and dark hair color. This not only revealed their beliefs in the genetic foundations of socially valued attributes such as intelligence, it also showed, yet again, their strategic choice of socially inconspicuous attributes. The fathers justified matching their own and the donors' skin and hair color by what they perceived as the need to protect their children from being too different from the majority of their peers.

> We chose an egg donor who would resemble the Spanish type of woman, and not someone with certain physical characteristics that are not common in our family, for example we didn't want a blond American woman. We didn't want to add extra difficulties for our son, like being very blond in a country where people are not so blond, or being Black when there are so few Black people in this country. I think by the fact of having two fathers and the fact of having been born through surrogacy, he is already different enough from his peers.

Even though most of the fathers aimed to achieve phenotypical similarity between themselves and their children, they reported this to be motivated by the objectives of social inclusion, claiming to regard the importance of genetic links to their offspring as secondary. They were aware that such links could have a potential impact on the social and legal recognition of their family relationships, and some thus resorted to strategies of counteracting or co-opting two-parent biology, such as creating two embryos, each with the semen of one of the fathers in a couple. Most of them, however, did not consider biological parenthood the major criterion in their choice of surrogacy.

Yet another family formation practice through which these fathers blended the innovative and the conventional was their interpretation of gendered parenting roles. All of them assumed household and childcare tasks traditionally associated with both mothering and fathering, despite the atypicality of men as primary caregivers in Spain (Smietana 2011). However, many of these fathers did not ultimately escape the context of gender, class, and national hierarchies, as they resorted to at least part-time babysitting by female and often immigrant nannies.

Mononormativity, Homonormativity, and the Politics of Normalization

Transnational surrogacy arrangements involving many parties imply that the available options for family formation have expanded beyond the normative household of two biological parents of two different genders within the legal context of Spain. Moreover, the men interviewed in this study assumed partially innovative interpretations of gender and sexuality identity scripts, in agreement with previous research on intentional gay father families (Biblarz and Stacey 2010).

Nonetheless, in family formation, they aimed to create rather conventional nuclear families: the surrogates and egg donors were not considered mothers, the fathers sought Spanish citizenship for their children, and they desired to be seen as no different from other families. Hence, compared to the gay and lesbian "families of choice" based on friendship ties that formed unconventional "experiments in living," described by Kath Weston (1991) or Jeffrey Weeks *et al.* (2001), the gay father families interviewed within this study appeared to have been working with more conventional family characteristics so as to navigate access and social acceptance. This normalizing process has also been captured by other studies of surrogacy and ARTs (Thompson 2005; Jadva and Imrie 2014), as well as gay parenting (Pichardo Galán 2009; Jennings *et al.* 2014), both in the USA and the UK as well as in Spain. This is not to say that all families created by gay men have become "conventional"; within the non-heterosexual population (as in the heterosexual one) a variety of family models co-exist. Yet, with the extension of relational and parenting rights, those gay men who opt to raise children are strategically incorporating and thereby slowly changing the normative kinship scripts.

The normative trait most emphasized by these gay fathers through surrogacy was nuclear parental exclusivity and legitimacy, which has also been reported as important to adoptive gay father families in different Western contexts such as the UK and Spain (Jennings *et al.* 2014; Smietana *et al.* 2014). Even though both of these family types rely on third parties in their family formation, and open as they may be to contact with those parties (particularly in surrogacy in the USA, where such contact is favored by social and legal circumstances), this does not infringe upon the nuclear family cornerstone. While subscribing to this family structure, the Spanish gay fathers through surrogacy did not view biological links to the children as an essential or unambiguous criterion in their choice of the path to parenthood; however, they did eventually co-opt the legal and social importance of their genetic ties to the child.

Similarly to adoptive gay father families, for these fathers through surrogacy, an important determinant in their choice of the path to parenthood was ease of access, as perceived by the men. In this process, surrogacy fathers avoided the regulating practices of state adoption agencies; instead, they became more immersed in social class dynamics, which permit surrogacy to parents from higher social classes in wealthy Western nations; thus, in Sarah Franklin's (2011) words, reproducing a traditionally stratified world (see also Vora and Iyengar, this volume). In contrast to the racially diverse Spanish gay father families through transnational adoption (Smietana 2011), in navigating social inclusion, the Spanish gay fathers through gestational surrogacy in the USA also reconstituted the dominant biopolitics of race and class, by a strategic matching with educated egg donors of white Mediterranean skin color.

New practices such as surrogacy and gay parenting were normalized by the men in this study through their interpretation of them as "new examples of old things" (Thompson 2005, 141), or, in the interviewees' own words, as "a family like we'd always known, but with two men." Still, even in the favorable Spanish social context "beyond the closet," the existence of these surrogacy families was not completely normalized, either socially or legally. Therefore, in challenging the taboos embodied by gay father surrogacy families, the interviewed men resorted to the identity politics of "normal families," in agreement with their aspirations and beliefs about what constitutes a family. In other words, to repair their parental identity, which in the majority society's view was not "normal," these fathers strategically inhabited and mobilized normative family scripts.

In counteracting the social ambiguity of surrogacy in Spain, the men also provided ethical justifications for their reproductive choices. Like other participants in technology-assisted family formation, for example in donor insemination (Tober 2001), these fathers subscribed to neoliberal values of free and global economic exchange in commodified reproduction, yet at the same time they self-regulated and justified their reproductive decisions with altruistic motivations, such as the exchange of life favors with empowered surrogates (for similar arguments in transnational egg donation see Kroløkke, and Namberger, this volume).

These gay fathers' narratives represent what queer scholars have called "mononormativity" (Kean 2015), whereby a monogamous family structure of two adults in a romantic and sexual relationship is seen as a coherent and privileged mode of relationality, as opposed to, for example, coparenting. This, in conjunction with the other normative family formation practices I have described in this chapter (the biopolitics of class and race, the identity politics of normalcy), allows one to state that these Spanish gay fathers through surrogacy comply with the structures and processes of "homonormativity" (Wiegman and Wilson 2015). In this way, gay positionalities are recoded in normative terms, and at the same time often in adherence to the reproduction of classed, gendered, and racialized hierarchies.

Yet, in order to interpret these gay fathers' narratives, it is important to understand the political and social pressures exerted on them. As a researcher, I faced the challenge of addressing the complexity of the existing power relationships within which my interviewees were immersed, without downplaying their egalitarian aspirations or causing harm to their parenting projects. As pointed out by Judith Stacey (2004), there has been social pressure for both lesbian and gay parent families and the research on them to prove that they are no different from their heterosexual counterparts, which demonstrates that social inclusion limits de novo definitions of family formation to the given gendered, classed, and racialized hierarchies and histories of particular jurisdictions. This normative pressure has been internalized by gay parents themselves, who often seem to view it as a way to fulfill their parenting aspirations, including gaining the privileges of social inclusion. As expressed by a member of a major Spanish LGBT family association whom I interviewed, "We don't have a moral duty to invent family forms that would challenge the norm."

Acknowledgments

Writing this chapter was possible thanks to funding from the Marie Curie International Outgoing Fellowship of the European Union (Grant Agreement no. 629341), which I received with the support of Professor Sarah Franklin at the Reproductive Sociology Research Group of the University of Cambridge, UK, and Professor Charis Thompson at the Department of Gender and Women's Studies of the University of California, Berkeley. The chapter's contents reflect only my views as the author. I carried out most of the empirical research discussed here in 2013 as part of the project "Adoptions and fosterages in Spain" within the research group AFIN at the Autonomous University of Barcelona, mentored by Professor Diana Marre. I am deeply grateful to my interviewees in Spain, many of whom were recruited with the help of the associations Son Nuestros Hijos and Familias de Lesbianas y Gays. I owe my gratitude for comments on earlier drafts of this chapter to this volume's editors, to Professor Charis Thompson, and to the scholars of the Beatrice Bain Research Group of the University of California, Berkeley, in spring 2015, in particular to Ingvill Stuvøy from the Norwegian University of Science and Technology.

Notes

1 The resources the interviewed fathers used to pay for surrogacy came from their earnings and savings, in some cases aided by bank loans they had taken out for that purpose or by family resources such as inheritance. Despite the existence of free health care and welfare benefits in Spain, no state subsidies were involved due to the lack of legal recognition of surrogacy.

2 This approximate price, quoted by my interviewees, included the total cost they incurred for surrogacy in the USA: the fees for the surrogate, egg donor, clinic, attorney, and agency, as well as health insurance, flights, and hotels.

3 All quotations are my translations from interviews, conducted in Spanish or Catalan with fathers through surrogacy, unless indicated otherwise.

4 For a debate on the extent of the agency and self-determination experienced by surrogates in the USA, see e.g., Twine 2015. I look at the experiences of surrogates and egg donors in the USA in the research project "SurrogARTs," see www.surrogarts.eu.

5 As this study did not include the surrogates themselves, I am not in a position to judge how accurate the fathers' assessments of their specific surrogates' situation were, either in India or the USA. Whilst the payment received by surrogates in India may significantly change their life prospects, they come from the lowest social classes and often lack full protection during the process (Sama 2013). With regard to gay fathers, in 2013 new Indian regulations limited access to surrogacy only to married heterosexual intended parents in whose home countries foreign surrogacy is legally recognized (Twine 2015). For a discussion of transnational surrogacy in India see also Førde, and Vora and Iyengar, this volume.

References

Berkowitz, Dana. 2007. "Gay Parenthood: A Sociohistorical Analysis of Gay Men's Procreative Consciousness." *Journal of GLBT Family Studies* 3 (2–3): 157–190. doi:10.1300/J461v03n02_07.

Biblarz, Timothy J., and Judith Stacey. 2010. "How Does the Gender of Parents Matter?" *Journal of Marriage and Family* 72 (1): 3–22. doi:10.1111/j.1741-3737.2009.00678.x.

Brunet, Laurence, Janeen Carruthers, Konstantina Davaki, Derek King, Claire Marzo, and Julie McCandless. 2013. *A Comparative Study on the Regime of Surrogacy in the EU Member States*. Brussels: European Parliament.

Franklin, Sarah. 2011. "Not a Flat World: The Future of Cross-Border Reproductive Care." *Reproductive BioMedicine Online* 23 (7): 814–816. doi:10.1016/j.rbmo.2011.09.016.

Goffman, Erving. 1963. *Stigma: Notes on the Management of Spoiled Identity*. New York: Simon and Schuster.

Jadva, Vasanti, and Susan Imrie. 2014. "The Significance of Relatedness for Surrogates and their Families." In *We are Family? Perceptions of Relatedness in Assisted Conception Families*, edited by Tabitha Freeman, Susanna Graham, Fatemeh Ebtehaj, and Martin Richards, 162–177. Cambridge: Cambridge University Press.

Jennings, Sarah, Laura Mellish, Fiona Tasker, Michael Lamb, and Susan Golombok. 2014. "Why Adoption? Gay, Lesbian, and Heterosexual Adoptive Parents' Reproductive Experiences and Reasons for Adoption." *Adoption Quarterly* 17 (3): 205–226. doi: 10.1080/10926755.2014.891549.

Kean, Jessica. 2015. "A Stunning Plurality: Unravelling Hetero- and Mononormativities through HBO's *Big Love*." *Sexualities* 18 (5/6): 698–713. doi:10.1177/1363460714561718.

Ley 13/2005, de 1 de julio, por la que se modifica el Código Civil en material de derecho a contraer matrimonio (13/2005 Act, dated July 1, through which the Civil Code is modified on the matter of the right to contract marriage). BOE – Boletín Oficial del Estado, n.º 157: 2 de julio de 2005.

Ley 14/2006, de 27 de mayo, sobre técnicas de reproducción humana asistida (14/2006 Act, dated May 27, on techniques of assisted human reproduction). BOE – Boletín Oficial del Estado, n.º 126: 27 de mayo de 2006.

Ministerio de Justicia. 2010. Instrucción de 5 de octubre de 2010, de la Dirección General de Registros y del Notariado, sobre régimen registral de la filiación de los nacidos mediante gestación por sustitución (Instruction from October 5, 2010, by the General Directorate of Registries and the Notary, on the register regime of the filiation of those born through surrogacy). BOE – Boletín Oficial del Estado, n.º 243: 7 de octubre de 2010.

Pichardo Galán, José I. 2009. *Entender la Diversidad Familiar: Relaciones Homosexuales y Nuevos Modelos de Familia* [*Understanding Family Diversity: Same-Sex Relationships and New Family Models*]. Barcelona: Bellaterra.

Sama: Resource Group for Women and Health. 2013. *Birthing a Market: A Study on Commercial Surrogacy*. New Delhi: Sama.

Smietana, Marcin. 2011. "Family-Based Affirmative Action? Subversion and Resilience Strategies of Gay Father Families." PhD diss., University of Barcelona.

Smietana, Marcin, Sarah Jennings, Cathy Herbrand, and Susan Golombok. 2014. "Family Relationships in Gay Father Families." In *We Are Family? Perceptions of Relatedness in Assisted Conception Families*, edited by Tabitha Freeman, Susanna Graham, Fatemeh Ebtehaj, and Martin Richards, 192–211. Cambridge: Cambridge University Press.

Stacey, Judith. 2004. "Marital Suitors Court Social Science Spinsters: The Unwittingly Conservative Effects of Public Sociology." *Social Problems* 51 (1): 131–145. doi:10.1525/sp. 2004.51.1.131.

Thompson, Charis. 2005. *Making Parents: Reproductive Technologies and Their Ontological Choreography*. Cambridge: MIT Press.

Tober, Diane M. 2001. "Semen as Gift, Semen as Goods: Reproductive Workers and the Market in Altruism." *Body & Society* 7 (2–3): 137–160. doi:10.1177/1357034X01007 00205.

Tribunal Supremo. 2015. Incidente de nulidad de actuaciones. Gestación por sustitución. Fecha de resolución: 02/02/2015, Nº Recurso: 245/2012. [Incident of nullity of actions. Gestational surrogacy. Resolution date: 02/02/2015, Appeal Nº: 245/2012]. http://goo. gl/26W8Yp.

Twine, France W. 2015. *Outsourcing the Womb: Race, Class, and Gestational Surrogacy in a Global Market*. New York, London: Routledge.

Weeks, Jeffrey, Brian Heaphy, and Catherine Donovan. 2001. *Same Sex Intimacies: Families of Choice and Other Life Experiments*. London: Routledge.

Weston, Kath. 1991. *Families We Choose: Lesbians, Gays, Kinship*. New York: Columbia University Press.

Wiegman, Robyn, and Elizabeth A. Wilson. 2015. "Introduction: Antinormativity's Queer Conventions." *Differences* 26 (1): 1–25. doi:10.1215/10407391-2880582.

4 Destination Spain[1]

Negotiating Nationality and Fertility When Traveling for Eggs

Charlotte Kroløkke

Introduction

Faced with long waiting lists for egg donation in Denmark, Lea and her husband googled egg donation and also talked to Danish fertility clinics about their options. They chose to visit IVI Valencia, a fertility clinic in Spain. Lea quickly became pregnant using a Spanish donor egg, which was fertilized by her husband's sperm. In her story, Lea emphasizes the joy associated with now having a family, as well as her plans for a future pregnancy using one of the leftover frozen embryos, although she does wonder about her son's biological connection to her. Yet, the fact that she carried him for nine months, shared her blood system with him, felt his kicks, gave birth, and nursed him, creates, she says, a biological connection between the two (Dahlgaard 2010).

Lea's story is by no means exceptional. The European Society of Human Reproduction and Embryology (ESHRE 2010) estimates that the multi-million dollar fertility industry now tailors its treatments to infertile individuals who are willing to travel in order to receive treatments that may be either unavailable or inaccessible at home. Legal barriers, along with the increasing privatization of infertility treatments, and long waiting lists, combined with new communication technologies that speed up communication among the various actors involved, are central to the emergent and growing trend of fertility travel. Key destination hubs, in terms of numbers of patients, include Spain, the Czech Republic, and South Africa for egg donation, Denmark for sperm donation, and India, Mexico, and the United States for commercial surrogacy (see, for example, Namberger, Adrian, Vora and Iyengar, this volume).

This chapter focuses on Danish women who choose Spain as a destination for egg donation and embryo implantation. Three scholarly questions are considered: What are the Danish and Spanish legal and ethical contexts? How do Danish recipients of donor eggs who travel to Spain for treatment construct fertility travel? How are motherhood and relatedness negotiated and redefined in the making of Danish babies using Spanish eggs?

Theoretical and Analytical Framing

Fertility travel is an emergent topic within feminist, sociological, and anthropological scholarship (e.g., Inhorn 2009, 2010). It involves individuals who cross national borders, as well as clinical expertise, cryopreservation technologies, and reproductive assistants such as international coordinators, egg donors, and surrogates employed within the fertility industry. Sociological and anthropological studies have theorized fertility travel and the movement of biogenetic substances as forms of reproductive flows (e.g., Inhorn 2009, 2010) and globalized biocrossings (e.g., Bharadwaj 2008). To Inhorn (2010), the concept of "reproflows" (ibid., 183) captures the transnational movements (flows) of technologies, bodies, knowledge, and body parts that cross national borders:

> Men and women "flowing" across transnational borders in search of reproductive "assistance"; and of reproductive "assistors" who "flow" and are "flown" to other countries in transnational reproductive networks.
>
> (Ibid., 184)

While Inhorn pinpoints the unpredictability of these flows, including the reproductive mobility of egg donors, she is not only talking about humans crossing national borders, but other crossings as well, in which biogenetic substances flow or cross between biology and machine, across commercial, ethical, and moral borders. Bharadwaj (2008) suggests the concept of "biocrossings" to indicate both how biological matter moves and the values that become assigned to it throughout the extractions and insertions of tissue that occur within the (trans) national fertility industry. For example, human eggs move from having little value (being rhetorically framed as "excess" or "waste" material) to having immense value ("intelligent" eggs) or potential (as "my future baby"). Consequently, eggs cannot be understood as stable entities. Rather, they are dynamic tissues imbued with varying and shifting values, as they cross not only time and space but also varying cultural terrains (Bharadwaj 2008).

Feminist scholars have noted how biological substances and genes frequently become both gendered and social signifiers when both donors and recipients make sense of their experiences in light of the intent to parent (e.g., Thompson 2005; Inhorn 2010). Thompson (2005) uses the term "strategic naturalising" to explain how recipients, or in this case fertility travelers, rhetorically make sense of assisted reproductive technologies and choreograph the process to fit their own desire for relatedness. Lea's story, presented in the introduction to this chapter, serves as a case in point. In her story, fetal kicks, the shared blood system, the birth, nursing, and caring for the baby all position her not as a gestational surrogate mother, but rather as a biological mother. Biological relatedness is separated from genetic relatedness and strategically adapted, in Lea's case, to intended parenthood. To Lea, shared substance and shared space form a more intimate biological connection than shared genetics.

Interestingly, strategic naturalizing is a rhetorical strategy that is also employed by egg donors. Spanish egg donors, for example, typically de-emphasize the importance of genetics and monetary compensation, while at other times stressing the gifting and the hard work involved in donating eggs (and, consequently, the willingness to be compensated) (Orobitg and Salazar 2005). Based on an interview study with Spanish egg donors, Orobitg and Salazar (2005) use the framework of the cultural bricoleur to illustrate how egg donors exert agency in their decision to donate and to show how egg donors "turn their individual and idiosyncratic experience into a new social reality" (ibid., 49). The authors conclude that egg donors are neither victims of a growing fertility industry who are entirely separated from the reproductive gifts that they bestow, nor solely identified with them.

Taken together, the prior research establishes a framework for understanding how identities such as gender, sexuality, and nationality intersect in the arena of assisted reproduction and fertility travel. To feminist scholars, globalized reproduction is intricately tied to clinical and biocapital networks. As noted by Namberger (this volume), the logic of global capitalism, in the specific case of South Africa, influences the way in which egg donation is organized and experienced by both donors and fertility travelers. In what follows, I briefly turn to the Danish and Spanish national legal contexts to illustrate how the legal infrastructure creates exits and entrances for transnational mobility.

Egg Donation in Denmark and Spain

The current Danish law on assisted reproduction permits gamete donation (by both anonymous and known donors) and fertility treatments for single women, lesbians, and heterosexual couples, while banning embryo donation, commercial surrogacy, double donation, and treatment for women who are older than 45 (Danish Law on Assisted Reproduction, 2015). The law exists not only in opposition to, but also in parallel with, notions of "natural" insemination, as new reproductive technologies and access are frequently evaluated on the basis of how well they mimic the "natural" process. Petersen (2009) illustrates this in his study of the Danish legal debates on lesbian women's access to assisted reproduction. In these debates, maternal abilities and ideals associated with the notion of a "suitable parent" effectively position lesbian women as already being potential mothers, while they effectively exclude other individuals, most notably gay men. Notions of the natural reappear in debates on maternal age. The fact that women older than 45 are denied treatment and that women's reproductive cells (unlike men's) can only legally be preserved for a five-year period, are justified using arguments about when individuals can "naturally" parent. As noted by the Ethical Advisory Board (2004, 12), "Individuals who are permitted to make use of reproductive technologies should represent the age corresponding to when one naturally has children." In Denmark, the right to motherhood expires when the woman turns 46, while the right to fatherhood never expires.

Altruism colors the Danish legal and ethical debates on gamete donation. In the particular case of egg donation, compensation in Denmark is approximately €300 per donation,[2] yet even this comparatively low figure is problematized and repositioned as a form of "reproductive prostitution" and "trafficking" in poor women's eggs (Skov 2010). The Danish Ethical Council (2012) seems to fear that compensation will lead to a change in women's motives and behaviors (potentially diminishing egg quality as a result). Moreover, in this scenario, compensation leads to a change in the societal values assigned to eggs, which may turn women into victims of an exploitative commercial system (ibid.). In general, the ethical debates illustrate a cultural discomfort associated with women's reproductive choices or, as noted by one of my informants, women's choice as egg donors to (like sperm donors) "spread their genes."[3] In this manner, the altruistic narrative reframes the potential monstrosities associated with "selling" maternal capacity into a narrative of the altruistic (good) woman, which is a more socially desirable feminine quality (Pollock 2003).

In sharp contrast to the Danish legal and ethical context, the Spanish debates center on "women helping women" and "solidarity with other women" as key slogans in the recruitment of egg donors. Egg donation is not only legal in Spain, but it is also one of the few Western European countries with short waiting lists. Unlike the Danish context, egg donation in Spain is exclusively an anonymous process. Yet, similar to Denmark, donors in Spain must be between 18 and 35 years of age and in good psychophysical health (Barcelona IVF 2015). While the altruistic context is highlighted in Spain, donors receive compensation of approximately €900.

Having children is recognized as a right by the Spanish constitution. The discourse of maternal "rights" redefines what could be seen as a monstrous act into an act of gifting or helping other women to achieve their fundamental right to motherhood. While no legal upper age limit for treatment exists, one of the leading Spanish clinics gives 51 years as the upper limit for women.[4] Egg donation is constructed as involving "excess"[5] tissue or tissue drawn from a "natural reserve"[6] of eggs that would otherwise have gone to waste. Although eggs are framed as key reproductive cells in the development of a child, an important and worthy contribution, in these Spanish biocrossings, attention is focused on the outcome of fertility treatments. Consequently, the narrative shifts from the egg as a carrier of various predispositions to the importance of pregnancy (shared nutrients), the immunological protection that the pregnant woman (the intended mother) grants the developing baby, and, importantly, maternal love (Clinica Eugin 2015).

Altruism, not commercial compensation, is stressed in both the cultural and the legislative context. Carlos Simon, director of IVI Valencia, frames egg donation in light of a "general" Spanish tendency to donate "excess" tissue or even organs.[7] While he acknowledges the fact that Spanish transplant law presumes consent unless otherwise stated and interprets this law and practice into a Spanish willingness to donate excess tissue (organs as well as reproductive cells), the compensation of approximately €900 is framed as covering trips to the clinic, missed time at work, transportation, and extra food expenses. However, the economic compensation is framed by some clinics as a reward, offering women the option to donate their compensation to a non-profit organization such as a home for children (ibid.). The "discourse of gifting" goes hand in hand with a "discourse of female solidarity" and a "discourse of specialness." In this context, egg donors are good women or, as noted in the online marketing material of IVI Spain, "Egg donors are very special people" (IVI Spain 2015).

Nowhere does the concern about reproductive prostitution or the fear that compensation may in fact reduce quality, which are dominant in the Danish cultural context, surface. This lack of attention, in a sense, allows egg donation to be positioned as an acceptable act and egg donors themselves as worthy of economic compensation (now redefined as a reward) while simultaneously positioning them as "good" women (and not reproductive prostitutes). While, in the Danish context, the desire for maternity is more likely to be framed as a cultural construction viewed alongside the values associated with a childfree life, in the Spanish context maternity is essentialized, positioning infertile women as rightfully in search of their "natural" fulfillment as mothers.

Having briefly introduced the two cultural and legal contexts, my attention now shifts to the empirical framework at hand.

An Ethnography of Traveling to Spain

My research and interest in fertility travel and egg donation led me to Spain. Not only did I discover early on that Spain is a popular fertility destination for Danish women and couples, I also learned that medical expertise is frequently shared between Spanish and Danish clinics. Through the sharing of knowledge, research, and ultimately patients, Spain is constructed by the Danish doctors to whom I spoke as being "most like" Denmark in terms of ethical and medical standards.

My research project is based on interviews with seven Danish women who had either already been to Spain, were at the time of the research undergoing treatment in Spain, or were in the process of considering different clinical options in Spain. The analysis also includes one visit to a Danish private fertility clinic[8] and a similar visit to a Spanish clinic to which Danish women frequently turn.[9] The seven interviewees came from a wide range of networks, including contacts made through a Facebook support group ("Egg donation can help many people"), members of the Danish Association for the Involuntarily Childless, word of mouth, and contacts made possible through the Danish private fertility clinic Trianglen, which is located in an upmarket neighborhood just north of Copenhagen. Each participant was promised anonymity. All of them emphasized the difficulties associated with going abroad for treatment, and several expressed anger that, due to Danish law or long waiting lists, they were forced to go abroad.

In what follows, I discuss how Danish recipients construct fertility travel and Spanish donor bodies, and I conclude by discussing how fertility travel and motherhood are negotiated and redefined in light of current Danish and Spanish law and ethics in the making of Danish babies through Spanish eggs.

Imagining Spanish Donors and their Eggs

When Rita embarked on her first trip to Spain for treatment at the age of 46, she was both outraged by the Danish law stipulating that she was too old for treatment and comforted by the fact that she had the financial means to pay for treatment in Spain. Five years later, at the age of 51, Rita became the mother of a baby girl, the product of her many trips to Barcelona and enabled by the Spanish law that allows double donation. In the interview with Rita, similar to the other women, she expressed curiosity about the imagined egg donor:

> They [the egg donors] come and go in the clinic just like we do. So we're all sitting in that waiting room, right. But you can clearly see that young Spanish women walk in one door and older European women walk in the other door [laughs]. I'm not at all in doubt about who is who when you walk in the door. And, funnily enough, sometimes you wonder: "Is she the one?" Well, of course she isn't because she's already been there and so on. None of them looked like they were dying of starvation or oppressed or anything. I remember one who came swaying through the waiting room with hips, big breasts, the whole nine yards, and the entire waiting room was like [shows her mouth dropping and laughs].
>
> (Interview, September 2010)

In Rita's account, the Spanish donor is imagined in terms of a well-known cultural stereotype as a sensuous and feminine woman. In the above narrative, the donor signifies fertility (wide hips and full breasts), and through this indication of fertility she comes to embody hope (a future child) while also exhibiting femininity in a highly conventional and distinctly "Spanish" manner. In several of the narratives, what gets constructed as a form of "Spanish" femininity (youthfulness, sensuality, and physical movement) is separated from and contrasted with "European" (older, infertile) recipient women. Labeling the "older" women "European" (although Spain is European as well), of course speaks to the fact that clients come from many different European countries (Britain, Germany, and Scandinavia in particular). In the narratives "European" exclusively comes to refer to the recipients, however, while "Spanish" is commonly, by the clinical staff as well as the recipient women, used to refer to the donors. This in spite of the fact that the donors may also arrive from Eastern Europe or South America to participate in this increasingly globalized economy in reproduction. In the case of Rita, she expresses that her own eggs have "expired," yet she feels that her fertility and her sensuality can receive new life from this younger fertilized egg, enabling her to perhaps mimic the ideal of the imaginary Spanish donor.

The interviews suggest that traveling for eggs is governed by an idea of the empowered Spanish donor. For example, Rita sees the imaginary donor walking through the door as an empowered woman, displayed in the way she walks ("swaying through the waiting room") as well as in the appearance of egg donors in general ("none of them looked like they were dying of starvation or oppressed or anything"). In a similar vein, another interview participant sees the smiles displayed by a Spanish woman at her chosen Alicante clinic as a sign of donor empowerment, while simultaneously also confirming her preconceived idea that Spanish people are friendlier than Danes. Donor friendliness is frequently used in the interviewees' understanding of compensation as a reward and egg donation, when undertaken in Spain, as an altruistic practice. Even the financial compensation is framed in terms of the mixture of empowerment and altruism, co-opting the clinical narrative and supporting the idea that Spanish women do not donate exclusively for money but deserve a reward for their work.

The narrative of empowerment is important throughout the interviews. Ruth prefers not only a Spanish donor but also "fresh eggs," as, she says, these are less likely to have been flown in from Eastern Europe. The distinction between "fresh" and "frozen" comes to signify not only "fertile" and "subfertile" genetic material, it also becomes a substitute for "empowered" versus potentially "exploited" and "Western" versus "Eastern." In the interview with Ruth, "freshness" becomes a stand-in for "Spanish," "empowerment," and "fertility," while it simultaneously mimics "natural" reproduction and grants the recipients a frame within which this particular procreation story can be told. Moreover, this construction positions Spanish donors as more empowered than Eastern European donors.

Imagining the Spanish donor helps the Danish recipients to make sense of transnational egg donation and their own fertility travel. The recipients, like the donors in Orobitg and Salazar's (2005) research, ponder what kind of reciprocity will exist. They engage in strategies of identification with and disassociation from the donor, while also constructing a creation story in which nurture and sociality are foregrounded and genetics is transformed and aligned with altruism as a prerequisite for motherhood. As noted by one of the interviewees:

RUTH: There's a woman who wanted to help another couple and I imagine someone who must have a lot of faith in people. So, of course, I will always, in some way, be indebted to this woman because, without her, it wouldn't be able to happen [emotional with tears]. But I see her more as a woman who chooses to help other people.

INTERVIEWER: Would you like to meet her if you could?

RUTH: No, I feel no need for that. And I'm also thinking that it wouldn't be very appropriate as far as the child is concerned but that's because I'm thinking that it's – that it's not like I'm thinking that to be a mother.... If it was adoption it would be entirely different because, then, she has carried the child and given birth to it. And then, the situation is entirely different. It also creates an emotional connection through the pregnancy, carrying it, whereas egg donation – the women who – well, I think the women who donate are not connected to their eggs in this way.

(Interview with Ruth, August 2011)

Ruth creates her potential maternity through the privileging of emotional connection and shared substance, created through pregnancy and birth. Egg donation, in her narrative, is a form of reproductive assistance made possible because a nice woman in Spain wanted to help other women and the intended mother desired a child so much. The donor is framed as a "gift giver" and not a "mother," while Ruth's motherhood is established through pregnancy and intent. In her narrative, Ruth even notes how the pregnant body is able to switch genetic predispositions in the fetus "on" or "off" and, thus, the recipient body is framed as not merely a vessel but rather as an active and purposeful agent shaping the future child. In the above narrative, the egg donor is clearly not a mother, but only a provider of necessary genetic material.

Intent is similarly used as the key marker of maternity in clinical practice. For example, the Spanish clinic uses the recipient woman's blood and serum to culture the fertilized eggs. While no clear clinical evidence exists that necessitates this practice, it deconstructs the otherness of the donated egg and contributes to a new creation story in which the intended mother, including her bodily fluids, takes center stage early on. In Spanish clinical practice, the fertilized egg is surrounded by the fluids (arguably representing love and care) of the recipient body, making her contribution – if not scientifically, then at the very least symbolically – important in embryonic development.

Throughout the interviews, the Spanish donor eggs are not only "mini-women," they also act as stand-ins for imagined national traits. Framed as voluptuous and empowered, Spanish donors carry with them traits conventionally seen as Spanish. Even the product of these travels, the baby, as in the case of Rita's six-month-old baby, is positioned as "just like that." The baby has "Spanishness" (warmth, charm, and friendliness) and, in this manner, Rita's baby possesses personal characteristics frequently assigned to Spanish women, even to the extent of enjoying specific physical contact such as kissing.

Consequently, eggs are positioned as influencing not only physical characteristics (hair color, height, eye color, etc.), but also social competencies (such as warmth, extroversion, etc.). The egg is not only a biological entity permitting Rita to have a child but, importantly, it is also a metaphor shaping such things as personality, identity, and even sociality. In this case, going to Spain involves not only choosing a clinic with high professional and ethical standards, but also the creation of a more capable, more socially competent, and lovable child. Interestingly, none of the Danish women made requests concerning the appearance of the donor. Nevertheless, resemblance in terms of basic physical characteristics (such as height), personality (such as extroversion), and intelligence is important to them. Ruth, for example, notes that Spain is a perfect choice for her because Spanish women tend to be shorter – just like her. Rita expresses no explicit wishes as far as appearance or socioeconomic status is concerned, yet recounts her conversation with the female Spanish fertility doctor in which she noted how important education was to her. Although Rita welcomed a more exotic child, or her "nougat baby" as she calls her, she is also interested in some degree of normalcy, namely education and the assumption of intelligence and class that comes with it.

Conclusion

Returning to the question of how Danish recipients construct fertility travel and how they negotiate and redefine motherhood and relatedness when traveling to Spain, this study has highlighted the work that goes into imagining the future baby as one's "own" child as well as the ethical work that Danish travelers do to make traveling for treatment a morally acceptable option. While the donor is largely imagined and narrated within a conventional understanding of Spanish women, the future child is always already positioned as "part" of the recipient or, by extension, someone to whom the recipient can relate. In traveling to Spain for treatment, the recipient is seeking a donor who is both familiar and foreign: Familiar because she is from a culture that is known and respected by the recipients, yet simultaneously different or, as noted in these interviews, an exotic gift giver of sorts. Similar to Namberger's study of South Africa (this volume), Spain becomes a top destination for those seeking egg donors in large part due to its appeal to Danish and other European recipients and due also to its cutting-edge medical facilities which, combined with a comfortable climate and tourist attractions, makes going to Spain a desirable choice.

The interviews demonstrate how maternity is positioned as involving intent, pregnancy, birth, and nurturing the baby. As a result, the ideal donor is only imagined and is purposely kept at arms-length. None of the interviewees expressed a desire to receive more information about the donor, yet they imagine that she is someone who is "kind," "warm," and "loving" – characteristics that they simultaneously see as embedded in Spanish culture. Lone, for example, applauds anonymity and is happy not to have a photo of the actual donor. Instead, she suggests that this lack of information permits her to see herself (and not the genetic mother) in her future child. In this manner, fertility travel materializes or (re)produces imagined national bodies and engages in both the de- and reconstruction of national and bodily boundaries. Moreover, the empirical material demonstrates that the indebtedness the recipients feel is not directed toward a specific Spanish woman but, in a more general sense, toward the place and the nation in which donation took place. Recipients stress empowerment and altruism as reasons for donating. They want to feel good about the creation story and, as noted by Pollock (2003), no one wants to tell their child that economic need was the driving force behind donation.

The material suggests that relatedness is brought into being by various discourses on imagined, idealized, and feminized Spanish donor bodies, while compensation is negotiated by recipients to fit Danish ideals of egg donation as an altruistic practice. Fertility travel involves the making of a procreation story in which love and the desire for a child pre-exist and are so strong that they unfold in a country with happy and forthcoming people. In these stories, the neoliberal reproductive flows involving transnational travel, exiting and entering new regulatory systems, and significant capital investment are replaced with narratives emphasizing and re-naturalizing maternal desire. The recipients enact new forms of relatedness and indebtedness. They engage in on-going translations of their experiences of traveling to Spain, their spiritual relatedness to Spanish people, and their continued hopes for pregnancy and the birth of their "own" child. Thus, similar to Førde's study (this volume), Danish fertility travelers call upon a mixture of gendered, sexualized, and nationalized discourses, yet make their fertility travel legitimate within a narrative of altruism and empowerment.

Notes

1 "Destination Spain" is also the title of two National Geographic videos on Spain (available on YouTube www.youtube.com/watch?v=oyXNducx4QQ) as well as the title of an article that was published in the British newspaper the *Guardian* on August 22, 2010.
2 The Danish compensation has increased from 500 Danish kroner in 2010 to 2400 Danish kroner in 2015.
3 Interview with Ruth, August 2010.
4 Interview with IVI personnel, October 2012.
5 Interview with Carlos Simon, Director of the IVI Fertility Clinic in Valencia, Spain, October 2010.
6 Interview with Carlos Simon, Director of the IVI Fertility Clinic in Valencia, Spain, October 2010.
7 Interview with Carlos Simon, Director of the IVI Fertility Clinic in Valencia, Spain, October 2010.
8 This interview was conducted at the Trianglen clinic with two of the main fertility doctors, April 2010.
9 IVI Valencia staff were interviewed over the phone, October 2010, while IVI Barcelona was visited, July 2011.

References

Barcelona IVF. 2015. "Donors: General Information Egg Donors." Accessed October 13, 2015. www.barcelonaivf.com.

Bharadwaj, Aditya. 2008. "Biosociality and Biocrossings: Encounters with Assisted Conception and Embryonic Stem Cells in India." In *Biosocialities, Genetics and the Social Sciences: Making Biologies and Identities*, edited by Sahra Gibbon and Carlos Novas, 98–116. Oxford: Routledge.

Clinica Eugin. 2015. "How Does Egg Donation Work?" Accessed October 13, 2015. www.eugin.net/en/fertility-and-infertility/egg-donation/12/188.html.

Dahlgaard, Mette. 2010. "Jeg føler, han er en del af mig" [I Feel He Is a Part of Me]. *Berlingske Tidende*, March 31. Accessed May 2, 2012. www.b.dk/danmark/jeg-foeler-han-er-en-del-af-mig.

Danish Council of Ethics. 2012. "Udtalelse om compensation for aegdonation" [Opinion on Compensation for Egg Donation]. Accessed February 10, 2012. www.etiskraad.dk/da-dk/Nyhedsarkiv/2013/februar/~/media/bibliotek/udtalelser/2013/DER-Udtalelse-om-kompensation-for-aegdonation.pdf.

Danish Law on Assisted Reproduction. 2015. Accessed September 1, 2015. www.retsinformation.dk/Forms/R0710.aspx?id=167647.

Ethical Advisory Board. 2004. "Kunstig befrugtning – Etisk set" [Artificial Insemination – Ethically Seen]. Accessed September 2, 2013. http://etiskraad.dk/~/media/publikationer/kunstig-befrugtning/kunstig-befrugtning-etisk-set/kunstig-befrugtning-etisk-set-2004.ashx.

European Society of Human Reproduction and Embryology (ESHRE). 2010. "Cross-border Reproductive Care in Six European Countries." Accessed March 2, 2013. http://humrep.oxfordjournals.org/content/25/6/1361.full.pdf+html

Inhorn, Marcia. 2009. "Rethinking Reproductive 'Tourism' as Reproductive 'Exile.'" *Fertility and Sterility* 92 (3): 904–906.

Inhorn, Marcia. 2010. "'Assisted' Motherhood in Global Dubai: Reproductive Tourists and Their Helpers." In *The Globalization of Motherhood: Deconstructions and Reconstructions of Biology and Care*, edited by Jane M. Maher and Wendy Chavkin, 180–202. New York: Routledge.

IVI Spain. 2015. Egg Donor Information. Accessed October 13, 2015. http://ivfspain.com/donors.html.

Orobitg, Gemma, and Salazar, Carles. 2005. "The Gift of Motherhood: Egg Donation in a Barcelona Infertility Clinic." *Ethnos* 70 (1): 31–52.

Petersen, Michael. 2009. "Fra barnets tarv til ligestilling: en queerteoretisk undersøgelse af Folketingets forhandlinger om kunstig befrugtning" [From the Best of the Child to Equality: A Queer Theoretical Examination of Parliamentary Debates on Artificial Reproduction]. *Kvinder, Køn og Forskning* (2): 30–42.

Pollock, Anne. 2003. "Complicating Power in High-Tech Reproduction: Narratives of Anonymous Egg Donors." *Journal of Medical Humanities* 24 (3–4): 241–263.

Skov, Maria. 2010. "Kvindeæg er blevet en værdifuld vare." [Women's Eggs Have Become a Valuable Commodity]. *Information*. Accessed March 12, 2012. www.information.dk/226974.

Thompson, Charis. 2005. *Making Parents: The Ontological Choreography of Reproductive Technologies*. Cambridge: MIT Press.

5 The South African Economy of Egg Donation[1]

Looking at the BioEconomic Side of Normalization

Verena Namberger

Introduction

"It used to be almost like a backstreet operation, like these shady deals, like a black-market baby stealing or something," says a donor from Cape Town, describing her perceptions of the early days of egg donation.[2] Today, egg donation in South Africa has left the shady backstreets and moved into shiny fertility clinics and donor agencies located in upmarket areas, materializations of a self-confident and booming fertility industry. A little world of its own has emerged, a world of agency offices filled with pink kitsch and cute baby pictures, anonymous donors and recipients exchanging curious looks in waiting rooms, online databanks of donors in all shapes and sizes just a click away, cool agency "gals" caring for the empowerment of their donors. Encountering this world challenged my (feminist) thinking more than once.

This chapter uses egg donation in South Africa as a case study to examine the way in which ARTs are changing from once highly contested into (almost) mundane practices. It begins with the observation that the country's infrastructure around the procurement of oocytes as well as the public acceptance thereof has grown rapidly over the last decade, making South Africa one of the global hotspots for fertility travel and a source of donor eggs for the surrogacy business in South Asia (see Vora and Iyengar, Smietana, and Førde this volume).[3] Both the signs and the catalysts of this development are egg donation agencies, which constitute key non-medical actors in the field. My hypothesis is that, in order to understand this "maturing" of egg donation, it is necessary to look not only at its social and cultural contexts but also at the economic dimension – a dimension that is often ignored in the social study of ARTs. Thus, on the one hand, this chapter contributes to one of the main aims of this volume, namely to gather more knowledge about how ARTs work in different places around the world as globally traveling technologies embedded in local socio-cultural contexts and power relations.[4] On the other hand, my account focuses on the *bioeconomic* dimension of egg donation as a normalized practice. With the global success story of IVF, it is not only medical procedures, regulations, and ideas about human reproduction that are changing, but economic infrastructures and business models are doing so as well. We thus cannot understand the socio-cultural normalization of reproductive technologies without considering the contemporary conjuncture of the life sciences and global capitalism – and *vice versa*. Avoiding the trap of economic determinism, which assumes a hidden capitalist rationale behind everything, I understand economic and socio-cultural processes as interrelated. It is these interrelations that I trace in the following pages with the intention of unfolding the logic(s) of value in the South African bio-economy of egg donation. My reasoning draws on work in science studies that seeks to theorize the economic value of the body or "life itself" at the intersection of biotechnologies and capitalism, coining terms like biocapital (Sunder Rajan 2006), biovalue (Rose 2007) or "life as surplus" (Cooper 2008). I argue that, in the face of established, (trans-)national markets for donor eggs, critical (feminist) research needs to do more than merely denounce egg donation as the exploitation of women's bodies under the guise of altruism.[5] It is time to understand egg donation as a paradigmatic site of biocapitalism, characterized by paradoxes and spatiotemporal varieties that need to be studied in detail. I will do so by analyzing the so-called "donation" of eggs as a form of naturalized labor, asking how the procurement of oocytes and their marketing is organized, regulated, and embedded in social (power) relations, and also how donors (stratified along lines of race, class, etc.) experience it.

Business Ideas Travel as well as Technologies

I want to start by briefly narrating the story of egg donation in South Africa – or rather one version of the story, which is dependent on my subjective perspective and access to the field as a white, female PhD student from Germany. The country's infrastructure around egg donation has undergone rapid development over the last ten years, from egg donation being very rarely practiced in the early 2000s to its becoming a routine medical procedure and a professionalized and booming industry today. So what has happened during the last decade? What has made this remarkable development possible? These questions were in my head as I flew to Cape Town, eager to understand the everyday realities of a practice that has sparked so many feminist debates, which continue until this day.

I was surprised to discover that in the South African case normalization began with an outright scandal. In 2002, Robin Newman, a woman from the United States who had experienced infertility herself and was looking for a promising business idea, opened the first egg donation agency in South Africa, offering "egg safaris" to infertile American couples.[6] She was entering unknown legal territory, and quickly sparked a public outcry about the "online sale of eggs" and "Bargain Babies in the Mother City" (Peters 2005). A major reason for this indignation amongst the medical community was that "the American" was copying the US model of agencies and "overpaying" the donors, offering compensation rates that were considered inappropriately high in the local context, or even "perverse," as one interviewee called them off the record. The Ministry of Health, fertility clinics, and IVF specialists, organized within the *South African Society of Reproductive Medicine and Gynaecological Endoscopy* (SASREG), were alarmed and in April 2004 the agency was closed down, albeit re-opening shortly afterwards.[7] Yet, this brief episode had profoundly changed the field. Clinics recognized the immense demand for IVF using donated eggs and the value of agencies in terms of donor supply, a time-consuming service that they could not offer themselves.[8] New agencies quickly copied the idea, "seeing that there is a business to be done"[9] – with the difference that they acted more carefully, especially with regard to compensation rates and the wording of advertisements. In addition, the broad media coverage gave the topic a degree of publicity that it had not had before, even though the headlines were predominantly negative. A self-perpetuating process had begun: More and more agencies were striving to find donors via advertisements or informational events (often on university campuses), which led to growing donor databases and a rising number of mostly international "fertility travelers" making use of donor eggs. With the increasing experience of egg donation cycles, medical procedures improved and became more standardized, and complications became quite rare, which in turn made it easier to find donors and foster public and governmental acceptance. Ethics played a decisive part in this process. Due to the lack of detailed legislation and the commercialization of the field being perceived as inappropriate, in 2008 SASREG published guidelines for gamete donation and additional ones for agencies four years later. Even though these SASREG guidelines are not mandatory but only a code of conduct by which clinics and agencies are expected to abide, they are an integral part of the professionalization and new image of the industry. The recommendations include the ideal age of donors (between 18 and 36), context-sensitive advertising and recruiting (which basically means avoiding statements about financial gain), screening of donors, anonymity of donation, disapproval of donors traveling abroad justified by medical concerns about disrupting the continuity of care, and the proposal to keep monetary compensation no higher than R7000[10] (R6000 until November 2014).

Today, the field of egg donation is structured around private IVF clinics and competing agencies as non-medical service providers. Between 60 and 80 percent of patients come from overseas (figures vary from clinic to clinic), the majority from Australia. South Africa is among the top destinations for so-called reproductive tourism, advertising its "large pool of racially diverse donors" immediately available, its "Western culture" and "first-world" medical facilities, favorable exchange rates and tourist attractions.[11] The cooperation between clinics and SASREG-listed agencies seems to run quite smoothly despite critique and discontent on both sides, mainly rooted in the different spheres to which the two actors belong: the world of medicine on one side and business and marketing on the other. All in all, we can speak of a well-established, ethically regulated and quite professional egg donation market. What should have become clear, however, is that its development does not correspond to an understanding of normalization as a slow process of changing norms and discourse that may go widely unnoticed and is only visible in the long run. Rather, it was the sudden confrontation with the "abnormality" of the US agency model that laid the foundations for the later success story of egg donation in South Africa. It was not legal, social, or scientific factors but rather accidental developments, an imported business idea, and the discovery of the new profitable business field it entailed that triggered the normalization of egg donation in South Africa.

Unraveling Egg Donation: Marketing, Logistics and Consumer Culture

Having briefly outlined the field, I now further examine the notion of "egg donation" by taking a closer look at the South African economy around the procurement and brokering of oocytes. I see egg donation not as a static and unchanging medical procedure but as formed by the socio-cultural context and – my main focus here – the logics of value in which it is embedded and by which it is driven. The following paragraphs illustrate how economic structures and practices shape what is commonly referred to as egg donation. These determine both how the market is organized and how it is experienced.

Considering ARTs as a burgeoning *industry* first enables us to see the ambiguous status of its ethics. While doctors and clinical staff emphasize the importance of SASREG in terms of securing medical and ethical standards, this association can also be seen as an instrument for market self-regulation and "national price-fixing through professional standards" (Krawiec 2009, 25). Even some of the physicians raised this point, describing the society of reproductive physicians' regulation of their own field of business as a slippery slope. Moreover, ethical regulations play a crucial role in marketing as they give SASREG-listed institutions market credibility and thus a competitive advantage. It is not my intention to denounce SASREG guidelines as arbitrary or useless, but to draw attention to the fact that there might not be a clear-cut boundary between ethics and economics, but instead a rather blurred line. Market forces and economic considerations – not only medical ethics – influence the way in which egg donation is regulated.

Furthermore, the process of donating has changed significantly, in terms of both the requirements and the actual meaning of being a donor, with the emergence of agencies. These changes are mainly due to the presence of a highly competitive agency business following the rules of neoliberal capitalism. Application forms for the best-known agencies are often 20 pages long, in most cases followed by a personal interview. Try to apply as a donor yourself (as I did) and you will realize that there is far more to it than simply selling your eggs. You are asked to trace your (medical) family history, to describe your personality, to answer open questions creatively and in addition you must be prepared to learn more – perhaps more than you would like – about your medical condition and genetic predispositions along the way.[12] Donors told me that it sometimes took days and a lot of effort to complete the form and that they were quite nervous during the whole application process. The results are very detailed profiles that intending parents can browse online, looking at pictures of the donor as a child and searching for specific physical features (race, hair and eye color, height) or more personal characteristics (religion, education, special talents).

Information about donors has thus risen in quantity and quality, offering recipients, otherwise known as customers, a high standard in terms of choice. As a result, the time and effort it requires to become a donor has increased as well, increasing the unacknowledged labor that donors invest, as I argue below.

At the same time, agencies follow a different marketing strategy from clinics, capitalizing on personal experience rather than medical expertise. Part and parcel of this image is a team built on friendship rather than working relations, and close relationships with donors. The latter is reflected in the fact that, for *some* donors, agencies become more than mere brokers. These donors appreciate the rather personal and informal relationship with "their" agency (which, by the way, are all run by women) or even become involved in the business, referring friends or organizing recruiting events. Some agencies invite their donors to events like "nail parties" or "pamper sessions," which are welcome treats and occasions to meet with other donors. Agencies and their business model hence set a different frame around what it *can* mean to be a donor. They give the medical procedure a marketable touch of friendship, fun and (depending on the agency) the image of cool, empowered women or of a pink fairytale world of "donor angels." Thus, clients not only purchase eggs but also buy (into) the affects deployed by the fertility business.

The above examples show that, even though technologies and medical procedures might have remained much the same over the last few years and might be similar around the globe, it is necessary to unravel the catch-all term "egg donation" in order to understand what it describes. It is becoming evermore important to consider the business dimension as it is likely that profit-orientated considerations, in combination with technological developments, will induce yet another change in the transnational fertility industry. According to one of the leading fertility specialists in South Africa, IVF success rates using "fresh eggs" are still higher than using "frozen eggs" and probably always will be, even though freezing technology has improved significantly. He nonetheless predicts that the future lies in frozen egg banks as it makes the logistics a lot easier in terms of timing (there is no need to synchronize the cycles of recipient and donor), traveling (donor and recipient do not need to be in the same place), and, moreover, it maximizes the business model of egg donation: "If you get an egg donor and you extract 15 eggs, then they will split five, five, five for each recipient. So they can make the most amount of money per egg donor."[13] This likely scenario would have an impact not only on the market structure but also on donors' experiences. The now anonymous, but still (imagined) existing relationship between donor and recipient – with both of them going through the process of injections, scans and emotional stress at the same time and in the same place – would become even less personal and "real." However, it is exactly this relationship that can make donating a rewarding experience, as I learned from donors' accounts. It is the news of their recipient being pregnant and a healthy baby being born that gives them the feeling of being more than just a supplier of genetic material.

It can thus be concluded that, to a considerable extent, an economic rationale and the logic of global capitalism influence the way in which egg donation is organized and experienced. However, it is not simply determined by cost-benefit calculations and economics in a narrow sense. The analytical challenge ahead is precisely to see the (market) value of egg donors/donations "not merely as a function of economic considerations but also as a function of desire, fantasy and imaginaries" (Waldby and Cooper 2008, 66) and thus as a truly *social* product.

Egg Donation and the Logic of Value

In order to understand the logic(s) of value in egg donation, one faces the challenge of overcoming the distinction between economic and cultural systems of signification. It is this challenge that recent literature on biocapital(ism) and biovalue addresses. What might look like a collective attempt of "(re)writing volume 1 of (bio)*Capital*" (Franklin and Lock 2003, 13) rather comprises diverse theoretical perspectives, bringing forth a variety of "species of biocapital" (Helmreich 2008) and different conceptualizations of the pathway from biology to biocapital. This lively interdisciplinary debate underlines the complexity of the question. A common ground is the insight that commodification is not a "generic social process" (Almeling 2011, 338), which is the understanding that one often finds in bioethical writing, "which essentially is that of a light switch: if money is exchanged, then there is commodification, and the author does not need to know much more than that to speculate about its objectifying, alienating, and dehumanizing effects" (ibid., 170). Looking at the case of egg donation in South Africa requires us to move beyond the mere observation that there is money paid for oocytes (even though it is called compensation) and that it is big business for clinics, agencies and indirectly also for the tourism sector, travel agents, and the pharmaceutical industry.

Among the different "species of biocapital," I find one line of thought particularly promising. I am referring to feminist work that analyzes egg donation, surrogacy, or participation in clinical trials as new forms of (gendered and/or racialized) reproductive or embodied labor under the guise of altruism – and thereby as a naturalized *conditio sine qua non* of bioeconomies (Cooper and Waldby 2014; Pande 2014). The concept of labor entails an important shift of perspective. It forecloses the possibility of imagining a "natural" value latent in the female body that only needs to be harnessed.[14] In addition, this approach recognizes donors as (re)productive laborers and thus as actors rather than mere victims of the fertility industry, albeit subjected to specific socioeconomic constraints, geopolitical positioning and "working conditions" (see Vora and Iyengar, this volume). This perspective reveals structural forms of exploitation whilst acknowledging the subjective experiences and decision-making processes of donors who might not feel exploited at all. Within this framework, it is worth asking what actually constitutes the commodity on the egg donation market. I follow Kristin Holster in her attempt to overcome the "debate between those who argue that in egg donation human eggs are being sold, and those who believe that the product is instead the time and effort of the donor" (Holster 2008, 62) by adding the donor's profile to the two above-mentioned dimensions:

"the donor profile may serve to embody the genetic material such that it is the personification of the egg and donor that the recipient is purchasing" (ibid., 63). This reasoning becomes especially relevant with the professionalization of agencies that operate primarily online. Part and parcel of their business model is to offer potential clients a donor pool that is as big and (racially) diverse as possible, comprising "good quality" donors with appealing profiles. Hence, donors' profiles themselves are valuable to the agency, which means that donors contribute to the realization of surplus value even before or without actually donating, providing data instead of bodily tissue. Considerations such as these underline the relevance of a contextual analysis of egg donation as a value-generating activity based on interwoven economic and cultural systems of signification. Even though I have only been able to touch upon some aspects here, it should have become clear that the logic of value in the bioeconomy of egg donation is not easy to grasp. Moreover, it is not a straightforward process but is embedded in social renegotiations of what is considered normal and valuable – and what is not.

(Not) a Business Like Any Other: The Politics of Normalization

One side of my reasoning has been to illustrate how the "maturing" of egg donation in South Africa has been shaped by economic considerations and market logic. The other and equally important side is to understand the apparent normality of the egg donation business as interrelated with existing norms and power structures, reiterating socioeconomic disparities, racialized differences and the gendered dichotomy of production/reproduction. To further delineate this point is the aim of the remainder of this chapter.

Given the dramatic gap between rich and poor in South Africa, which still mainly runs along racial lines with more than 90 percent of the poor being Black (Lehohla 2014), the question of normalization arises anew. As all major infertility clinics are privately run and IVF treatment is not covered by medical aid, in practice what is normal, and for whom, is ultimately also a question of money. It is not simply a matter of culture, as I was sometimes told with regard to "Black culture," then associated with backwardness and mistrust of (Western) technology. Considering that approximately three-quarters of recipients come from abroad, one should hesitate to speak of egg donation as a rather normal local practice.

Against this background, I want to come back to the foundational feature of the egg donation business, namely the euphemistic signifier "donation" as a prerequisite for its cultural normalization. While having a drop-down menu to select a donor, or in other words the genes of one's future child, seems to be widely accepted, the idea of women earning money or *working* as donors is a cultural taboo. This is not only true for South Africa, as studies on the US context and European countries show (Pollock 2003; Orobitg and Salazar 2005; Boulay 2008; Kroløkke, this volume). Egg donation is discursively excluded from the realm of economic activity, money, commodities and wage labor, in marked contrast to the market for donor sperm (Rubin 2008; Almeling 2011; Adrian, this volume). The hegemonic frame is that of motherhood, gift-giving and female solidarity, reiterating the historical association of women with nature, emotions and reproduction. Given the reality that egg donation is a booming and highly competitive market, such a framework enfolds a paradox. Many of the professionals I interviewed were struggling to find the right words to describe the features of the field and their work. They used terms like industry, supply, selling, profits, competition and marketing while expressing their discomfort with this "business language," often putting the words in "quotation marks" while talking. Even though egg donation itself is regarded as a rather normal practice, this is not true for associated forms of economic activity and relations of (re)production that challenge not only norms of gender, race and kinship but also those of (paid) labor. The intersection of race and class in this unacknowledged labor market is becoming evident as the demand for Black donors increases with more and more affluent recipients from African countries beginning to seek treatment. Most agencies struggle to meet the demand, stating that it is quite difficult to recruit Black donors. One reason might be a lack of knowledge and the resulting misconceptions (like the fear of not being able to conceive afterwards), as one Black African donor, who had become active as an "ambassadress" for egg donation in the Black community through her agency, explained to me.[15] However, a lack of internet access also represents an obstacle for socioeconomically deprived women, as some of the well-known agencies require applicants to have an email address and/or to apply online. Other agencies offer the option to fill out the application on paper and only expect a working mobile phone as a minimal technical requirement, thereby enlarging the pool of potential donors. It is thus likely that a stratified labor market is emerging, brought about by different barriers to entrance, and strongly intersecting with the applicants' socioeconomic status.

At the same time, online databases representing donors as mere bundles of (genetic) information and combinations of social categories from which intending parents can choose, have become a rather uncontested feature, entailing amongst other things a "routinized reinscription of race at the genetic and cellular level" (Almeling 2011, 337). Moreover, some agencies offer "package deals" that comprise all treatment-related services for a fixed price and are sometimes even tailored to address recipients of a specific nationality, thereby mimicking the business model of other service industries. The routine embedding of these devices is based on a strategy of copy and paste. Agencies, and to some extent clinics as well, make use of "discourse templates" provided by adaptations of a global consumer capitalism that, "organize novel or exotic information in ways that are highly familiar to an audience" in order to "create comfort zones and mitigate the strangeness of the new market" (Schmidt and Moore 2007, 559). As I would argue further, the strangeness of the market for donor eggs only becomes socially acceptable through its philanthropic and comforting framing, which also reconciles the sphere of technology with ideas of motherhood, natural procreation and kinship through the concept of "giving nature a helping hand" (Franklin 1997, 103). Donors' motifs play a key role in this narrative. Agency websites, adverts, ethical regulations, and interviews with professionals reflect the industry's (and society's) consensus that egg donors should be motivated primarily by altruism and the wish to help infertile women rather than by monetary incentives. The liberal market in some US states, with compensation rates of up to $50,000, is often referred to as a negative example whilst South Africa is represented as having chosen a different path. A major reason for this insistence on egg donors being altruistic angels is a globalized customer demand: most (international) "fertility customers do not want egg donors who reveal monetary motivations for the desire to donate" (Krawiec 2009, 68). These social norms and ethics represent a cultural medium that has not only enabled the growth of the South African egg donation economy but has actually become endemic to its business strategy.

Not surprisingly, all the donors I met admitted (and I am using this term deliberately) that financial compensation was, at the very least, an important incentive for becoming a donor. While my small sample is by no means representative, it corresponds with the estimate of an egg donation coordinator at a large clinic that about 80 percent of donors "do it for the money."[16] This fact again underlines the necessity of analyzing egg donation as labor and thus as an income-generating activity, even though donors themselves do not frame it in those terms and money might not be their only motive. Most donors stressed that they were *also* driven by the desire to do something good and by a feeling of pity for infertile women, and described the donation process as fulfilling. It is hard to tell the extent to which the social desirability of being altruistic influences these accounts. Agencies and clinics understood as Foucauldian disciplinary institutions might also play a role in producing the ideal donor subject (Pollock 2003), especially in cases where women are "in the business" for a longer period of time. "If I listen to the different donors from the different agencies, I can hear other people's voices because I know how they explain it to their donors," a psychologist recounts with a laugh, referring to the answers she gets when asking "Why do you want to donate?" during the routine psychological screening.[17] The coexistence of monetary and non-material motives represents a contradiction that South African society finds hard to face and donors hard to negotiate – and that the fertility industry is taking advantage of. This is one of the many paradoxes and fault lines of the egg donation economy that has, in some respects, become appallingly normal while also reiterating existing norms of what is *not* normal.

Conclusion

I have argued in this chapter that the social study of ARTs needs to pay more attention to its *bioeconomic* dimension – not only as a context in which socio-cultural renegotiations of these technologies are taking place, but also as a driving force. To exemplify this hypothesis, I took a closer look at the development and organization of the South African economy around the provision of donor eggs. Empirical data shows not only that the professionalization and normalization of egg donation was triggered by business considerations but also that today's infrastructure, standardized procedures, ethics, and donors' experiences of the practice are heavily influenced by market logic and neoliberal consumerism. My focus on the economic dimension circled around the question of how to conceptualize the production of surplus value in this context. I do not pretend to have a comprehensive answer to this question. Yet, the above reasoning delineated some directions for further thought based on an analysis of egg donation as a form of labor, which is embedded in context-specific social relations, desires, discourses, technological settings, and politics of normalization. The picture I sketched is inevitably a partial one. From here the aim must be to add more layers of analysis, identifying further interrelations between intersecting categories of power, cultural norms, technologies, and the logic of biocapitalism. This is the task at hand in order to make sense of the present conjuncture of ARTs and capitalist modes of (re)production and accumulation.

Notes

1 As it is the dominant signifier in the public and medical discourse I use the term "egg donation" while at the same time criticizing it for obscuring the transactional nature of the provision of eggs.
2 Interview with donor, November 2014. In the text, all interviewees remain anonymous except when they explicitly agreed to their full names being used.
3 While SASREG ethical guidelines (see below) do not approve the practice of South African women traveling to places like India or Nepal to provide oocytes for transnational surrogacy arrangements, it is not prohibited by law and seems to be widespread.
4 My empirical data is based on 24 qualitative face-to-face interviews with IVF specialists, staff in fertility clinics, agency owners and donors during field research in South Africa in November/December 2014, and additionally collected material (Skype interviews, newspaper articles, websites, radio features).
5 This does *not* mean we should stop criticizing the notion of "donation" as an ideological misnomer. See also Sourbut 2009.
6 Skype interview with Robin Newman, October 2014.
7 See Elsabé Brits, "Site Selling Egg Cells 'Frozen'", *News24*, April 24, 2004.
8 Previously, they had relied on patients finding their own donors among relatives or friends, or on very small local pools of donors.
9 Interview with fertility specialist, November 2014.
10 Which is about €460 at the current exchange rate (October 2015).
11 "India" is often referred to as a negative example in this context, symbolizing exploitation and dubious ethical standards (see Førde, this volume).
12 Donors are genetically screened for more and more factors. With genetic panels soon to be commercially available very cheaply, the importance of genetics is likely to increase dramatically, impacting upon both the selection criteria for donors and the "side-effect" of finding out about one's genetic predispositions.
13 Interview with fertility specialist, November 2014.
14 This discourse can be found, for example, in OECD and EU policies designed to foster the bioeconomy as a scenario for future economic growth.

15 Interview with donor, November 2014.
16 Interview with egg donation coordinator, November 2014.
17 Interview with psychologist, December 2014.

References

Almeling, Rene. 2011. *Sex Cells: The Medical Market for Eggs and Sperm*. Berkeley: University of California Press.

Boulay, Kate. 2008. "Embodied Value: Egg Donation, Visuality and Cyberculture in the United States." *Atlantis* 33 (1): 103–113.

Cooper, Melinda. 2008. *Life as Surplus: Biotechnology & Capitalism in the Neoliberal Era*. Seattle and London: University of Washington Press.

Cooper, Melinda, and Catherine Waldby. 2014. *Clinical Labor: Tissue Donors and Research Subjects in the Global Bioeconomy*. Durham: Duke University Press.

Franklin, Sarah. 1997. *Embodied Progress: A Cultural Account of Reproduction*. London: Routledge.

Franklin, Sarah, and Margaret Lock. 2003. "Animation and Cessation: The Remaking of Life and Death." In *Remaking Life & Death: Toward an Anthropology of the Biosciences*, edited by Sarah Franklin and Margaret Lock, 3–22. Santa Fe: School of American Research Press.

Helmreich, Stefan. 2008. "Species of Biocapital." *Science as Culture* 17 (4): 463–478.

Holster, Kristin. 2008. "Making Connections: Egg Donation, the Internet, and the New Reproductive Technology Marketplace." In *Patients, Consumers and Civil Society*, edited by Susan M. Chambré and Melinda Goldner, 53–73. Bingley, UK: Emerald Group Publishing Limited.

Krawiec, Kimberly D. 2009. "Sunny Samaritans and Egomaniacs: Price-Fixing in the Gamete Market." *Law and Contemporary Problems* 72 (3): 59–90.

Lehohla, Pali. 2014. "Poverty Trends in South Africa. An Examination of Absolute Poverty between 2006 and 2011." 10–03–06. Pretoria: Statistics South Africa. Accessed April 15, 2015. http://beta2.statssa.gov.za/publications/Report-03–10–06/Report-03–10–06March2014.pdf.

Orobitg, Gemma, and Carles Salazar. 2005. "The Gift of Motherhood: Egg Donation in a Barcelona Infertility Clinic." *Ethnos* 70 (1): 31–52.

Pande, Amrita. 2014. *Wombs in Labor: Transnational Commercial Surrogacy in India*. New York: Columbia University Press.

Peters, Melanie. 2005. "Bargain Babies in the Mother City", *IOL News*, August 20. www.iol.co.za/news/south-africa/bargain-babies-in-the-mother-city-1.251276.

Pollock, Anne. 2003. "Complicating Power in High-Tech Reproduction: Narratives of Anonymous Paid Egg Donors." *Journal of Medical Humanities* 3 (4): 241–263.

Rose, Nikolas. 2007. *The Politics of Life Itself: Biomedicine, Power, and Subjectivity in the Twenty-First Century*. Princeton: Princeton University Press.

Rubin, Caroline. 2008. "The Gendered Language of Gamete 'Donation.'" Accessed April 2, 2015. https://stuff.mit.edu/afs/athena.mit.edu/org/w/wgs/prize/cr08.html.

Schmidt, Matthew, and Lisa J. Moore. 2007. "Constructing a 'Good Catch', Picking a Winner: The Development of Technosemen and the Deconstruction of the Monolithic Male." In *Beyond the Body Proper: Reading the Anthropology of Material Life*, edited by Margaret Lock and Judith Farquhar, 550–566. Durham: Duke University Press.

Sourbut, Elizabeth M. 2009. "Property in Reproductive Body Parts." PhD diss., University of York.

Sunder Rajan, Kaushik. 2006. *Biocapital: The Constitution of Postgenomic Life*. London: Duke University Press.

Waldby, Catherine, and Melinda Cooper. 2008. "The Biopolitics of Reproduction: Post-Fordist Biotechnology and Women's Clinical Labour." *Australian Feminist Studies* 23 (55): 57–73.

Part II

Perplexed State Regulations, Legal Inconsistencies and Cultural Tricksters

6 Governing New Reproductive Technologies Across Western Europe

The Gender Dimension

Isabelle Engeli and Christine Rothmayr Allison

The Regulatory Challenge Posed by ARTs

The rapid development of ARTs has raised major regulatory challenges for governments across Western Europe since the end of the 1970s. In addition to cutting-edge infertility treatments, ARTs also provide technological support for the development of new forms of parenthood (Bryld 2001). For example, gay couples can access parenthood through surrogacy and single women or lesbian couples can rely on sperm donation. These new forms of parenthood call into question the predominance of the traditional heterosexual family, and confront governments with complex new questions about family law, legal access to parenthood, and filiation. Regulatory responses to the challenge of ARTs vary greatly across Western Europe. Some countries, such as Switzerland and Germany, have adopted very restrictive policies that drastically limit medical autonomy to practice ARTs and restrict ART treatment to heterosexual couples. In contrast, the United Kingdom and the Netherlands have opted for permissive regulations that grant broad autonomy to both the medical community and patients in opting for ARTs.

To explain these regulatory divergences across Western Europe, we first argue that ART policies are multi-dimensional. The regulatory challenge of ARTs not only raises the issue of deciding what physicians can and cannot do regarding treatments, it also raises the question of defining who shall and who shall not be permitted to access ART treatments and, ultimately, become parents. In this chapter, we argue that failing to take into account the multi-dimensionality of ART policies, and in particular the gender dimension, inhibits a full and systematic explanation of the regulatory variation across Western Europe. We then discuss the main explanations offered in the literature and show how gendered societal hierarchies have played a major role in shaping regulatory answers to the challenge of ARTs in Western Europe.

Women's social roles have traditionally been linked to their reproductive capacity; this biological differentiation was in turn used to legitimize the assignment of differentiated social roles to women and men. Governmental responses to the regulatory challenge of ARTs constitute a valuable analytical perspective for capturing the ongoing transformation of gendered social roles in Western

Europe. We show that a strong consensus within the medical community and a strong presence of Christian Democrats in the party system explain a great deal of the regulatory variation across Western Europe. However, when confronted with public controversy, physicians have more often than not been forced to accept compromises with their critics by forging alliances either with women's movements or religious actors.

Gendering ART Regulations Across Western Europe

To assess the permissiveness of ART regulation, most comparative research considers the medical community as being the main target group of ART policies, and thus focuses only on the professional autonomy of physicians. However, ART regulation not only addresses the degree of freedom granted to physicians to resort to ARTs, but also defines categories of patients/recipients. Consequently, ART policies determine who can access ARTs and under what conditions. As a result, when regulating the field of human biotechnology, governments also have to define their position on three separate but interrelated issues: (1) To what extent should the field of ARTs be left to self-regulation by the medical community? (2) What kind of parental model(s) should be promoted? (3) Should the state finance ART treatment or should it be left to private financial resources?

These three dimensions of the ART issue do not necessarily follow a linear regulatory pattern and they can be combined in multiple ways. Indeed, several regulatory regimes in Western Europe grant broad autonomy to physicians while strictly limiting patient access to heterosexual couples and those who can afford the financial cost of such treatments. From a gender perspective, such policies cannot be considered as being in any way permissive, because they impose heteronormative standards on access to treatments and reinforce existing sexual orientations and socio-economic discrimination. We argue that failing to acknowledge the multi-dimensionality of ART regulation, and in particular the gender dimension, prevents us from fully understanding the puzzle of regulatory variation across Europe. Accordingly, we propose a comparison of ART policies in Western Europe across three dimensions: (1) the autonomy granted to the medical community to practice ARTs; (2) the constraints imposed upon access to treatment; and (3) the availability of healthcare coverage for fertility-related treatment.

The Analytical Dimensions of ART Policies

These three analytical dimensions highlight the key actors involved in the regulatory process: physicians, governments, and citizens in general – and more particularly, women and same-sex couples.

The medical community constitutes an important policy target group and has been heavily involved in the regulation of ARTs (Engeli and Rothmayr 2015). Developments in ARTs have opened up promising fields of medical activity, such as sterility treatments, gene therapy, and stem-cell research, and regulation of ARTs impacts upon the autonomy of the medical community to practice (Bleiklie *et al.* 2004). The second analytical dimension focuses on access to ARTs. Regulation may entitle single women, post-menopausal women, and same-sex couples to access ARTs, thereby enabling diversity in parenthood. Alternatively, regulation can reinforce the heteronormative features of the traditional family model and impose restrictive criteria regarding marital status, age, and sexual orientation. The third analytical dimension of ART policies addresses the level of financial coverage for treatment. Feminist scholars have emphasized the importance of financial coverage in reproductive rights (Yishai 1993). To really reflect a permissive approach, formal access has to be supplemented by financial coverage. Financing ART treatments is expensive; leaving it dependent upon the financial resources of patients creates serious socio-economic inequalities in accessing ARTs.

Our approach qualitatively evaluates each dimension, and then aggregates them into an index that classifies ART regulations along a continuum running from "permissive" to "restrictive" (Engeli 2009).

Permissive Policy – Permissive policies grant the medical community and any category of recipient full access to ART treatments. Doctors are not constrained in their use of ART treatments, and patients are entitled to access ARTs regardless of their personal circumstances, marital status, or sexual orientation. In addition, the reimbursement of treatment costs is guaranteed by means of state funding or private medical insurance.

Restrictive Policy – In sharp contrast, restrictive policies impose severe restraints on each of the three dimensions. Medical autonomy is strictly limited by constraints or even bans on the use of ART techniques. Restrictive policies limit ART access to heterosexual couples and exclude single women and same-sex couples. In addition, they do not include broad financial coverage for treatments. As a result, lower socio-economic groups may find themselves excluded from fertility-related treatments.

Intermediate Policy – Regulation of the three dimensions does not necessarily follow a uniform pattern. An intermediate policy, therefore, combines characteristics of the restrictive and permissive dimensions. For instance, an intermediate policy may grant patients broad formal access to treatments, regardless of individual characteristics, but may not cover the cost of such treatments. Another example of an intermediate policy would be one that gives the medical community a high level of autonomy to resort to ARTs, but also strictly limits access to only heterosexual couples.

The Evolution of ART Policies Over Time Across Western Europe

Table 6.1 maps out ART policies in 15 Western European countries over time along our three analytical dimensions.[1] It reveals two striking spatial and temporal variations in the degree of regulatory permissiveness. First, it is clear that

Table 6.1 Evolution of ART Policies in Western Europe Over Time

Permissive	Intermediate	Restrictive
• Broad patients' access, *and* • Broad medical autonomy, *and* • Full/quasi-full reimbursement	• Patients' access under conditions, *or* • Limited medical autonomy, *or* • Low or no reimbursement	• Patients' access under conditions, *and* • Limited medical autonomy, *and/or* • No or low reimbursement
No major regulatory change over time		
Belgium (1999, 2007)	Portugal (2006)	Germany (1985, 1990, 2011)
The United Kingdom (1990, 2008)	Spain (1988, 2003, 2006)	Switzerland (1992, 1998)
The Netherlands (1989, 1993, 2002, 2007)		Austria (1992)
Finland (2006)		Norway (1987, 1994, 2003, 2007)
Major regulatory change over time		
France (1988) →	France (1994, 2004, 2011)	
	Italy (1985, 1987) →	Italy (2004)
Sweden (2016) ←	Sweden (2006) ←	Sweden (1985, 1988)
Iceland (2009) ←	Iceland (1996)	
Denmark (2007) ←	Denmark (1992, 1997, 2004)	

Sources: Bleiklie *et al.* 2004; Engeli *et al.* 2012.

Note
Ireland has not enacted any regulation.

national regulatory patterns diverge *in the overall degree of permissiveness*. Second, there is clear variation across dimensions *within these national patterns*.

First, Belgium, Finland, the United Kingdom, the Netherlands and more recently Denmark, Iceland, and Sweden, all govern ARTs in a permissive way (for Finland see Eriksson, this volume). Each of these countries has developed policies that, explicitly or implicitly, entitle a broad range of "patients" – heterosexual couples, lesbian couples, and very often single women as well – to access ART treatments.[2] These policies also grant the medical community broad autonomy to use ART techniques. For the most part, they only impose licensing and reporting procedures and do not impose substantive restrictions on the use of ART techniques that would interfere with the practice of ARTs. In addition, treatment costs are fully covered by health insurance schemes, at least for the first series of treatment cycles.

In contrast, since the beginning of the development of ARTs, Austria, Germany, Switzerland, and Norway have adopted drastically different regulatory approaches (for Norway see the contributions of Spilker and of Melhuus, this volume). In 2004, Italy joined this set of restrictive countries, after having initially been very permissive in its policies. All these countries ban a number of core techniques associated with ARTs, such as surrogacy or egg and embryo donation. In addition, they impose severe restrictions on how the techniques that are permitted can be used. As a result, many types of infertility cannot be treated, and this has led to a significant wave of fertility travel, with a large number of patients traveling to get the ART treatments they require in more permissive countries such as Belgium or Spain (see e.g., Kroløkke, this volume). In addition to these strict limits on medical autonomy, this second group of countries severely restricts access to ARTs. On the one hand, access is restricted to heterosexual couples, with Germany and Switzerland even requiring couples to be married for sperm donation. On the other hand, financial coverage is, at best, only partial. Switzerland, for instance, only provides coverage for artificial insemination (which is less and less practiced) while Germany covers just half the cost of treatment. This restrictive regulatory approach increases inequality between heterosexual and same-sex couples, as well as between socio-economic classes.

Finally, a third group of countries has developed an intermediate regulatory approach and these show striking variation across the three regulatory dimensions. Portugal, France since 1994, Iceland, Spain, Denmark until 2007, and Sweden until 2010, have all imposed similar heteronormative standards on access to ARTs as the restrictive group of countries, restricting access to heterosexual couples, who have to show some evidence of a long-standing relationship. Spain does not explicitly discriminate against patients according to their sexual orientation, but there are still obstacles for gay couples who want to become parents (see Smietana, this volume). However, in contrast to the restrictive group, the intermediate countries show more permissiveness along other dimensions. For instance, France, Sweden, Iceland, and Denmark have offered generous coverage for treatment costs while Italy, until 2004, was providing physicians and patients with broad autonomy but only a very low level of subsidies.

Patterns of policy change over time show a second puzzling variation. In some cases, such as Germany, Switzerland, the United Kingdom, and the Netherlands, initial regulation has been confirmed and reinforced by subsequent regulation. In these countries, strong path dependence is at work and regulatory approaches have not deviated over the last several decades, regardless of the level of permissiveness (Engeli and Rothmayr 2013).

In contrast to the path dependence in these four cases, major changes in the direction of public policies have occurred in other countries. France has become more restrictive over time, while Denmark and Sweden have progressively liberalized their regulation by softening the restrictions imposed on the medical community and enlarging access to same-sex couples. Italy has probably deviated the most from its initial regulatory path over time. For two decades, the field of ARTs in Italy was regulated by just two administrative circulars (addressing the prevention of HIV transmission through sperm donation). As a result, virtually any and all ART practices were de facto allowed. The 2004 law on assisted reproduction dramatically changed the situation and provided Italy with one of the most restrictive regulatory regimes across Western Europe to date (for an extended discussion of the Italian case, see Perrotta, this volume).

Explaining ART Policy Variation Using a Gendered Perspective

Comparative research has failed, so far, to fully explain these puzzling variations in the regulatory approaches adopted by Western European countries to tackle the complex issue of ART development. Most comparative research concentrates on the variation in the degree of autonomy granted to the medical community and does not pay attention to two other important actors in the field of reproduction (Latham 2002; Bleiklie *et al.* 2004; Engeli 2009): women's movements and religious actors. This disproportionate focus has left the variations in individual access to ARTs largely unexplained.

In contrast, we argue that the gender dimension of ART policy is key to fully understanding regulatory divergences across Western Europe. Medical actors do not constitute the sole target group of regulation; we argue that regulating ARTs also means regulating access to parenthood and, more generally, addressing the definition of gendered social roles (Bryld 2001; Lie 2002; Michelle 2006). Women have traditionally been defined according to their biological reproductive capacity. This biological differentiation has in turn been used to legitimize the contrasting social roles assigned to women and men in the public and private spheres, with maternity constructed as the natural feminine vocation. The development of ARTs has enabled a dissociation of the different reproductive functions and has thus offered new reproductive possibilities. The genetic mother no longer necessarily coincides with the gestational mother or the social mother. Sperm donation allows single women and lesbian couples to access parenthood without being involved in a heterosexual relationship, while surrogacy provides gay male couples with an alternative to adoption. Policies that impose restrictions on individual access to ART treatments actually legitimize specific forms of motherhood and family structure (Michelle 2006). As Bryld (2001) shows for the Danish case, the exclusion of same-sex couples in the initial phase of regulation was strongly influenced by the willingness of the majority in Parliament to reaffirm the pre-eminence of the traditional family and heteronormative social rules. Initial policy excluded lesbians as *unnatural mothers.*

The Unlimited Power of the Medical Community?

The impact of the medical community has been the focus of most comparative research on ART policy. Physicians are pivotal actors in the reproductive field, enjoying social prestige and professional authority. Engeli and Rothmayr (2013) argue that a high level of congruence in interests among ART physicians may lead to comprehensive self-regulation, which in turn impacts strongly upon state regulation. ART breakthroughs, with their implications regarding human embryos, have posed major regulatory challenges to governments. Self-regulation by the medical profession provides the government with some "ready-to-use" regulatory approaches whose efficiency has already been demonstrated.

The case of the UK is particularly illuminating in this respect. Medical associations developed voluntary self-regulations that were progressively accepted by the whole medical community and also became valued by public opinion in general. In drawing up the relevant law, the government relied heavily on self-regulatory mechanisms to craft its proposal. The legitimacy of this voluntary self-regulation exerted a clearly discernible influence on the development and evolution of the UK regulatory regime over time. It reflected both the efficacy and efficiency of such voluntary authority. It provided the government with some evidence of the success of license-based regulatory approaches, which facilitate scientific advances while allowing little, but key, scientific gatekeeping in the "command and control" features of the regulatory regime.

While strong and cohesive medical communities such as that in the UK have a clear and convergent impact on ART regulations, fragmented and weak medical communities tend to produce divergent policy responses. In Belgium, Schiffino and Varone (2004) emphasize that the division among physicians did not inspire the public authorities to comprehensively tackle the ART issue; rather they were content to merely regulate the licensing of medical centers without banning any specific medical techniques (with the sole exception of reproductive cloning). However, the Italian case tends to contradict this argument. In Italy too, the medical community was very fragmented over the issue, torn between Catholic doctors defending a restrictive policy that would allow only basic ART techniques for married couples, and doctors working in the private sector offering fertility treatments to post-menopausal women, which were regularly reported in the media (Fenton 2005). In this case, fragmentation within the medical community did not result in a permissive policy, as in Belgium, but rather in one of the most restrictive among Western European countries. The inability of Italian physicians to speak with one voice prevented them from establishing comprehensive self-regulation and containing the ART issue within the medical community. Rather, the media devoted a lot of attention to post-menopausal treatments and the ART issue became highly controversial in the public sphere. As Fenton (2005) showed, Catholics and pro-life actors successfully challenged the professional authority of doctors by extending the debate to the sanctity of life and the moral dimension of ARTs.

In sum, in the absence of public controversy, doctors prove to be powerful actors, who may succeed in keeping decision-making in the hands of the medical community. In turn, the resulting policies tend to address *only* medical issues as they relate to the regulation of the medical profession. However, in the face of public controversy, the medical community's impact on regulation will be moderated, and it is obliged to compromise with competing powerful actors in the field, such as women's movements and pro-life movements.

The Moderate Impact of Women's Movements

Women's movements have introduced a gender-conflict dimension to the debate, seeking changes in gendered social roles. Just as much as the liberalization of abortion, developments in the field of ARTs have challenged traditional gender roles. Restricting access to ARTs to heterosexual couples, as is the case in Italy, France, Germany, and Switzerland, reinforces the supremacy of the heterosexual family structure, in which women are responsible for nurturing and caring. Any assessment of the impact of women's movements on ART policy is complicated by the fact that, in some countries, the issue of ARTs deeply divides activists and does not command a high priority on the agendas of most women's movements in the countries under study. In addition, the transformation of women's movements by the end of the 1970s and their weakened mobilizing capacity complicates comparison across policy issues.

Among the women's movements that have emphasized the issue of ARTs, however, one can still observe great differences in terms of policy goals and impact on ART regulation. In Great Britain and Italy, for instance, women's movements chose to secure the liberalization of abortion by promoting a permissive position on ARTs, opposing pro-life attempts to impose the pre-eminence of the protection of the human embryo (Latham 2002). In these countries, feminists opted for a liberal position on reproductive technologies and framed the ART issue as part of the debate on the key reproductive rights to which every individual (in this case women) should be entitled. If they had some concerns about surrogacy and the potential commercialization of women's bodies, they nevertheless maintained a liberal stance on all components of the debate. They promoted permissive regulation that would respect the dignity of women and diversity in reproductive choices; namely, full access to ARTs without any discrimination related to civil status or sexual orientation, and the development of precise guidelines to monitor surrogacy practices.

In contrast, the German and Swiss women's movements pursued a very different approach in framing the gender dimension of ARTs (on Germany, see Bock von Wülfingen, this volume). Rather than emphasizing women's reproductive freedom, many feminist groups adopted an ecofeminist standpoint (Engeli 2009). They framed the ART issue along the nature-nurture nexus and linked the medical exploitation of women to male exploitation of the environment. Within this frame, feminist movements in Germany and Switzerland were strong advocates of restrictive ART policies that would protect women from scientific and patriarchal abuse.

Finally, some feminist movements failed to reach an internal consensus on how to deal with the issue of ARTs, which in turn contributed to their progressive exclusion from the policy-making process. In France, the feminist movement was clearly divided into two opposing camps over the issue. Part of the movement adopted a liberal stance and favored permissive regulation that would guarantee women's reproductive freedom. In complete contrast, the radical side of the movement was firmly opposed to ART development and mobilized around a total ban. Although the feminist movement was well integrated into the public debate over ARTs during the 1980s and mid-1990s, their disagreements prevented them from speaking with one voice and they collectively failed to inject a gender perspective into the debate. As a result, the feminist movement was progressively excluded and remained outside the policy-making process.

In addition to the salience of ARTs on feminist agendas, the success of women's movements seems to depend strongly on their policy allies. A weakened Italian movement fought alone against the pro-life movement, and failed to block restrictions on patient access, while the internal divisions among French feminists prevented any alliances (Fenton 2005). In contrast, the UK, Swiss, and German movements successfully benefited from important political allies that overcame their decreased capacity for mobilization.

In the UK, the women's movement forged a successful strategic alliance with the medical community against the pro-life movement to ensure women's freedom of choice regarding ARTs (Latham 2002). In Germany and Switzerland, the alarmist discourse of feminists on ARTs coincided perfectly with the critical stance adopted by the Social Democrats and the Greens. Their alliance with the left wing compensated for the weakness of the movement and provided them with a key ally in the decision-making process that sustained the political resonance of their frame. Indeed, the Social Democrats and the Greens became the official mouthpieces of feminist concerns during the parliamentary debates on the issue. As a result, the Swiss and the German parliamentary debates on ARTs integrated a gender perspective in a more significant way than in France.

The Defensive Role of the Christian Democrats

Turning to the impact of party politics on the regulation of ARTs, the findings of public policy research are more nuanced (Bleiklie *et al.* 2004; Engeli, Green-Pedersen, and Larsen 2012). On one hand, issues related to reproduction tend to engender heated public controversies that cut across political cleavages and internally divide political parties. On this basis, some authors argue that reproduction-related issues are no-win issues in electoral competition and therefore do not attract the attention of political parties (Burns 2005). However, Engeli *et al.* (2012; Engeli, Green-Pedersen, and Larsen 2013) argue instead that the way in which the religious cleavage structures the party system is a key factor in understanding political conflicts over the issue of ARTs.

The presence or absence of Christian Democrats in the party system generates different agenda-setting patterns and conflicting definitions of ARTs. For instance, Christian Democrats in Germany, Switzerland and the Netherlands greatly contributed to the politicization of the issue (Engeli *et al.* 2012). In order to sustain their electoral appeal in the face of a strongly secularizing environment, Christian Democrats had previously adopted an unsecular strategy in maintaining their appeal to their core religious voters (Engeli *et al.* 2012). Given the challenge of adapting to the process of secularization without losing their religious identity or core electoral base, the issue of ARTs provided Christian Democratic and other religious parties with an opportunity to revitalize their religious identity and draw renewed attention to religious themes.

At first sight, empirical analysis shows a contrasting pattern in terms of the impact of Christian Democratic parties on the regulation of ARTs. The strong mobilization of Christian Democrats does not necessarily result in ART policies that protect "the beginning of life" and preserve the traditional heteronormative family model. For instance, Belgian and Dutch regulations are much more permissive than those of Switzerland, Germany or Norway. Investigating the policy process in each case provides us with a more fine-grained picture of the impact of the Christian Democrats on the regulation of ARTs, as a comparison of the role of Christian Democrats in Germany, Italy and the Netherlands shows. In Germany, ART policy – specifically, the 1990 law on embryo protection – was adopted under a coalition government of Christian Democrats and Liberals. Drawing on the 1975 decision of the Federal Supreme Court to strike down the abortion law, the Christian Democrats advocated for protection of the human embryo. Their position was strengthened by the presence of a heterogeneous coalition of actors, all promoting different values, but all seeking very restrictive policies. Indeed, Christian Democratic opposition to ARTs was fueled by similar opposition from the left wing. The left feared that ARTs would open the door for eugenics – with all of the negative historical and cultural connotations that go with it – and were therefore in favor of banning IVF. Furthermore, mobilization against ARTs was equally motivated by distrust of the scientific and political elite that characterized the active German social movements of the 1980s. In Italy, the repetitive attacks of religious actors against the initial permissive regulation systematically failed during the 1980s and 1990s. Weakened by the disintegration of the Christian Democratic Party, religious actors lacked strong institutional support and failed to impose any restrictive regulation. Berlusconi's re-election and his electoral strategy of strongly pursuing the Catholic vote provided religious actors with a real opportunity to have an impact on the regulation of ARTs. Indeed, in 2004, under pressure from Catholic interest groups and the Vatican, the Italian government eventually revised its policy on ARTs and met most of the pro-life movement's policy goals – i.e., banning all techniques that involve the destruction of human embryos (Fenton 2005).

Both in Italy and Germany, the Christian Democrats and other religious actors needed some institutional support and allies to block permissive ART regulation, but even so they did not manage to impose a total ban. In contrast, in the Netherlands political parties were reluctant to put on the agenda any issue that could relaunch the controversy over abortion. The issue of ARTs was quickly depoliticized and relegated to science-related venues and specialized advisory bodies (Timmermans and Scholten 2006). During the 1980s and 1990s, the government refrained from any substantive intervention in the field. Instead, it simply issued procedural decrees – mainly imposing licensing procedures for ART centers in 1989, 1998 and 2000 – with the broad support of the medical community. Nevertheless, breakthroughs in embryo-related research during the 1990s put the issue back on the political agenda. The exceptional absence of the Christian Democrats from the government coalition between 1994 and 2002 allowed the formation of a secular coalition that was ready to address how best to substantively govern the ART field (Engeli *et al.* 2013). The resulting 2002 Embryo Act is one of the most permissive regulations in Europe regarding human embryonic research. While it imposes a temporary ban on the creation of embryos for research purposes and therapeutic cloning, the Act provides the medical community with wide autonomy in conducting research on embryonic stem cells derived from embryos that have not been used, once the treatment has been completed or interrupted. The reintegration of the Christian Democrats into the government coalition in 2002 did not result in any major revision of prior regulations; however, it has rendered it unlikely that the ban on embryo creation for research purposes will be removed in the near future.

Conclusion

Governing the field of ARTs has proven to be a very contentious issue in most Western European countries. This has resulted in a wide variation of regulatory approaches, ranging from allowing broad medical autonomy and unlimited patient access on the one hand to restricting access to ARTs to heterosexual couples and banning some important ART techniques on the other. Countries such as Italy and Switzerland ban same-sex couples' access to ARTs and impose severe constraints on heterosexual couples' access as well. Other countries, such as the Netherlands and the UK, do not impose any restrictions on ART access and grant the medical community broad autonomy in practicing ARTs. Investigating the regulation of ARTs across Western Europe over time, this chapter has shown that the gender dimension of such regulation is a key element to take into account. Such policies not only address medical autonomy in the practice of ART techniques, but also determine what kinds of parenthood are deemed socially legitimate. The issue of ARTs is thus best apprehended through three analytical dimensions: the autonomy granted to the medical community, the constraints imposed upon patients' access to ARTs, and the availability of healthcare coverage for ART treatments.

In regulating the field of ARTs, the medical community has played an important role. When physicians support congruent interests, they have, to a large extent, succeeded in imposing their policy preferences. However, medical authority has proven to be less influential when the ART issue is exposed to heated public controversy. Indeed, the multi-dimensionality of this issue often catalyzes intense public controversy that mobilizes numerous and divergent interests – among them, women's movements and pro-life actors representing strongly competing interests.

Women's movements generally bring a gender perspective to the debate, arguing in favor of women's rights and seeking changes in gendered social roles. However, as we have noted, women's movements have faced some difficulties in mobilizing and reaching a common position on the issue of ARTs. Where this is the case, it has weakened their impact on the regulatory process. Their success is strongly dependent on their ability to work with specific policy allies. Movements which succeeded in fostering strategic alliances with either the medical community or the political left were more likely to succeed in adding a gender perspective to the general debate. These alliances compensated for the possible weakness of the movement itself and acted as allies for feminist policy positions in the decision-making process.

Finally, a strong mobilization of Christian Democrats and the pro-life movement has not *necessarily* resulted in more restrictive ART policies, those that would protect the human embryo and preserve the heteronormative family model. Nevertheless, in some countries, religion-based opposition has resulted in higher levels of politicization of the conflict and retardation of the policy-making process. Just as women's movements have tended to be more successful in influencing the policy-making process and injecting their policy positions when they are able to forge strategic alliances, so too have religious actors been more likely to have a determining role in that process when they have formed policy alliances with those sympathetic to their values, notably right-wing parties.

To summarize, this chapter makes three major claims about the processes by which ART regulation has been developed in a Western European context and about its relationship to existing gendered and heteronormative structures. First, under conditions in which the medical community is highly cohesive, there may be little politicization of the issue and thus no debate or challenge to prevailing standards. Second, where the state does become more heavily involved (i.e., when the medical community fails to contain the scope of the conflict), the presence of Christian Democratic parties in government may lead to the issue being perceived in a more value-oriented way and thus a path may be opened up for actors from civil society to become heavily engaged in the policy process. Third, when those actors do become engaged (whether in challenging or maintaining existing gendered and heteronormative biases), their ability to act in alliances with political parties and/or the medical community – itself largely dependent upon their cohesiveness – will determine the extent to which they are able to exert an influence over policy outcomes.

Notes

1 This analysis does not include surrogacy legal arrangements.

2 Access to ART treatments for male same-sex couples at domestic medical facilities depends on national regulations regarding surrogacy. Some permissive countries allow for forms of altruistic surrogacy, for example the UK, Belgium, Greece or the Netherlands, while other countries ban any form of surrogacy within the domestic healthcare system such as Iceland and Sweden.

References

Bleiklie, Ivar, Malcolm L. Goggin, and Christine Rothmayr, eds. 2004. *Comparative Biomedical Policy: Governing Assisted Reproductive Technologies*. London: Routledge.

Bryld, Mette. 2001. "The Infertility Clinic and the Birth of the Lesbian: The Political Debate in Assisted Reproduction in Denmark." *European Journal of Women's Studies* 8 (3): 299–312.

Burns, Gene. 2005. *The Moral Veto: Framing Contraception, Abortion, and Cultural Pluralism in the United States*. Cambridge: Cambridge University Press.

Engeli, Isabelle. 2009. "The Challenges of Abortion and Assisted Reproductive Technologies Policies in Europe." *Comparative European Politics* 7: 56–74.

Engeli, Isabelle, and Christine Rothmayr. 2013. "Diverging Against all Odds? Regulatory Paths in Embryonic Stem Cell Research across Western Europe." *Journal of European Public Policy* 20 (3): 407–424.

Engeli, Isabelle, Christoffer Green-Pedersen, and Lars Thorup Larsen, eds. 2012. *Morality Politics in Western Europe: Parties, Agenda, and Policy Choices*. Basingstoke: Palgrave Macmillan.

Engeli, Isabelle, Christoffer Green-Pedersen, and Lars Thorup Larsen. 2013. "The Puzzle of Permissiveness: Understanding Policy Processes Concerning Morality Issues." *Journal of European Public Policy* 20 (3): 335–352.

Fenton, Rachel Anne. 2005. "Catholic Doctrine versus Women's Rights: The New Italian Law on Assisted Reproduction." *Medical Law Review* 14: 73–107.

Latham, Melanie. 2002. *Regulating Reproduction: A Century of Conflict in Britain and France*. Manchester: Manchester University Press.

Lie, Merete. 2002. "Science as Father? Sex and Gender in the Age of Reproductive Technologies." *European Journal of Women's Studies* 9 (4): 381–399.

Michelle, Carolyn. 2006. "Transgressive Technologies? Strategies of Discursive Containment in the Representation and Regulation of Assisted Reproductive Technologies in Aotearoa/New Zealand." *Women's Studies International Forum* 29 (2): 109–124.

Schiffino, Nathalie, and Frédéric Varone. 2004. "Art Policy in Belgium: A Bioethical Paradise?" In *Comparative Biomedical Policy: Governing Assisted Reproductive Technologies*, edited by Ivar Bleiklie, Malcolm L. Goggin, and Christine Rothmayr, 21–41. London: Routledge.

Timmermans, Arco, and Peter Scholten. 2006. "The Political Flow of Wisdom: Science Institutions as Policy Venues in the Netherlands." *Journal of European Public Policy* 13 (7): 1104–1118.

Yishai, Yael. 1993. "Public Ideas and Public Policy: Abortion Politics in Four Democracies." *Comparative Politics* 25 (2): 207–228.

7 Norwegian Biopolitics in the First Decade of the 2000s

Family Politics and Assisted Reproduction Understood through the Concept of the Trickster

Kristin H. Spilker

> A child is born. The happy "uterus-mother" rejoices together with the legal father. The biological mother died three years ago, and no one knows who the biological father is. This is not the introduction to a science-fiction story, but a situation that is far from unique in many countries, and which we might also have had in Norway if the social committee had not drawn a line.[1]

The above quotation was taken from the political debates over Norway's latest amendments to the Act on Biotechnology (*Bioteknologiloven* 2003), and demonstrates the fear and sense of risk attached to ARTs as well as a belief in Norway as a country that stands out in its willingness to govern. The quote contains several words that refer directly to the human body: uterus, biological mother and biological father. But it also mentions "the legal father," a phrase that refers directly to the Act. The national public debates on the definition of parenthood frequently refer to bodily material, as well as to social institutions such as the Act, or more fuzzy social entities, such as custom and tradition. The concept of biopolitics refers to the complex ways in which human life and relations between humans, or in relation to human tissue, are regulated, either legally or by means of other normative tools (Foucault [1976] 1998; Rose 2001; Foucault [2004] 2009; Lemke 2011).

The purpose of this article is to analyze some of the elements and paradoxes that make up Norwegian biopolitics. In 2003, Norway enacted what, in the media, was labeled "The world's strictest act on biotechnology," and, at the same time, a White Paper on the Family (*St.meld. nr. 29 2002–2003*) was presented that was supportive of family values in general, and the traditional heterosexual family in particular. Nevertheless, only five years later, Norway was one of the first countries in the world to enact a gender-neutral Marriage Act (Lov 2008–12–19, nr 112), which meant that, as married couples, lesbian couples also had access to assisted reproduction according to the Act on Biotechnology (*Bioteknologiloven* 2003). How could this movement happen so fast, indeed, historically, almost simultaneously? If one follows the ideological lines of party politics, the obvious answer is that there was a change of government in 2005, when the Conservative government, led by the Christian Democrats, was replaced by a Socialist government, led by the Labor Party. However, this chapter seeks to explore a different route, one that hopefully sheds light on the way in which processes of social change are infiltrated by unruly concepts and unruly technologies.

By applying Donna Haraway's concept of the trickster (Haraway 1992), I seek to tell a more complex story, one that speaks to unruly technologies as well as unruly concepts. The mythological figure of the trickster is an inspiring tool for analyzing biopolitics. It creates space to include actors of different sorts: technologies, language and humans can all be ascribed trickster qualities or act like tricksters. This further implies that the trickster works simultaneously as a methodological and analytical tool.

The argument is composed of textual analyses of the parliamentary debates on the Act on Biotechnology (*Bioteknologiloven* 2003), the White Paper on the Family (*St.meld. nr. 29 2002–2003*) and the Marriage Act (Lov 2008–12–19, nr 112), as well as a qualitative interview with a same-sex couple who have become parents to twins, but whose parenthood is simultaneously both included and excluded by the Norwegian state.

The Trickster at Work: Enrolling Technologies and Concepts

The figure of the trickster is theoretically grounded within science and technology studies. A fundamental tenet within this tradition is that technologies, cultural codes and language work together as a network of actors. What is different and controversial about this approach to social theory is its insistence on the agency of nonhumans. This insistence is made because it allows an analysis of the relations between nonhumans and humans, or the material and semiotic (Haraway 1991, 1992). This line of thought is akin to Bruno Latour's (2005) argument for the need to "re-assemble the social"; that is, not to see social phenomena as stabilized entities, but to seek to trace the connections of which they are made at a certain time and in a certain place. This implies that "social phenomena" are seen as co-constructions of different kinds of human and nonhuman agents, such as for example concepts and technologies, which, in joint action, are doing work that helps to stabilize or destabilize these phenomena.

In social studies of bioscience, this approach has been applied to show how bodily processes, technology and bioscientific language interact (Oudshoorn 1996; Rose 2001; Smelik and Lykke 2008). In the particular empirical field of assisted reproduction, it has contributed by revealing the ways in which new techno-medical devices are part of a cultural dialogue on sexuality and parenthood (Franklin 1997; Lie 2002; Thompson 2005).

Donna Haraway's concept of the cyborg has been a major contribution to the field of science and technology studies, and is especially inspirational for studying the relationship between the body and technology (Haraway 1991, 1992; Lykke and Braidotti 1996). The metaphor of the cyborg challenges the ways in which we think of the human body and its natural boundaries, and also how we conceptualize techno-medical interventions such as assisted reproduction. But in this analysis I make use of another, less familiar, concept from Haraway's writings: the trickster. Before analyzing Haraway's concept of the trickster, I explore the connotations of this concept, outlining the ways in which it adds value as an analytical and methodological tool for this particular empirical material.

The trickster, first and foremost, refers to a mythical character found in folk tales and legends worldwide. The trickster is described as a spirit or a god, and often as an anthropomorphic animal that plays tricks or otherwise disobeys the rules of "normal" behavior. The trickster deity breaks the rules of the gods of nature, sometimes maliciously, but usually with positive effects. Its actions are often in the form of tricks, but also thievery. Tricksters are sometimes described as sacred figures themselves, or as playing with the sacred. The Greek Titan Prometheus, who stole fire from the gods to give to humans, offers one example of how tricksters have been shown to play with the sacred (Lock 2002; Grassie 1996).

Tricksters can be cunning or foolish, or both; they are often funny, even when considered sacred or when they are performing important cultural tasks such as those involving reproduction. It is remarkable how often the trickster acts as an equalizer, plays with gender and, sometimes, has the capacity to change gender.

An internationally known example of a Norwegian trickster is the Norse God Loki, who is the god of misfortune, accident or unfortunate incidents (Ashram 1995). For Norwegians, a more familiar and contemporary example is Mikkel Rev – or Mike the Fox. He appears in Norwegian fairy tales as a "Luring" – that is, a sneak, or the sly fox. Mikkel Rev often operates in disguise, and his actions create consequences and alter situations in unexpected ways.

The primary motivation for Donna Haraway's use of the trickster concept was to say something about knowledge production and the problems that arise from treating the world and the things in it as parts of nature, or passive resources. Haraway explains that she wants to point out how worldly things are produced out of connections – connections and enrollments.

She further comments that "Feminist objectivity makes room for surprises and ironies at the heart of all knowledge production; we are not in charge of the world" (Haraway 1991, 199). A few pages later, she elucidates this idea further: "Perhaps the world resists being reduced to mere resource because it is – not mother/matter/nature – but coyote, a figure for the always problematic, always potent tie of meaning and bodies" (Haraway 1991, 201).

Following Haraway's reminder that we need to see the world as a collection of connections and enrollments, I explore how assisted reproduction is connected to the wider field of family politics, and follow parts of the knowledge production that took place within this field in Norway during the first decade of the twenty-first century.

Norway: A Modern Welfare State with the World's Most Restrictive Act on Biotechnology?

In Norway, human biotechnology has, for several decades, been a highly politicized field; this dates back to the very first national legislation on assisted reproduction in 1987. Regulation of ARTs has not only been prominent in public debate, but has also entered party politics and been central in marking political divides (Brekke and Sirnes 2011, 359). According to Brekke and Sirnes, the restrictive line that has been taken toward biotechnology has been grounded partly in religion, but also in what they label "a critique of instrumentalisation." In a previous study of the Norwegian debate (Spilker and Lie 2007), we found that the defining ideological pillars supporting the debates about ARTs in Norway are gender equality, technology and the welfare state. These pillars are framed as interconnected by some participants in the debate, in the sense that, given the technological possibilities, the modern welfare state of Norway has the responsibility to offer reproductive technologies for the advancement of gender equality.

The Labor Party has historically been the biggest political party in Norway, and also the party that has had the strongest position and the most prime ministers during the post-war period. My assertion is that the Labor Party's identity is still deeply rooted in the decades following the Second World War, the late 1940s and 1950s. In retrospect, the Labor Party has received much of the honor for developing Norway as a modern welfare state during this period, and for building it up as a social democracy with the ideal that everyone should have access to common goods. What is relevant in this context is that the Labor Party can be summed up as modernist, in the sense of being positive or even positivist, toward science, technology and new knowledge. This is illustrated by the following quote from a parliamentary debate on assisted reproduction, by the Labor representative:

> The Labour Party sees it as a goal to help women who are involuntarily childless and who are infertile. We see this as a medical condition [...] and hence when we have the knowledge, and given our society and health service, we have the responsibility to offer these women treatment.
>
> (Spilker and Lie 2007, 333)

In 1997, for the first time, Norway elected a prime minister from the Christian Democrats. He led a Conservative coalition government including the Right and the Centre Party, which, with a short break, governed until the election in 2005. During these years of government, a new Biotechnology Act and a new White Paper on the Family were prepared. As exemplified by the quote in the introduction, much of the debate on assisted reproduction has concerned the desire to govern this area and, moreover, the desire to "draw a line." Furthermore, there were some concepts that were particularly important in framing the Norwegian discussion, the most important of these being: "the sanctity of human life," "the precautionary principle," "the sorting society" and "the best interests of the child" (Melhuus 2005; Solberg 2009).

When Norway's Act on Biotechnology was approved in 2003, the actual techno-medical fertility treatments discussed were egg and sperm donation. The Act retained the prohibition on egg donation, and also repealed the right to sperm donation from an anonymous donor. Sperm donation from the public health service could, from that point on, only be obtained if the donor were picked from the public sperm bank, which gave the eventual child the right to identify the donor when that child reached 18 years of age. At that time, egg donation was accessible in most European countries, and likewise sperm donation from an anonymous donor. As a consequence, the new Act was referred to as "the world's strictest act on biotechnology" in the Norwegian media and, later, in the international media.

So how did it come about that, in 2008, Norway was among the first countries to pass a new Marriage Act allowing same-sex couples the right to assisted reproduction?

The First Trickster: The Concept of the Family

The introduction to the White Paper on the Family is entitled: "The value base of family politics," and describes the value of the family in society: "The family is the fundamental unit of society; the most important arena for belonging, intimacy and community. The family is the meeting point between the individual and society" (*St.meld. nr. 29 2002–2003*, 5).

Here, "the family" is referred to in the singular and portrayed as a stable unit. Furthermore, the family unit is given the status of being fundamental to both the individual and society, and the site where the values of society meet the needs of the individual self. According to this perspective, the government, led by the Christian Democrats, legitimizes the importance of "active" family politics. But just a few paragraphs below, the concept of the family becomes less stable and is given extensive clarification: "The family comprises married couples with or without children, cohabitants with or without children, single parents living with children, parents with 'visiting systems,' families with foster children and single persons, and persons living alone" (*St.meld. nr. 29 2002–2003*, 5).

Here, "the family" is still designated in singular form, but it is carefully described to make family politics relevant to all Norwegian citizens. The following pages of the White Paper on the Family clarify that families with children are the main focus of policy development, and that, even though there are many types of family, not all of them provide the same qualities for children:

> At the same time we can say that not all kinds of cohabitation give children the same amount of security. When both parents are present and live in a stable, binding and enduring relationship, it will increase the child's experience of security. This safety also encompasses the parents' sexuality and loving relations. A secure sexuality that includes the psychological, social

> and biological dimensions and makes up a mature and lasting relationship, will affect the children in the family positively.
>
> (*St.meld. nr. 29 2002–2003*, 8)

These excerpts show, first, an attempt to be inclusive and to make family politics relevant to all, and thereby an attempt to legitimize this inclusivity in national party politics. On the other hand, the second excerpt illustrates a notion of the family that creates a hierarchy between families. Altogether, the three excerpts point to a number of contradictions and tensions in the definition of family and the connections from which it is made: Should it include marriage and the law? Should it include children? Need these be genetically related children? Must they live in the same household? Is each and every one of us a family in our own right?

Looking at the concept of "the family" as a trickster, we see that at the outset, it is stable, a little bit conservative and a solid building block for society. The second time it appears, it gives another impression: unstable and a character with many faces. Then, by its last appearance, it is much more firm and eager to tell right from wrong – or at least, to give some clear advice about best practice. This last visit from the trickster also indicates that possibly it wants to exercise some power. So, in other words, what at first seems to be a concept designating a quite clear assemblage of men, women and children who are connected in specific ways, turns out to be a rather unstable and vague conceptual construction – perhaps even a myth.

In the same year as the White Paper on the Family was launched, Norway also adopted a new Act on Biotechnology (*Bioteknologiloven* 2003). This is another document in which it is possible to follow movement and instability.

The Second Trickster: Assisted Reproduction

In the Act on Biotechnology (*Bioteknologiloven* 2003), it is made explicitly clear that all fertility treatment should be reserved for medically infertile heterosexual couples, and should contribute to making families of a specific kind: "Assisted conception can only be carried out when a woman is married to, or lives with, a man in a marriage-like relationship" (*Bioteknologiloven* 2003, §2–2).

Here, assisted reproduction is clearly restricted to contributing to the production of families consisting of one man, one woman and one or more children. At the same time, it shows that there is actually a need for explicit clarification. *Who* should have access to assisted reproduction? This marks an important point: this paragraph in the Act on Biotechnology is not concerned with regulating techno-medical methods, per se, but with trying to stabilize, and at the same time destabilize, certain assemblages of technologies and human units of flesh and blood. This concern is very much in line with what seems to be the aim of the trickster figure in the previous section.

Throughout the 2000s, ARTs were no longer solely discussed as new techno-medical practices or simply as forms of biotechnology. Assisted reproduction had become a vital issue in what became open political controversies about the connections between reproduction, heterosexuality and parenthood. The 2005 general election resulted in a change of government, and, after two periods of Conservative rule led by the Christian Democrats, a Socialist government was elected, led by the Labor Party with support from the Socialist Left. This government soon started work on what was to become a new and gender-neutral Marriage Act.

In the preparations for what was to become the new Marriage Act (Lov 2008–12–19, nr 112), it is possible to follow the ambivalence about reproduction and what issues reproductive technologies should address. The White Paper on the Family that constituted the preparation for the new Act came from the Ministry on Children, Equality and Inclusion. This chapter shows that the issue of whether infertility among same-sex couples should be equated to medical infertility was acknowledged as a relevant question:

> Whether one should equate medical reasons with other reasons for not being able to have children in the normal way, is a question. This has been emphasized by several bodies in the public hearing. A major argument for allowing assisted reproduction for lesbians is that this will lead to equal treatment, and thereby equal rights, between heterosexual and homosexual couples who live in stable relationships. In connection with this we refer to The Norwegian Centre for Human Rights, which in the hearing expresses: "[...] the opinion that this proposition will contribute to increased equality, tolerance and respect, aims that are promoted through the Convention on Human Rights."
>
> (Barne-, likestillings- og inkluderingsdepartementet 2007)

Norway was the sixth country in the world to adopt a gender-neutral Act on Marriage (Lov 2008–12–19, nr 112). The new Act was passed by Parliament in June 2007, and became operative in 2008. It brought along with it changes to three other laws: the Act on Biotechnology (*Bioteknologiloven* 2003), the Children Act and the Act on Adoption. The Act on Biotechnology now gives equal rights to assisted reproduction for heterosexual and same-sex couples, the Children Act establishes legal parental rights for co-mothers in lesbian couples and the Act on Adoption gives lesbian and homosexual couples access to adoption.

This section has highlighted the way in which ARTs have shifted in character, from techno-medical practices assisting bodily dysfunctions to techno-medical practices addressing differences based on gender or sexual orientation. Thus, the right to seek methods that are legal and available within the Norwegian health-care system has been equalized. In principle, the right to seek sperm donation and IVF treatment have become established as new rights for lesbians and single women. However, men without a female partner still have no opportunities to access reproductive assistance.

Tricksters of Flesh and Blood

This last empirical section does not deal with white papers or legislation, but with the story of a male couple who, in 2007, became fathers through a specific assembly of human and techno-medical resources. I interviewed the couple in late autumn 2007, during the period when the new Act on Marriage was being prepared and lesbians' right to seek assisted reproduction was attracting much support.

The couple are parents of two children who were conceived in California by gestational surrogacy. This arrangement involves one woman donating an egg, which is then implanted in another woman, who subsequently becomes pregnant and gives birth to the child. In this specific case, the donor eggs were fertilized with sperm from the two men. Consequently, the children have the same genetrix but different genitors, and one surrogate carried them through as a "twin" pregnancy. Asked why they chose gestational surrogacy, one father answered: "We wanted to make a twist, to make it a bit easier to create a distance, both biologically and socially." In California, both fathers were noted on each child's birth certificate, and the family of four traveled home to Norway. But back in Norway they found that their family constellation was not compatible with the Norwegian state's definition of the family. This was made clear when the fathers attempted to inscribe their children in the National Register. At the registration office, forms do not provide room for the signatures of two fathers for the same child, and when the fathers used the "mother" column for one of their names, they afterwards received a letter informing them that this was not acceptable. The children were entered in the National Register – but without parents.

The authorities then suggested a solution, wherein both fathers could take DNA tests to define genetic paternity and give them legal paternity to one child each. Later, they could apply for adoption of each other's child. But the fathers did not approve of this solution; as one father expressed it: "We did not want to be picked apart by DNA tests, and then later be pieced together in a new way, and in a way that society finds suitable."

This example clearly shows that the question of men becoming parents is not necessarily limited by bodily or techno-medical constraints. Quite the contrary, as certain methods of assisted reproduction involving combinations of bodily capacities and techno-medical practices make it possible. The difference between surrogacy and other forms of assisted reproduction lies, rather, in the connection between bodies and technologies and, possibly, the lack of stabilization and involvement of the "mother" concept. This assumption is substantiated by the fact that a number of heterosexual couples have applied the same ART practices and inscribed their children in the National Register without further hindrances.

Conclusion

The actual historical course of ARTs in Norway during the first decade of the 2000s reveals the ways in which the regulations and distribution of technologies have comprised examples of time- and space-specific "assemblages of the social." Certain conceptual framings of the family and certain techno-medical practices came together and became vital actors in Norwegian biopolitics, in a way that human actors might not have foreseen. Politicians, bureaucrats and various interest groups that were involved in the field of family politics worked with unstable concepts and unruly technologies. This is why I chose to employ the concept of the trickster – to make visible how these different nonhuman and human actors all played a part in the story, and also made themselves useful, as both allies and competent opponents.

The trickster showed up during several stages of the transitions that took place during this decade. The first trickster appeared in the concept of the family as outlined simultaneously in the White Paper on the Family and the Act on Biotechnology of 2003. "The family" was, first, the fundamental building block for both the individual and society. There, the trickster's performance shone through, for what happens when we have already been told that we are all part of (or are) families, and that families are defined as "the most important arena for belonging, intimacy and community?" Is it then possible, in the next round, to argue that someone is not family, or should not be allowed access to technology to create the families they want – and are able – to create?

The second trickster became visible in §2–2 of the Act on Biotechnology (*Bioteknologiloven* 2003), which stated two things at once: first, that ARTs must be reserved for heterosexuals; second, that these technologies have wider potential. Even if ARTs were originally developed and framed as a solution for medically infertile heterosexual couples, they also provide possibilities for other groups of people, such as homosexuals and single people.

Laws are textual entities, but consist of powerful linguistic constructions that distribute rights and duties amongst citizens. When ARTs were first discussed in relation to legislation in 1987, they were discussed as part of new biotechnologies; that is, in relation to genetic engineering or even cloning. However, the trickster became of crucial importance: from that point on, ARTs were no longer discussed within the frame of new technologies, but within the frame of equal rights. This particular shift implies that ARTs changed from being techno-medical devices assisting bodily dysfunctions to technologies addressing differences based on gender or sexual orientation. This is underlined by the fact that the latest change in the legislation on assisted reproduction came about from the field of family politics and the Act on Marriage, not from political processes concerning biotechnology. This development exemplifies how legislation connects and enrolls entities of different orders; through the law, technologies, humans and inherent cultural values are organized, re-assembled and, possibly, stabilized.

The above analysis shows, however, that both the concept of the family and the concept of ARTs fit the description of the trickster and, thus, are not easily stabilized. The family is described in paradoxical ways: a building block for society, an arena for feelings and a unit of children and parents. ARTs also have different agendas and, even if they first came along exclusively to assist heterosexual couples, they almost simultaneously revealed their potential to assist more people. And this potential, in turn, implied that the concept of the family was further destabilized; the question of which bodies and which connections make up a viable concept of "the family" became relevant once again.

In 2008, with the new legislation on marriage and the amendments to the Act on Biotechnology, lesbian couples became enrolled in the family of families. At the same time, sperm donation and IVF treatment transformed from techno-medical practices addressing medical conditions into solutions to inequality based on gender and sexuality. Still, this new connection between ARTs and gender equality did not generate a viable solution for how to stabilize the paradoxical concept of the family. Even though more people were now included in the definition of family, there was still a huge group excluded, their potential and connections not even discussed by Parliament or legislative authorities. This group, comprised of men without a female partner, remains huge.

The third empirical section dealt with a male same-sex couple and described how they conceived their own family of flesh and blood. Their case illustrates the way in which power is also enacted outside legislation and institutions. These fathers illustrate that people do not necessarily think and act in the ways that legislation or other normative powers suggest, but, rather, according to their own horizons of possibility. As Marilyn Strathern poignantly formulates: people simply do what they think can be done.

> [S]ocial change sometimes comes about in a very simple way. As far as English culture is concerned, all that is required is what (middle-class) people do all the time, namely that they do what they think can be done. Put into action, this becomes an effort to promote and implement current values. Values are acted upon: implicit assumptions become explicit, and that includes rendering culturally visible what may be perceived as a natural process.
>
> (Strathern 1992, 44)

This last story, about the family of four, exemplifies the most current open controversy in Norwegian family politics: that of surrogacy as a method of building Norwegian families. The techno-medical practices included in traditional or gestational surrogacy cannot separately be rendered as new – it is the combinations making up gestational surrogacy that are relatively new. I would like to emphasize this point: that it is first and foremost the connections, the relations and the (perhaps missing) enrollments that make this techno-medical practice so controversial.

The concept of the trickster might help to dissolve and destabilize pre-set connections between concepts, technologies and human actors in relation to ARTs and family politics in Norway. ARTs have largely been normalized and integrated into society by processes of adaptation to already-existing cultural values. But the trickster shows that these processes of integration are neither linear nor predictable, and that technologies can sometimes enter into or constitute new and unforeseen alliances. This is similar to Latour's reminder not to see "the social" as something already designated, but rather as time and space connections out of which "the social" is made.

Note

1 This statement was made by a representative of the political party, The Right, and was made in a meeting in which Parliament was addressing assisted reproduction as regulated by the Act on Biotechnology (*Bioteknologiloven* 2003); Parliamentary meeting June 17, 2002, case no. 4, "Recommendation from the social committee on the medical use of biotechnology."

References

Ashram, Andrew. 1995. "Power and Invisibility. Introduction: Obsolete Bodies, Ancient Cyborgs." Koni VI. Accessed February 5, 2008. www.koni.ch/cyborg/cyborg.html.

Barne- , likestillings- og inkluderingsdepartementet [Ministry of Children and Equality] 2007. *White Paper on the Family*.

Bioteknologiloven. 2003. www.lovdata.no/all/nl-20031205–100.html.

Brekke, Ole Andreas, and Thorvald Sirnes. 2011. "Biosociality, Biocitizenship and the New Regime of Hope and Despair: Interpreting 'Portraits of Hope' and the 'Mehmet Case.'" *New Genetics and Society* 30 (4): 347–374.

Foucault, Michel. [1976] 1998. *The History of Sexuality Vol. 1: The Will to Knowledge*. London: Penguin.

Foucault, Michel. [2004] 2009. *Biopolitikkens fødsel. Forelesninger på Collège de France 1978–1979*. København: Hanz Reitzels Forlag.

Franklin, Sarah. 1997. *Embodied Progress: A Cultural Account of Assisted Reproduction*. London: Routledge.

Grassie, William. 1996. "Donna Haraway's Metatheory of Science and Religion: Cyborgs, Tricksters and Hermes." *Zygon* 31 (2): 285–304.

Haraway, Donna. 1991. *Simians, Cyborgs and Women: The Reinvention of Nature*. New York: Routledge.

Haraway, Donna. 1992. "The Promises of Monsters: A Regenerative Politics for Inappropriate/d Others." In *Cultural Studies*, edited by Lawrence Grossberg, Cary Nelson, and Paula Treichler, 295–337. New York: Routledge.

Latour, Bruno. 2005. *Re-Assembling the Social: An Introduction to Actor-Network Theory*. Oxford: Oxford University Press.

Lemke, Thomas. 2011. *Biopolitics: An Advanced Introduction*. New York: New York University Press.

Lie, Merete. 2002. "Science as Father: Sex and Gender in the Age of Reproductive Technologies." *European Journal of Women's Studies* 9 (4): 381–399.

Lock, Helen. 2002. "Transformations of the Trickster." *Southern Cross Review*. www.southerncrossreview.org/18/trickster.htm.

Lov 2008–12–19, nr 112. *Ekteskapsloven* [The Marriage Act]. Last accessed January 2009. www.regjeringen.no/en/dokumenter/the-marriage-act/id448401/.

Lykke, Nina, and Rosi Braidotti, eds. 1996. *Between Monsters, Goddesses and Cyborgs: Feminist Confrontations with Science, Medicine and Cyberspace*. London: Zed Books.

Melhuus, Marit. 2005. "'Better Safe than Sorry': Legislating Assisted Conception in Norway." In *State Formation: Anthropological Perspectives*, edited by Christian Krohn-Hansen and Knut Nustad, 212–233. London: Pluto Press.

Oudshoorn, Nelly. 1996. "The Decline of the One-Size-Fits-All Paradigm, or, How Reproductive Scientists Try to Cope with Postmodernity." In *Between Monsters, Goddesses and Cyborgs: Feminist Confrontations with Science, Medicine and Cyberspace*, edited by Nina Lykke and Rosi Braidotti, 153–169. London: Zed Books.

Rose, Nicholas. 2001. "The Politics of Life Itself." *Theory, Culture & Society* 18 (6): 1–30.

Smelik, Anneke and Nina Lykke, eds. 2008. *Bits of Life: Feminism at the Intersections of Media, Bioscience and Technology*. Seattle and London: University of Washington Press.

Solberg, Berge. 2009. "Getting Beyond the Welfare of the Child in Assisted Reproduction." *Journal of Medical Ethics* 35 (6): 373–376.

Spilker, Kristin, and Merete Lie. 2007. "Gender and Bioethics Intertwined: Egg Donation within the Context of Equal Opportunities." *The European Journal of Women's Studies* 14 (4): 327–340.

St.meld. nr. 29. 2002–2003. www.regjeringen.no/nn/dokumenter/stmeld-nr-29–2002–2003-/id471301/.

Strathern, Marilyn. 2002. *After Nature: English Kinship in the Late Twentieth Century*. Cambridge: Cambridge University Press.

Thompson, Charis. 2005. *Making Parents: The Ontological Choreography of Reproductive Technologies*. London: MIT Press.

8 Bringing It All Back Home

Cross-Border Procreative Practices. Examples from Norway

Marit Melhuus

Framing the Issue

Transnational procreative practices, and in particular cross-border surrogacy, are a challenge to the authorities in Norway, as elsewhere (Inhorn and van Balen 2002). In Norway, surrogacy is not permitted. This not only has to do with a reticence against commercialization of reproduction and concern for the best interests of the child, it is also a question of ascribing proper filiation. This in turn revolves around shifting notions of maternity, paternity, and parenthood; in short, family formation. The nexus for these disputes, I argue, is the significance attributed to biology as a particular kind of truth knowledge (Salazar 2009), in establishing certain relations. As a reproductive practice, surrogacy works differently for men and women: a man can be accorded paternity if he can prove his biogenetic link to the child. However, this is not the case for women.

The following example, which mobilized the Norwegian public, illustrates the point (see also Kroløkke 2012). In January 2010, an Indian surrogate mother gave birth to twins for a Norwegian woman. Both donor sperm and donor eggs had been used to conceive the two children. The intending mother – Kari Ann – proceeded to apply to the Norwegian authorities for the right to adopt the twins. When she initially stated that the children were biogenetically hers, it seemed that the adoption process would go smoothly. However, at a later date it was revealed that Kari Ann was not their biogenetic mother. Her application was denied on August 4, 2010 as was her appeal. A year later, Kari Ann was still in India, living with the twins in Goa. Not only was she an illegal resident, but her children were also without papers. They were undocumented and in fact stateless. The Norwegian authorities claimed that the children were Indian (having been born to an Indian woman), whereas the Indian authorities insisted that they were Norwegian.

In the meantime, Kari Ann had engaged a lawyer and Norwegian politicians had become involved with her case. In her local community, a support group of grandmothers started a fundraising campaign for Kari Ann and her twins. By April 2011, the Norwegian authorities had worked out a solution and the children were finally able to travel to Norway, having been granted a residence permit. Once in Norway, it was the responsibility of the Office of the Public

Guardian (*Overformynderiet*) to find a suitable guardian for the twins, who were in theory without parents. Thereafter it was the job of the Child Welfare Authorities (*Barnevernet*) to find a permanent solution.

It is important to keep in mind that it is not illegal for Norwegian citizens to enter into cross-border surrogacy contracts. The issue is how to bring the children legally to Norway. This, in turn, has to do with filiation and the proper ascription of motherhood and fatherhood. It is apparent, at least in the case of Kari Ann, that it is no easy task to establish legal parenthood of children born to a foreign surrogate abroad. Many different people, including the authorities, were enrolled in order to find a solution. Procreative intent is not enough to justify legal parenthood in Norway, all the more so if there is no proof of a biogenetic connection between the intending parent and the child. However, there is another point to be made. In the case of Kari Ann, it is the way in which the children have been brought into being that challenges her parenthood. They are (by the Norwegian authorities at least) viewed as the product of an illicit exchange. And it is the character of this exchange that creates the problem (more on this below).

Norwegian law defines the mother as the one who gives birth, irrespective of whether or not the genetic material is hers. It also prohibits egg donation. This has several ramifications. For example: a Norwegian woman in need of an egg may make use of such a service at a fertility clinic abroad. Because she gives birth, she will be considered the mother of the child, despite the fact that the genetic material is not hers. The same holds true for a woman who makes use of anonymous donor sperm. As Norway prescribes the use of known donor sperm, those who prefer an anonymous donor must travel abroad. Again, her maternity will not be questioned. In both situations, the actual genetic make-up of the child is ignored, as birthing is privileged over other (f)acts. The only other way to obtain legal maternity is through adoption. Hence, a Norwegian woman making use of a surrogate – even if, unlike Kari Ann, she has used her own eggs – is precluded from claiming motherhood. Her eggs don't count. Reproductive intent is not accepted as a legal ground for establishing parenthood.

Norwegian citizenship is based (primarily) on *jus sanguinis*. This implies that children with either a Norwegian mother or father will automatically gain Norwegian citizenship. There is thus a link between filiation, the ascription of paternity and maternity, and obtaining citizenship. This link is activated in transnational reproductive practices. As Kroløkke states: "Biogenetic substances become the building blocks for such fundamental cultural structures as kinning and citizenship" (Kroløkke 2012, 320).

In this chapter, I focus on some of the dilemmas that have emerged as a result of surrogacy practices. To begin with, I will, albeit briefly, discuss some salient aspects regarding the legal incorporation of reproductive technologies in Norway.[1] I am concerned with two particular developments in the biopolitical domain. The first is the increasing biocentrism or privileging of biological connectedness, with regard to filiation. The other concerns the ways in which maternity and paternity are differently ascribed, and the shifting grounds of proof to establish the facts of procreation (Strathern 1999). These two developments are intimately connected and may perhaps be seen as a response to the uncertainties that reproductive technologies provoke regarding fundamental notions of kinship and relatedness.

However, these tendencies are primarily articulated through – and hence derived from – public discourse and practices such as the legislative process. Those making use of assisted conception may certainly attach other meanings to such procreative events (Melhuus 2007). In other words, there is a tension between what the law permits and what some people actually do. Or, in the words of Campbell, a contrast between "the governance of reproductive intimacy ... [and] its vernacular negotiation" (Campbell 2007, 98). This discrepancy is made explicit by the existence of a transnational space within which assisted reproductive practices can potentially occur, by the legal void that (at least until 2011)[2] makes such practices possible, and by the public debates surrounding them. Regarding the latter, there is no doubt that the media plays – and has played – a significant role in drawing attention to surrogacy practices and the ethical dilemmas these entail. In fact, the media represents an important platform for the many voices concerned with surrogacy, not least for some of the parents of children born to surrogates (e.g., Fosse *et al.* 2011).

Legal Framework – The Context

The law regulating assisted conception in Norway has been based on the precautionary principle: "Better safe than sorry." This has implied restrictive regulation. However, the regulatory regime of biotechnologies is not fixed, but has been subject to renewed enactments as the biopolitical landscape and the alignments within it reconfigure. Initially, assisted conception was only offered to married heterosexual couples; this was later expanded to also allow treatment for heterosexual couples living in stable partnerships. Finally, the amendment to the Marriage Act in 2008 (Lov 2008–12–19, nr 112), granting same-sex couples the same rights as heterosexual couples, extended access to infertility treatment to these couples as well.[3] In practice, this only benefits lesbian couples, as Norwegian regulations do not permit forms of assistance – such as surrogacy – that would enable male same-sex couples to have children (see also Spilker, this volume).[4]

Underpinning the legislation is not just a concern with infertility and public health. The legislation is framed – and held in place – in terms of ethics. This was explicitly stated in relation to the first Act relating to artificial procreation (Lov 1987–06–12, nr 68. *Lov om kunstig befruktning*). Two overriding concerns were expressed regarding the aim of the legislation: to secure the best interests of the child and to ensure the interests of society, by preventing selective human breeding and the commercialization of reproduction (Innst. O. nr 60–1986–87: 2). Thus two significant elements are introduced: one articulates concern for the child, the other concern about practices that violate human dignity. In addition to setting the best interests of the child as the primary consideration, it is the idea of the instrumentalization of human life, through the commercialization of certain reproductive practices, that grounds the ethical reflections. Within such a frame, the idea of reproductive choice is perceived (by some) as problematic and one intention of the law is precisely to curb individual choice in these matters.

Since 1987, Norwegian legislation has permitted sperm donation. Until 2003, donors were anonymous. The anonymity clause was repealed in the Biotechnology Act of 2003 (Lov 2003–15–05, nr 100 §2–3 to §2–10), which granted a child the right to obtain information about the donor upon reaching the age of 18, on the basis that a child has the right to know its biological origins. However, the law does not oblige parents to tell a child about the nature of its conception. Meanwhile, egg donation has been consistently prohibited. According to the law, fertilized eggs can only be implanted into the woman from whom the egg cells were taken (Lov 2003–15–05, nr 100 §2–15). Although both these provisions invoke biology, they do so in different ways. Whereas the use of a known sperm donor underscores the significance of biogenetic relatedness, the prohibition of egg donation indicates the significance of maintaining a non-fragmented motherhood, insisting on the unity between conception, pregnancy and birth. These provisions in the Biotechnology Act, in conjunction with the gender-neutral Marriage Act, can be read as discriminatory in terms of gender equality (see Eriksson, this volume, for a discussion of equality principles in the Finnish case). Until recently, however, such arguments have gained little purchase.[5]

Surrogacy not only challenges established notions of motherhood, it also allows for same-sex male parenthood. As such, surrogacy sets a different agenda, one that initially was not even contemplated by Norwegian legislators.[6]

Proof of Parenthood

In her discussion of the role played by knowledge in creating relationships, Strathern points out the two ways in which procreative parenthood was traditionally established: mother through birth and body issue; father through presumed coitus with mother (Strathern 1999, 78). She goes on to say:

> These two routes to knowledge supposed two kinds of linkages.... The mother's biological tie to the child is at the root of her social obligation to it; the father's social tie to the mother is at the root of his knowledge of the biological connection with the child. In other words, in pre-technology Euro-American systems, motherhood and fatherhood required different kinds of proof to establish the facts of procreation. And fatherhood appeared to require more proof than motherhood.
>
> (Ibid., footnotes deleted)

This way of tracing parent-child linkages finds parallel expression in two principles that have, historically, and until this day, been central to European notions of procreative parenthood. They have to do with legally ascertaining paternity and maternity. The first of these is: *Pater vero est quem nuptiæ demonstrant* – the true father is established through marriage. This rule is often referred to as *pater est*. The other, *mater sempre certa est* (the mother is always certain), implies that motherhood is established through giving birth.

The first principle is dependent on marriage. Recognizing the uncertainty of paternity, it stresses the significance of the conjugal tie. Marriage ensures the legitimate status of the child.[7] The second principle, however, is perceived as an undisputable biological fact. No matter what the status of the child (whether legitimate or illegitimate; that is, born in or out of wedlock), the mother is always known, as she is by definition the one who gives birth. It is also this principle that underpins the legal definition of motherhood in Norway. In fact, until 1997 (with effect from 1998), Norway did not have a specific clause defining maternity. At that time, and as a result of the debates about reproductive technologies and assisted conception and the potential fragmentation of motherhood, the following provision was added to the Children's Act: "the woman who gives birth to a child is considered its mother" (Lov 1981–04–08, nr 09, Chapter 1 A §2).[8] Until 1997, motherhood was by definition a fact that did not need to be defined or made explicit. Giving birth was proof enough.

These two principles rest on what have been seen as indisputable biological facts: that paternity is always uncertain and that there is no doubt about who the mother (really) is. However, both these principles are, albeit in different ways, undermined by the advent of reproductive and other technologies. DNA testing has altered the "proof basis" of paternity, making fatherhood a potentially certain category, while reproductive technologies have complicated the ascription of motherhood. Whereas anonymous sperm donation is subsumed under the rule of *pater est* (as long as the intending couple are married) both egg donation and surrogacy challenge the prevailing notions of motherhood.

It seems that, within the legal framework, it is the "truth" of biologically based relatedness in identifying relations of filiation that has come to represent the "proof" of these same relations. Knowledge of our genes or of our birth constitutes knowledge of who we are, and where we come from. It is these ties – or at least the possibility of and belief in the necessity of establishing such ties – that frame the legislation, irrespective of whether they ground the actual relations that constitute a family. Family relations can take many forms, many of which are not based on biological connectedness (such as adoptive families, families that have made use of sperm or egg donors, reconstituted families and homoparental families; see Cadoret 2009). In some cases, knowledge of the presence or absence of a biogenetic tie is known – and shared – among members of the family. In other cases, such knowledge is intentionally withheld, and the family appears to be based on biological connectedness. However, there are some family forms where it is impossible to hide the fact of reproductive intervention. These latter family constellations represent a particular challenge for the authorities, especially in those situations where a surrogate has been used (in contrast to adoption).

Practices of Surrogacy

Surrogacy is gaining a place in Norwegian society, as more and more people are choosing this option and their choices inform Norwegian *offentlighet* through the media. Although transnational surrogacy is contested, it is, as I have noted, not illegal, but it may be (by some) considered illicit. It is therefore of interest to note that, in 2011, a man married to another man, who together have two children born to a surrogate using donated eggs, was appointed Director of Police in Oslo. There was much publicity surrounding this appointment, especially focusing on the fact that the Director of Police had circumvented Norwegian law.[9]

Surrogacy enables same-sex male parenthood that is not based on transnational adoption. Many of those who enter surrogacy arrangements travel to the USA, as several US states permit surrogacy and have extensive legal regulatory systems. Lately, India (and the Ukraine) has also become popular, mainly due to the lower costs involved (see also Vora and Iyengar, and Førde, this volume). In legal terms, cross-border surrogacy arrangements are particularly complicated. They involve other national legal systems as well as Norwegian legislation, including Norwegian citizenship laws and laws on legal parenthood. As mentioned above, according to Norwegian law, a person gains Norwegian citizenship if either mother or father is a Norwegian citizen. Hence, filiation is decisive. The ascription of legal parenthood is regulated by the Children's Act (Lov 1981–04–08, nr 07, §85). It is this regulation that underpins citizenship.[10] Thus, in cases of surrogacy, an unmarried man can claim paternity by acknowledging the child as his. If the surrogate is married, however, a DNA test is required, in addition to written consent from the surrogate's husband, relinquishing his paternity. A married heterosexual couple can also contract a surrogate, and if the husband claims paternity, the child will be registered as his. His wife can adopt her husband's child at a later date, and thus become its legal mother. However, for a woman, the situation is different. Even if she has used her own egg cells, adoption is the only vehicle for granting legal motherhood. In other words, motherhood must be transferred and this can only be done through adoption. If not, she has no legal recourse and the children cannot be considered Norwegian. This was the situation in the case of Kari Ann.

Adoption is also prescribed to establish legal fatherhood in the case of male homosexual couples. However, these provisions do not necessarily meet the aspirations of intending parents. Hence, surrogacy may also challenge the assumptions of legal fatherhood, insofar as this is framed in terms of biogenetic relatedness. This has been the case for several homosexual couples who have had children by employing a surrogate in the USA (see Spilker, this volume).

Briefly, the situation can be summed up as follows.[11] In certain US states (notably California), the birth certificate allows the registration of two fathers for a child. This is not legally tenable in Norway. A child can only have one father (and one mother). Thus, to solve the problem of paternity (for these cases), the Norwegian authorities proposed a solution: that each (registered) father take a DNA test in order to identify the biological father. Further, they proposed that the non-biological father proceeds to apply for step-adoption of the child of his spouse (as in the case of heterosexual couples). However, for some of these couples, this solution was unacceptable. Step-adoption would (in their eyes) undermine their mutual project of parenthood, as it does not recognize that the child belongs equally to both of them, despite having a biological tie to only one.

The authorities will accept a single ("known") father but cannot accept two "unknown" fathers. And the question turns on what "known" means. For these couples, all the children need to know is that they are the children of two fathers born to a surrogate in the USA. Thus, while excluding a mother, they nevertheless confirm the traditional attitude to paternity: that it is inevitably uncertain. In a sense, we could say that such couples are inadvertently invoking *pater est* (but with a twist), in demanding that each spouse be recognized as the father of their child or children. However, to the authorities it is a matter of knowing who the "real" father is in order to ascribe proper filiation. They need proof of fatherhood, and that can only be achieved through establishing a biogenetic connection. And they also need adoption so as to regulate an "irregular" procreative practice.

In these cases of same-sex male couples, their marriage is legal but their procreative practice is not, quite. Although their parenthood is based on biogenetic connections, not only is this partial, it is also in a sense uncertain as they do not wish to specify which of them is the biological parent of a given child. By refusing to accept the authorities' demand, they not only upset the drive for certainty that underpins Norwegian legislation, they also reject the notion that knowledge of biogenetic origin is fundamental to the identity of a child and to the establishment of fatherhood. Hence, they disagree with the authorities on what constitutes meaningful relatedness in family formation; the children are inscribed in local kin relations whether these are officially recognized or not. By insisting on being recognized as a family with two "unknown" (yet nevertheless biogenetically related) fathers, they are not only creating new forms of relatedness, they are also reconfiguring kinship practices, creating new social forms. Moreover, these practices also, and perhaps more significantly, produce effects that may not only confound but also actually subvert the current tendency (in law) to privilege biological forms of belonging over social ones.

Planned Parenthood? Bringing It All Home

There is in Norway a certain reticence around surrogacy. I have suggested that one issue of significance in this regard has to do with ascribing proper filiation. I have also intimated that children born through a surrogacy arrangement may, in Norway, be viewed as the product of an illicit exchange. This problem has to do with identifying legitimate kin relations, as a basis for establishing legal kin relations. It also has to do with obtaining the required documents or documentation of legal status. Marriage has been – and to a certain degree still is – the institution that has endorsed legitimate kinship relations.

Nevertheless, in Norway, as elsewhere, significant changes have taken place. Whereas in the past (at least up until the late 1950s) children born out of wedlock were considered illegitimate (a Norwegian term for an illegitimate child is *uekte barn*, connoting that the child is not "authentic") and unwed mothers were stigmatized, this is no longer the case. Procreation is no longer regulated through such moral categories. As I have argued elsewhere (Melhuus 2001), in Norway the distinction between legitimate and illegitimate children no longer carries any meaning; the categories as such are obsolete. The fact that this distinction is not culturally relevant can be seen as an expression of the shifts that have occurred in both the perception and organization of the relations between men and women, as well as the relations between men and women and their children. In many ways this loss of meaning sums up a series of other socio-cultural changes that have occurred in Norwegian society. It articulates an interface where the relations between sexuality, procreation, and morality meet. It is, I argue, also a precondition for the socio-cultural acceptance of assisted conception, capturing the move from a preoccupation with sex without procreation to procreation without sex.

Today, it appears that there is another shift taking place in the relation between sexuality, procreation, and filiation. Assisted conception – be it through egg donation or practices of surrogacy – throws up another configuration of procreative exchange that is morally contested. It is not a question of illicit sexual activity and its potential results. In fact the illicitness is not about sex at all (or marriage). On the contrary. It is, rather, about the absence of (procreative) sexuality. It is the non-sexual exchange that is problematic, in which procreative intent has replaced sexual activity as the ethically contested category. But this is not all. The illicit nature of the exchange can be understood as being about the absence of proof of biogenetic relatedness – the very possibility of establishing a definite connection between parent and child. This is the situation for both women and men, albeit in different ways.

The illicitness, in particular with regard to surrogacy, is also about the introduction of money, of paying for a gestational service that results in the birth of a child (for a somewhat related discussion of egg donation as a bioeconomic transaction, see Namberger, this volume). In a certain sense, the child and the service are conflated: paying for a womb is like paying for a child. This takes on the semblance of an instrumentalization of life and as such is morally objectionable. It is seen as a violation of human dignity and is considered not to be in the best interests of the child. According to some. Finally, and perhaps most significantly, commercial surrogacy raises the issue of unequal exchange, of the possible exploitation of poor women. Taken together, these factors compound and exacerbate the illicitness of the exchange. Again: for some people.

These issues hinge on the question of reproductive choice and hence on reproductive intent; and on the fact that Norwegian legislation explicitly rejects certain reproductive practices and thus reproductive choice more generally. Nevertheless, the global infertility market makes reproductive choice – and new forms of planned parenthood – a real possibility, for Norwegians along with everyone else. The law does not forbid either egg donation or the use of a surrogate if carried out abroad. However, with egg donation, as argued above, there is no (legal) problem: through giving birth to a child, a woman will be recognized as its mother. The genetic contribution is irrelevant. The problem (for women) arises with the use of a surrogate, especially if the entire exchange is based on donor gametes.

By entering into surrogacy arrangements, Norwegians – single or couples – are bringing this problem home. Literally. The child is to be brought to Norway. Sometimes this occurs without any obstacles. However, Norwegian authorities have as yet not found ways to handle all such cases in a satisfactory way. They are not able to classify the child – to decide to whom it belongs – in a way *that is meaningful for all those concerned.* And that is the significant point.

To those involved in surrogacy, or other forms of reproductive practices that are not allowed in Norway, there is nothing "illicit" in their actions. On the contrary. My intention in evoking the term "illicit" is to draw attention to the concerns that surrogacy and other ART-related practices raise – for the intending parents, the authorities and not least the child – and the way in which these concerns are articulated. The legal complications are only one aspect. The ethical, moral, and emotional concerns are others.

In this respect, the media cannot be ignored. Media events play a significant role not only in framing these issues but also in making them public. In fact, the media, in their own way, have also been instrumental in bringing this practice home. Within a global context, they set a local agenda. This agenda is not unidirectional; it reflects the lack of consensus on these issues in Norway. Nevertheless, the publicity surrounding what are often presented as sensational cases of surrogacy is reminiscent of earlier circuits of gossip: they serve not only to make intimate relations and personal preoccupations public but also to make them a moral matter of public concern.

Conclusion

In this chapter, I have shown how biology is put to work within a legislative framework with regard to assisted conception and reproductive technologies in Norway. I have also argued that the basis of proof for both maternity and paternity is shifting. Maternity is becoming more complicated and less certain, whereas the opposite holds for paternity. The tendency to privilege biogenetic relatedness contributes toward this trend, as does the emphasis on the separate relations of mother–child, father–child in ascribing filiation. At the same time, the privileging of giving birth works to conceal the actual genetic make-up of the child. Moreover, the global infertility market makes possible procreative practices that not only undermine the significance of biology, but also activate other principles – such as equal rights (in terms of access to assisted conception), children's rights and the best interests of the child, and the question of ethics regarding commercial surrogacy (Humbyrd 2009). These different principles work in different directions and it is not at all clear which will eventually prevail.

An attempt to bring them together (as the insistence that it is in the best interests of the child to know its biological origins) is not necessarily a viable solution. Moreover, such reproductive practices make visible a paradox around contemporary notions of maternity and paternity.

Surrogacy arrangements, it appears, are legally less complicated for men than they are for women. This is true insofar as the man involved is the biogenetic father of the child, and that proof of this connection is made available in some form. A woman, however, who makes use of a surrogate will necessarily have to become involved in an adoption process, even if the child is biogenetically hers (that is, the egg comes from her). Motherhood must be transferred from the woman who gives birth to the woman who has provided the eggs. If the biogenetic link is absent, the intending mother, according to Norwegian law, actually has no claim to the child whatsoever as long as reproductive intent is not recognized as legitimate. It is thus, in certain respects, easier for men to become fathers than it is for women to become mothers, as a woman has no "proof" (beyond her desire) to offer the authorities. Yet, a woman can make use of donated eggs, and become a legal mother through birth: no proof of genetic connection is required. Thus, reproductive technologies work to displace some certainties while creating others.

Contemporary biopolitics is undoubtedly a morally charged domain. Reproductive technologies and their accompanying practices have impacted on regulatory regimes worldwide (Inhorn and Tremayne 2012). Attempts to come to (legal) terms with the present reconfiguration of family relations that these technologies generate have proved complicated in Norway, as elsewhere. This complexity will prevail as long as it is possible to circumvent national regulations and people are willing to travel abroad to do what is not permitted at home. The transnational space within which reproductive technologies are embedded provides opportunities that some people are able to exploit. In doing so, they bring these procreative practices home, which in turn have varying effects. One possible effect is a shift in the regulatory regime – both in Norway and elsewhere – changing the premises not only of what is allowed, but also of what is possible.

Notes

1 This chapter draws on arguments that have been put forward elsewhere. For a much broader discussion of these issue within an ethnographic framework see Melhuus 2012. See also Engeli and Rothmayr Allison (this volume) for a comparison of European legislation.

2 The Norwegian government has since addressed some of these legal issues. See Melhuus and Syse (2016); this chapter also addresses the question of gender discrimination regarding sperm and egg donation.

3 Infertility treatment is covered by the public health system, with certain limitations (Romundstad and Sunde 2012).

4 However, male same-sex couples do have the right to adopt – but many of the countries that offer children up for transnational adoption do not grant homosexuals this possibility, and very few children are available in Norway.

5 See Hellum 2011; also *Bioteknologinemda (Bioteknologinemdas uttalelse om eggdonasjon)* (2011b). In 2014 the Norwegian Biotechnology Council changed its name to the Norwegian Biotechnology Advisory Board.

6 See the Commissioned report to Parliament on fatherhood, motherhood and changes in parenthood (NOU 2009, 5).

7 In addition to *pater est*, in Norway paternity can be established through recognition of the child or by legal conviction (with the use of DNA).

8 This provision excludes surrogacy arrangements as a legal practice in Norway. Nevertheless, the Act explicitly states that "An agreement to give birth to a child for another woman is not binding" (Lov 1997–06–13, nr 39. Amendments to the Children's Act). To give birth for a man is not even mentioned.

9 The summer of 2011 also showed an increased interest in surrogacy among Norwegian newspapers, as the result of an attempt by the Norwegian authorities (through the National Register) to uncover wrongly registered parents – that is children registered with two fathers. In 2011 Bioteknologinemda (2011a) delivered a statement on surrogacy, discouraging the government from permitting this practice.

10 See NOU 2009, 5; Barne-, likestillings- og inkluderingsdepartementet 2010; and Helsedirektoratet 2011, Rapport 15–1897. See also the website of the Royal Norwegian Embassy in India (2015); there is a special section on surrogacy and Norwegian legislation. Norwegian authorities advise against transnational surrogacy arrangements for people living in Norway, stating that the child may fail to obtain legal attachment to a Norwegian parent, and hence not be granted Norwegian citizenship or residency rights in Norway.

11 For a concrete example see Melhuus 2011.

References

Barne-, likestillings- og inkluderingsdepartementet [Ministry of Children, Equality and Inclusion]. 2010. *Rapport fra en interdepartemental arbeidsgruppe om håndtering av surrogatsaker* [*Report from an Inter-Departmental Workgroup Concerning Surrogacy Cases*]. Oslo.

Bioteknologinemda [The Norwegian Biotechnology Advisory Board]. 2011a. *Bioteknologinemdas uttalelse om surrogati* [*Statement on Surrogacy*]. March 23.

Bioteknologinemda. 2011b. *Bioteknologinemdas uttalelse om eggdonasjon* [*The Advisory Board's Statement on Egg Donation*]. November 22.

Cadoret, Ann. 2009. "The Contribution of Homoparental Families to the Current Debate on Kinship." In *Kinship in the Age of Biotechnology*, edited by Jeanette Edwards and Carles Salazar, 79–96. Oxford: Berghahn.

Campbell, Ben. 2007. "Racialization, Genes and the Reinventions of Nation in Europe." In *Race, Ethnicity and Nation: Perspectives from Kinship and Genetics*, edited by Peter Wade, 169–186. New York: Berghahn.

Fosse, Synnøve Skeie, Amalie Kvame Holm, and Eivind H. Natvig. 2011. "Tjenestepikene." [The Service Maids]. *Plot* (April/May): 12–40.

Hellum, Anne. 2011. "The Global Equality Standard Meets Norwegian Sameness." In *From Transnational Relations to Transnational Laws*, edited by Anne Hellum, Shaheen Sardar Ali, and Anne Griffiths, 71–92. Farnham: Ashgate.

Helsedirektoratet [Ministry of Health]. 2011. *Evaluering av bioteknologiloven. Status og utvikling på fagområdene som reguleres av loven* [Evaluation of the Biotechnology Act. Status and Development]. Rapport 15–1897. Oslo.

Humbyrd, Casey. 2009. "Fair Trade International Surrogacy." *Developing World Bioethics* 9 (3): 111–118.

Inhorn, Marcia, and Frank van Balen, eds. 2002. *Infertility around the Globe: New Thinking on Childlessness, Gender and Reproductive Technologies*. Berkeley: Berkeley University Press.

Inhorn, Marcia, and Soroya Tremayne, eds. 2012. *Islam and Assisted Reproductive Technologies: Sunni and Shia Perspectives*. New York: Berghahn.

Innst. O. nr 60–1986–87. *Innstilling fra sosialkomitéen om lov om kunstig befruktning.* [Recommendation to Parliament from the Social Committee on the Act of Artificial Procreation].

Kroløkke, Charlotte. 2012. "From India with Love: Troublesome Citizens of Fertility Travel." *Cultural Politics* 8 (2): 307–325.

Lov 1981 04–08, nr 09. *Lov om barn og foreldre* (*barneloven*). [Act 1981–04–08, no. 09. Children's Act].

Lov 1987–06–12, nr 68. *Lov om kunstig* (*befruktning*). [Act 1987–06–12, no. 68. The Artificial Procreation Act].

Lov 1997–06–13, nr 39. *Lov om endringer i lov av* 8.april 1981, no. 7. [Amendments to the Children's Act].

Lov 2003–15–05, nr 100. *Lov om humanmedisinsk bruk av bioteknologi m.m.* (bioteknologiloven). [Act 2003–15–05, no. 100. Act Relating to the Application of Biotechnology in Medicine etc. (The Biotechnology Act)].

Lov 2008–12–19, nr 112. *Ekteskapsloven.* [Act 2008–12–19, no. 112. The Marriage Act].

Melhuus, Marit. 2001. "Kan skinnet bedra? Noen meninger om assistert befruktning." [Is Seeing Believing? Some Notions of Assisted Conception]. In *Blod – tykkere enn vann? Betydninger av slektskap i Norge* [*Blood – Thicker than Water? Meanings of Kinship in Norway*], edited by Signe Howell and Marit Melhuus, 45–72. Bergen: Fagbokforlaget.

Melhuus, Marit. 2007. "Procreative Imaginations: When Experts Disagree on the Meanings of Kinship." In *Holding Worlds Together: Ethnographies of Knowing and Belonging*, edited by Marianne Lien and Marit Melhuus, 37–56. Oxford: Berghan.

Melhuus, Marit. 2011. "Cyber-Stork Children and the Norwegian Biotechnology Act: Regulating Procreative Practice – Law and its Effects." In *From Transnational Relations to Transnational Laws*, edited by Anne Hellum, Shaheen Sardar Ali, and Anne Griffiths, 51–70. Farnham: Ashgate.

Melhuus, Marit. 2012. *Problems of Conception: Issues of Law, Biotechnology, Individuals and Kinship.* New York: Berghahn.

Melhuus, Marit, and Aslak Syse. 2016. "Reproductive Surrogacy in Norway." In *Handbook of Gestational Surrogacy*, edited by Eric Sills. Cambridge: Cambridge University Press.

NOU [Official Norwegian Report]. 2009. *Farskap og annen morskap. Fastsettelse og endring i foreldreskap* [*Fatherhood and Different Motherhoods: Ascription of and Changes in Parenthood*]. Oslo: Barne-og likestillingsdepartementet.

Romundstad, L. B., and Arne Sunde. 2012. "Assistert befruktning – hva skal staten betale?" [Assisted Conception – What Should the State Pay?]. *Tidsskrift for Den norske legeforening* [*Journal of the Norwegian Medical Society*]. Accessed October 7, 2015. http://tidsskriftet.no/article/2254261. Doi: 10.4045/tidsskr. 12.0394.

Royal Norwegian Embassy, India. 2015. Accessed September 28, 2015. www.norwayemb.org.in/Norsk/Tjenester-for-nordmenn/Surrogati/#.VgpmOueWmqI.

Salazar, Carles. 2009. "Are Genes Good to Think With?" In *European Kinship in the Age of Biotechnology*, edited by Jeanette Edwards and Carles Salazar, 179–96. Oxford: Berghahn.

Strathern, Marilyn. 1999. *Property, Substance and Effect: Anthropological Essays on Persons and Things*. London: The Athlone Press.

9 Finland as a Late Regulator of Assisted Reproduction

A Permissive Policy under Debate

Lise Eriksson

Introduction

Finland's first Act on Assisted Reproduction (1237/2006) became law in 2007, which is much later than the other Nordic countries.[1] The legislative process began in the 1980s and went on for a couple of decades. During this time there was much debate across society on the need to impose limits on the liberal reproductive practices in Finland (Malin and Burrell 2004). This chapter will focus on three themes that appeared in policy documents and political debates on ARTs in the *Eduskunta* (the Parliament of Finland) prior to the changes in the law in 2007: (i) childlessness as a medical problem, (ii) religious arguments, and (iii) perceptions of fatherhood in relation to sperm donation and donor anonymity. All three themes were part of the negotiations on ARTs related to notions of gender, sexuality, and families. Restrictive standpoints constructed the image of ARTs as primarily a means for infertile heterosexual couples to have children. These positions relied on ideas of a natural order and the nuclear, heterosexual family as superior to other family forms. Other parliamentarians defended the permissiveness of the Government bills, advocating all women's equal right to access ARTs.

The concept of "equality" will be given particular attention in my analysis. In the context of policy proposals, equality can be defined as the result of the elimination of discrimination, and as equal rights or equal opportunities. In the field of ARTs, equality can refer to eligibility to access ARTs, and to equal access to both public and private clinics, or to economic equality between patients. The equal subjects may be all women, women in comparison to men, or same-sex couples and single people in comparison to heterosexual couples.

In the field of ARTs, Finland is a late regulator with a permissive policy (see Engeli and Rothmayr Allison, this volume). The country offered one of the most permissive regimes in Europe regarding ARTs when it lacked specific legislation on the issue (Malin and Burrell 2004, 88–89). According to Isabelle Engeli (2009, 60), a policy within the field of reproduction is permissive if (1) medical autonomy and patient access are regulated by light policy instruments or not regulated at all; (2) all categories of patients have access to abortion and ARTs regardless of personal circumstances, civil status or sexual orientation;

and (3) treatment costs are met by state funding or private medical insurance. I would characterize the Finnish Act on Assisted Reproduction as a relatively light policy, since it did not greatly change the liberal practice at clinics. It gives women the right to ARTs regardless of personal circumstances, civil status, or sexual orientation, but with some limitations. Treatment costs are reimbursed for heterosexual couples, but not for single women or lesbian couples.

The main principle during the process of drafting the law in Finland was: "Why change something that works?" The practice at fertility clinics had become normalized. Clinics could determine their own rules while ARTs were unregulated. According to Engeli and Rothmayr Allison (this volume), medical self-regulation often provides governments with efficient regulatory options. During the 1990s and early 2000s, some private clinics in Finland provided a wider range of treatments than most other Nordic countries. Heterosexual couples, lesbian couples, and single women could all receive ART treatment. Egg donation, embryo donation, and so-called altruistic surrogacy were all practiced until 2007. The liberal practices of clinics were incorporated into the law, with a few exceptions. The most important changes in 2007 were that surrogacy became forbidden and that donors of gametes or embryos were no longer permitted to be anonymous. Surrogacy became forbidden because of a political compromise. The Act on Assisted Reproduction had been in preparation for a long time, and the Government wanted it to finally be approved in Parliament. As Elly Teman (2010, 6–7) points out, surrogacy is often perceived as the least acceptable of the reproductive technologies (see also Melhuus, this volume). The public representation of surrogacy as a "cultural anomaly," as Teman describes it, may be the reason why the Government thought it was easier to abstain from the issue, and perhaps raise it separately later.

This chapter will examine how the process of drafting the law and the political debate differ from the permissiveness of the previous situation. The political debate in Finland oscillates between a liberal standpoint and one in which religious arguments play a central role, and in which the importance of equality is challenged.[2]

Theoretical Framework, Method and Material

In this chapter I conduct a rhetoric and discourse analysis of the policymaking process and political debates on ARTs in the *Eduskunta*. Discourse analysis involves the study of social phenomena or social categories, while also problematizing these categories, their contents, and effects (Börjesson 2003, 19). Since the material consists of political debates and policy documents, I regard rhetoric as an important aspect of the analysis, which I will conduct through quotations from policy documents and debates. Critical incidents and discontinuities in the text are principles for the selection of quotations (Fairclough 1992, 230). I will select quotations that are either representative of the material, or critical incidents that bring something different to the text, and represent a boundary or an interruption in the debate.

A working group at the Ministry of Justice delivered the first draft of a Bill on ARTs in 1988. Expert advisors were divided in their opinions about the contents of the draft, and it did not result in a Bill. In 1990, 1993, and 1997, working groups published new reports on ARTs (Malin and Burrell 2004). The first Bill (HE 76/2002), which was presented to the *Eduskunta* in 2002, was the result of many years of negotiations within Parliament and the Government. Unlike previous reports, this Bill proposed that surrogacy should be prohibited. However, the Government withdrew the Bill, because two issues created controversy in the Legal Affairs Committee in Parliament. The committee proposed that donor anonymity should be abandoned, and that only married or cohabiting heterosexual couples should have access to treatments (Malin and Burrell 2004, 82–88). However, the improvement of same-sex couples' rights was on the Government's agenda. The Act on Registered Partnership came into force in 2002, which may have contributed to the withdrawal of the Bill, because, on the one hand, it made the question of same-sex couples' right to reproduction via ARTs very urgent, while, on the other hand, Conservative parliamentarians did not want to engage with this issue. The second Bill on ARTs (HE 3/2006) was presented to the *Eduskunta* in 2006. Again, problems arose in the Legal Affairs Committee, which suggested that access to ARTs should be limited to heterosexual couples. The *Eduskunta* finally voted in favor of the Bill in October 2006.

This chapter's empirical material consists of the two Bills on ARTs from 2002 and 2006, law drafting reports, and the parliamentary proceedings of the plenary sessions. The parliamentary proceedings are transcribed political speeches made in Parliament, which are available to the public on the parliamentary website.

The chapter's theoretical framework concentrates on how problems are represented in policy proposals and political debates. Carol Bacchi and Joan Eveline (2010) have developed analytical principles for policy studies with a gender perspective. In studies of policy proposals one should ask: "What is the problem represented to be?" The researcher should study the meanings that a problem is given, and how it is discursively constituted in the policy or policy proposal (Bacchi and Eveline 2010, 114).

Through their effects, policies can reinforce social categories based on, for example, sexual orientation, class, or gender (Bacchi and Eveline 2010, 112). Against this background, this chapter studies how problems are represented, and how problems associated with ARTs are discursively and rhetorically produced. I will also study how childless people and gamete donors are categorized and represented.

The Representation of Childlessness as a Medical Problem

The introductions to the two Bills represent involuntary childlessness as a problem due to biological or medical factors, and emphasize female infertility (HE 76/2002, 5; HE 3/2006, 4).

> Involuntary childlessness has become increasingly common in recent years, and is estimated to affect about 15 percent of married or cohabiting couples of childbearing age in Finland. Female infertility increases with age, and the higher average age of first-time mothers clearly increases the difficulty of becoming pregnant, and the need for assisted reproduction.
>
> (HE 3/2006, 4)[3]

This representation of childlessness in the Bill does not mention social causes, e.g., civil status or sexual orientation.[4] In my opinion, a discourse that strongly emphasizes the belief that reproductive treatments should be received on medical grounds may be regarded as an expression of medicalization. Peter Conrad defines medicalization as follows: "a process by which nonmedical problems become defined and treated as medical problems, usually in terms of illness or disorders" (Conrad 1992, 209). According to Arthur L. Greil (2002, 102), through medicalization, childlessness and infertility have been defined in the context of the biomedical model and its perspectives on health, illness, and sick role. The concept "sick role" was created by the functionalist sociologist Talcott Parsons. It refers to the social role of being sick, and the rights and responsibilities of the patient, e.g., the sick person should try to get well. Medical specialists are perceived to have authoritative knowledge about infertility, and hold the exclusive right to treat it, while the infertile person accepts the role of patient.

Medical infertility is the focus of both Bills, but they also mention other situations in which ARTs can be applied. These exceptions include single women and lesbian couples, and cases where there is a risk of a serious genetically transmitted disease. One of the consequences of the representation of childlessness as primarily due to medical infertility is that the physician receives decision-making power over access to treatment. Engeli and Rothmayr Allison (this volume) describe a policy on ARTs that addresses only medical aspects as the typical result of a policy model that gives the medical community decision-making power. According to the Bill HE 3/2006, a prerequisite for treatment is that the person receiving assisted reproduction can ensure that the child receives a balanced upbringing, i.e., the physician should ensure that the child's best interests are taken into account. The Bill also states that it is the physician's responsibility to determine whether the woman's age is a health risk. The Bill mentions no age limit for the woman, nor does the Act on Assisted Reproduction. The previous Bill, HE 76/2002, proposed 46 years as an age limit for women. Neither of the Bills proposed age limits for men.

Other consequences of the focus on medical infertility concern financial compensation, treatment eligibility, and differences between ART procedures at public and private clinics. ART treatments are provided at both public hospitals and private clinics in Finland. Public district hospitals offer basic investigations, medication, and surgery, while the five public university hospitals in Helsinki, Turku, Tampere, Kuopio, and Oulu offer a wider range of ART procedures (Malin and Burrell 2004, 73–74). There are 13 private clinics in Finland that offer ART treatments on a fee-paying basis (Yli-Kuha 2012, 23). However, the national health insurance scheme reimburses some of the costs. A central difference between the public and private sectors is that private clinics are less bureaucratic than the public sector, and more liberal in regard to the woman's age and the number of treatment cycles that are offered. The procedures of egg and embryo donation were first introduced at private clinics during the 1990s (Malin and Burrell 2004, 73–74). Single women and lesbian couples are also referred to private clinics. The main reason for this practice is the distinction between involuntary childlessness, which is defined medically, and childlessness due to other causes.

Surrogacy arrangements occurred on a limited scale at four clinics in Finland during the period 1991–2007. Three of the clinics were private, and one was public.[5] The intending parents were in all cases heterosexual couples. In most cases the woman had no uterus – or a non-functional uterus – either from birth or as a result of a gynecological disease or childbirth complications. The surrogate mother was usually a close relative or friend of the couple. The arrangements were represented as altruistic and non-commercial. Children born through these surrogacy arrangements were in most cases the couple's genetic children (gestational surrogacy) (Söderström-Anttila *et al.* 2002, 748–750).

During the parliamentary debates, the relationship status of recipients of ARTs was often represented as a problem. The standard term for single women and lesbian couples in the Bill HE 3/2006 is "women who are not living in a relationship with a man." The relationship status of lesbian couples and single women is thus defined by the absence of a man. The legal purpose of this terminology was to ensure equality between women. However, it is also a neutralizing rhetoric, which avoids explicit talk of same-sex couples' desire to have children, which was represented as a problem both in the *Eduskunta* and in media debates about the proposed legislation (Kanckos 2012). The following quotation is from a plenary debate on the Bill HE 76/2002.

> Should medical reasons be the key criteria in health care and medical services? In my opinion, yes. What does it lead to, if medical evaluation is also removed in a wider sense from the evaluation of health-care services? A single person's or same-sex couples' infertility is not due to medical reasons. The world has been built and constructed in such a way that a woman and a man are required for the creation of life. In my view, nobody's rights are violated if ARTs are provided for medical reasons.
>
> (Sakari Smeds, Christian Democrats, PTK 198/2002)

This quotation shares the Bills' representation of childlessness as a medical problem, but goes even further. The speaker presents the world as being organized along a natural order, in which reproduction is based on heterosexual relationships. This quotation is an example of how arguments about nature can operate in medicalizing terms. The MP claims that medicine should serve to maintain the natural order. The traditional ideal of the nuclear family was justified in the debates by reference to biology, nature, medicine, tradition, or religion, which are typical authority arguments.

According to the Bill HE 3/2006, the people who are entitled to receive financial compensation for treatment are those who have a diagnosed medical cause for their infertility, which means that lesbian couples and single women are not compensated by the national health insurance. Treatment costs have also increased significantly since the law took effect in 2007. Another consequence of the emphasis on medical infertility is that a woman is not entitled to economic compensation if the cause of infertility is a reduced number of oocytes because of her age. It is recommended that couples who already have two biological children, people with an infectious disease (e.g., HIV), and sterilized individuals do not receive assisted reproduction within the public health-care system (HE 3/2006, 7–8).

In an interview published by several Finnish newspapers in July 2005, Minister of Justice Johannes Koskinen, who was responsible for the drafting of the legislation, declared that although lesbian couples and single women would not get health insurance reimbursement for ARTs, no one is entirely excluded from treatments (Koskinen 2005). In saying this, Koskinen defended the policy proposal's representation of childlessness, which gives priority to medical infertility. This representation of childlessness is based on a specific understanding of equality, and is based on exclusions. He introduces an idea of equality that refers to access to treatment at private clinics, rather than economic equality, or equal access to treatments within the public health-care system.

In sum, the representation of childlessness as primarily medical infertility in the Finnish ART policy documents has legal, practical, and financial consequences.

Religious Views on Changing Family Norms

Religion may impact upon people's attitudes to ARTs, in particular in a situation of moral uncertainty (Inhorn 2003). At the end of 2014, 74 percent of the Finnish population belonged to the Evangelical Lutheran Church of Finland, although active Church members represent only a small minority (Evangelical Lutheran Church of Finland 2015). As the majority Church, it may have an essential impact on political debates that concern moral or religious issues.

The debate on ARTs is also a good example of how the Christian Democrats have acted as defenders of conservative Christian family values in *Eduskunta*. The Bill's suggestion that single women and lesbian couples should have the right to receive ART treatments was often represented as a problem by the representatives from the Christian Democratic Party.

> One should not start artificially producing situations where the child does not have a dad. Nevertheless, in our society, regrettably many children grow up suffering from the lack of a father. I had also hoped that the petition, which the Church released two months ago, would have been considered in the bill. [The petition] also came to all MPs, and it suggested that fertility treatments should be limited to married couples.
>
> (Päivi Räsänen, Christian Democrats, PTK 76/2002)

ARTs are here represented as an artificial form of reproduction, and as a practice that should be limited by legislation. The chairman of the Christian Democrats, Päivi Räsänen, repeatedly emphasized the Church's position on ARTs. The Church was used as a moral authority. In the quotation above, she presents the lack of a father as a problem, and suggests that the decision makers should limit access to ARTs in accordance with the Church's proposal. This proposal was an informal petition that was sent to all Members of Parliament before the debate in 2002, suggesting that only married, heterosexual couples should have the right to treatment. The institution of heterosexual marriage was represented as threatened when other family forms become visible in society. The importance of marriage was often emphasized in the debates through references to religion.

Church statements were often referenced; for example, a statement made in 2005 by the Church Council of the Evangelical Lutheran Church.[6] This emphasized that ARTs should be restricted to heterosexual couples, and that only the spouses' own gametes should be used in the treatments (Church Council 2005). Many MPs who supported all women's equal right to ARTs also used religious arguments, or positioned themselves as members of a Christian community. The speaker in the following quotation legitimizes his view on equality through religion, while simultaneously drawing limits to the extent to which he can identify with the Church: "I would like to say that I perceive myself as a Christian, I am a member of the Evangelical Lutheran Church, but I feel alienated from such a Church that does not approve of equality between people" (Jouni Backman, Social Democrats, PTK 100/2006). Opinions about eligibility criteria for reproductive treatments were not only divided between parties, but also within parties. Members of Parliament were allowed to vote according to their own beliefs, which was an exception to the general rule of following voting decisions within parliamentary groups. This exceptional voting procedure is practiced in the *Eduskunta* on issues which are considered to concern personal values, e.g., alcohol, nuclear energy, religion, the family, and sexual orientation (Kanckos 2012, 110–111). This voting procedure probably contributed to an increased focus on personal values and religious beliefs in the debates on ARTs. Religion may have an impact on party politics in Finland not only through the personal beliefs of MPs, but also through the influence of religious institutions and organizations, such as the Evangelical Lutheran Church of Finland and the Christian Democratic Party (see Engeli and Rothmayr Allison, this volume).

Sperm Donation and Donor Anonymity

In the Finnish political debate, fatherhood was represented as a problem in relation to lesbians and single women who have children through ARTs. The sperm donor was represented by some speakers as a neglected biological father. Thus, the issues of sperm donation and donor anonymity were part of negotiations around notions of gender, sexuality, and families.

The Swedish model of registering the identity of gamete donors has been applied in many countries – including Finland – since Sweden paved the way in

1985 (Nordisk kommitté för bioetik 2006, 17, 46–47, 52). In accordance with the Act on Assisted Reproduction in Finland, since 2007 the identities of those who donate sperm, oocytes, or embryos have been registered by Valvira, The National Supervisory Authority for Welfare and Health. Children who are born as the result of ARTs with donor gametes or embryos may receive information about the donor's identity after they have turned 18.

The debate on anonymity for gamete and embryo donors clearly revolved around perceptions of differences between social and biological parenthood, as illustrated by the following quotation.

> If we approve of gamete donation, then we should ask whether we have thoroughly thought it through. For my own part, whenever we begin expecting a baby in the family, we already have in mind what kind of child it is, what kind of children are born to us. If it does not match our expectations, will our affection be just as robust as if it had been a genuine biological event within the family?
>
> (Hannu Aho, Centre Party, PTK 76/2002)

This MP suggests that genetic ties to both parents mean that the baby is authentic. He questions whether an affectionate family relationship can be formed if the child has its origin in donated gametes. However, a more common view was that families do not depend on biological ties, and that the love between parents and children is more important. This is exemplified in the following quotation, which denies that there is a contradiction between good parenting and the lack of a father. The child's best interests were used in the debates both for and against lesbian or single women's rights.

> I do not believe that such a contradiction exists. The best interests of the child and good parenting are based on a situation where a person has the desire to become a parent, and when she has this desire, it will give her the conditions to also ensure the child's best interests.
>
> (Anni Sinnemäki, Greens, PTK 13/2006)

In analyzing a political debate on egg donation in Norway, Kristin Spilker and Merete Lie (2007, 329–330) noticed that egg and sperm often metonymically referred to women and men. As a consequence, the debate concerned gender and family relationships, sexuality and heteronormativity. The importance of parenthood and equality was emphasized even at the level of cells. I have noticed a similar tendency in the Finnish debates. Some speakers felt it to be important that the child should have the opportunity later in life to meet its biological parent. The determination of paternity played a central role in the Finnish debates, but the discussion mainly concerned a defense of fatherhood at the symbolic level: "Equality between women is emphasized, but the equality between men and women is completely forgotten in this context. The man has no rights. Is it not irresponsible to enact a law in which we forget the role of fathers?"

(Nils-Anders Granvik, Swedish People's Party, PTK 100/2006). This MP believes that fatherhood is threatened when women who do not live in a relationship with a man receive the right to access ARTs. The quotation suggests that the emphasis on equality has focused on equality between women at the expense of the role of fathers. This quotation includes an understanding of equality as that between men and women. The MP is probably referring to sperm donors when he speaks of "fathers" and "men." Sperm donors were represented in several speeches as having an ambivalent relationship to fatherhood: He is the biological father, but his fatherhood is disregarded.

Some speakers mentioned the risk of children being exposed to bullying at school if they do not have two parents of different sexes.

> We imagine a lesbian couple's child, little Jussi, who attends kindergarten, and people asking him what kind of family he comes from. He says, "I have two moms, a lot more than other people." But then people ask him, "what about the father?" "Well, my father is a bank, a sperm bank. Dad thrives in cold conditions, apparently in the freezer." One can imagine what this would actually cause. There will be a black hole for the child until the age of 18, a black hole, when he does not really know his background, whatever he says there. What has been said about school bullying is likely; we cannot do anything about it, because schools are in any case rather rough places. Neither the teachers nor the parents, or anyone at all, can handle this situation. If we know of a situation like this, little Jussi will surely become bullied at school.
>
> (Esa Lahtela, Social Democrats, PTK 13/2006)

In this quotation, donor sperm metonymically refers to the father of the child (see Spilker and Lie 2007, 329). The anonymous sperm donor is represented as an absent father, who is also described as a sperm bank and a black hole. The imagery is powerful, the speaker using irony and humor as rhetorical tools. Using the metaphors of the sperm bank and the black hole, this MP suggests that lesbian couples who have children through ARTs depreciate the biological father. The child in the story speaks of his father as if he does not know what a father is. I consider these metaphors, and the talk about school bullying, to be a critical incident in the debate. The speech gave rise to strong reactions from other speakers. The argument about school bullying was considered offensive to same-sex parents and their children, and was called "by far the worst point" in the debate (Pertti Salovaara, Centre Party, PTK 13/2006).

The representation of the sperm donor as a father has several discursive and practical effects. It suggests that a single mother or two lesbian mothers cannot constitute a genuine family. The law enables registration of the sperm donor's paternity in cases where a single woman or a lesbian couple receives ART treatment. However, very few sperm donors have agreed to become registered as the father. There was a decrease in sperm donations immediately after the Act on Assisted Reproduction became law, which suggests that some potential donors were scared off by the compulsory registration of their identity. However, the

Act does not seem to have resulted in any long-term decrease in donor treatments. To date, about half of all sperm donors are foreign (*Assisted Fertility Treatments 2013–2014* 2015).

Couples whose embryos are left over from ART treatments may donate them to other couples. However, there was hardly any discussion about the importance of parenthood in relation to donated oocytes and embryos. Sperm donors were emphasized as father figures, while oocyte donors were apparently considered less important as mother figures. The reason for this absent discourse is most likely the cultural and legal determination of motherhood as adhering to the woman who gives birth to the child.

Conclusion

I would characterize the Finnish policy on ARTs as permissive (see Engeli 2009). The Act on Assisted Reproduction was prepared over the course of two decades. A consequence of this slow legislative process is that clinics had the opportunity to develop liberal reproductive practices, which included oocyte and embryo donation, altruistic surrogacy, and women's access to treatment regardless of civil status or sexual orientation. Surrogacy still remains an unresolved issue in Finland, and the policymaking process has continued since it was prohibited in 2007 (see Eriksson 2016).

Even though the Finnish case is permissive, it is not merely characterized by a secular bioethical discourse with statements on rights, consequences, and justice. There is a difference between the government bills, legislation, and liberal practices at clinics, which are permissive, and the political debate, which often exhibits discontent with this permissiveness.

The debates in Parliament reflect the post-secular situation of Finnish society, which includes voices in support of liberal practice, voices that support traditional family values, and conservative religious views. A post-secular situation is characterized by ambivalence, because distinctions between religious and secular spheres are blurred. Religious discourse is provided space in a society that has undergone a secularization process (Kanckos 2012). This chapter has examined the reasons behind and the effects of the Finnish ART policy proposals' representation of childlessness as a problem that primarily concerns medical infertility. I have argued that this representation undermines the importance of the social dimensions of childlessness. This representation has legal, practical, and financial consequences. For example, lesbian couples and single women are not compensated by the national health insurance scheme, and they are referred to private clinics. The Finnish debates indicate that assisted reproduction challenges many of the norms regarding parenting, gender, and sexuality that were previously taken for granted, but at the same time they illustrate that it can also be used to reinforce the norms of a society.

Notes

1 The Swedish Insemination Act, which came into force in 1985, was the first of its kind, and several countries have used this law as a model for developing their own legislation. The Norwegian Act on Artificial Procreation (68/1987) came into force in 1987. Iceland and Denmark passed laws on assisted reproduction in the 1990s: Iceland in 1996 and Denmark in 1997 (Nordisk kommitté för bioetik 2006).
2 This chapter summarizes some of the most important results of my doctoral dissertation. The dissertation examines the Finnish parliamentary debates on ARTs during the 2000s, and how these debates relate to changes in values and religious norms in society (Kanckos 2012).
3 All quotations have been translated from Finnish by the author.
4 Spilker (this volume) discusses perceptions of ARTs as techno-medical practices addressing medical infertility in comparison to lesbian couples' use of ARTs.
5 The total number of IVF treatments with surrogacy arrangements begun at Finnish fertility clinics during this period was 46, which resulted in 14 clinical pregnancies, and a total of 12 babies (*Assisted Fertility Treatments 2009–2010* 2011, Appendix Table 2; Kanckos 2012, 201; Söderström-Anttila *et al.* 2002, 748–751).
6 I have analyzed the impact of Church statements on the debate in another article (Eriksson 2016).

References

Assisted Fertility Treatments 2009–2010. 2011. Statistical Report 15/2011, Official Statistics of Finland. Helsinki: THL. Accessed October 13, 2015. http://urn.fi/URN:NBN:fi-fe201205085053.

Assisted Fertility Treatments 2013–2014. 2015. Statistical Report 9/2015, Official Statistics of Finland. Helsinki: THL. Accessed October 13, 2015. http://urn.fi/URN:NBN:fi-fe201504297845.

Bacchi, Carol, and Joan Eveline. 2010. "Approaches to Gender Mainstreaming: What's the Problem Represented to Be?" In *Mainstreaming Politics: Gendering Practices and Feminist Theory*, edited by Carol Bacchi and Joan Eveline, 111–138. Adelaide: University of Adelaide Press.

Börjesson, Mats. 2003. *Diskurser och konstruktioner. En sorts metodbok.* [*Discourses and Constructions: A Kind of Method Book*]. Lund: Studentlitteratur.

Church Council. 2005. "Lausunto oikeusministeriölle ja sosiaali- ja terveysministeriölle hedelmöityshoitolain valmistelusta." [Statement to the Ministry of Justice and the Ministry of Social and Health Care about drafting the law on assisted reproduction]. Case number 2005–00426.

Conrad, Peter. 1992. "Medicalization and Social Control." *Annual Review of Sociology* 18: 209–232.

Engeli, Isabelle. 2009. "The Challenges of Abortion and Assisted Reproductive Technologies Policies in Europe." *Comparative European Politics* 7 (1): 56–74.

Eriksson, Lise. 2016. "Finnish Legislation on Assisted Reproductive Technologies: Comparison of Church Statements." In *Reconsidering Religion, Law, and Democracy – New Challenges for Society and Research*, edited by Anna-Sara Lind, Mia Lövheim, and Ulf Zackariasson, 139–155. Lund: Nordic Academic Press.

Evangelical Lutheran Church of Finland. 2015. "Kirkko numeroina." [The Church in Figures]. Accessed October 13, 2015. http://evl.fi/EVLfi.nsf/0/68ED832793E78AF5C22575EF003AD029?OpenDocument&lang=FI.

Fairclough, Norman. 1992. *Discourse and Social Change*. Cambridge: Polity Press.

Greil, Arthur L. 2002. "Infertile Bodies: Medicalization, Metaphor, and Agency." In *Infertility around the Globe: New Thinking on Childlessness, Gender and Reproductive Technologies*, edited by Marcia C. Inhorn and Frank van Balen, 101–118. Berkeley, Los Angeles, and London: University of California Press.

HE 76/2002. Hallituksen esitys eduskunnalle laeiksi sukusolujen ja alkioiden käytöstä hedelmöityshoidossa ja isyyslain muuttamisesta. [The Government's Bill to *Eduskunta* Proposing an Act on the Use of Gametes and Embryos in Assisted Reproduction and an Amendment of The Paternity Act].

HE 3/2006. Hallituksen esitys eduskunnalle laeiksi hedelmöityshoidoista ja isyyslain muuttamisesta. [The Government's Bill to *Eduskunta* Proposing an Act on Assisted Reproduction and an Amendment of The Paternity Act].

Inhorn, Marcia C. 2003. *Local Babies, Global Science: Gender, Religion and In Vitro Fertilization in Egypt*. London and New York: Routledge.

Kanckos, Lise. 2012. "Barnets bästa i politikens främsta rum. Finlands riksdags debatt om assisterad befruktning." [The Best Interests of the Child in the Main Chamber of Politics: The Finnish Parliamentary Debate on Assisted Reproduction]. PhD diss., Åbo Akademi University.

Koskinen. 2005. "Koskinen: Naisparien hedelmöitys-hoidoille ei Kela-korvausta." [Koskinen: No Insurance Reimbursement for Female Couples' ART Treatments]. *Helsingin Sanomat* 25 July.

Malin, Maili, and Riitta Burrell. 2004. "Unregulated Practices, Familiarity and Legality." In *Third Party Assisted Conception across Cultures: Social, Legal and Ethical Perspectives*, edited by Eric Blyth and Ruth Landau, 73–93. London and New York: Jessica Kingsley Publishers.

Nordisk kommitté för bioetik. 2006. *Assisted Reproduction in the Nordic Countries: A Comparative Study of Policies and Regulation.* TemaNord 2006:505. Copenhagen: Nordic Council of Ministers. Accessed October 13, 2015. http://ncbio.org/nordisk/publikationer/.

PTK 76/2002 Parliamentary Proceedings June 10, 2002.

PTK 198/2002 Parliamentary Proceedings February 7, 2003.

PTK 13/2006 Parliamentary Proceedings February 23, 2006.

PTK 100/2006 Parliamentary Proceedings October 12, 2006.

Spilker, Kristin, and Merete Lie. 2007. "Gender and Bioethics Intertwined: Egg Donation within the Context of Equal Opportunities." *European Journal of Women's Studies* 14 (4): 327–340.

Söderström-Anttila, Viveca, Tom Blomqvist, Tuija Foudila, Maritta Hippeläinen, Henri Kurunmäki, Rita Siegberg, Maija Tulppala, Merja Tuomi-Nikula, Sirpa Vilska, and Outi Hovatta. 2002. "Experience of *In Vitro* Fertilization Surrogacy in Finland." *Acta Obstetricia et Gynecologica Scandinavica* 81: 747–752.

Teman, Elly. 2010. *Birthing a Mother: The Surrogate Body and the Pregnant Self.* Berkeley and Los Angeles: University of California Press.

Yli-Kuha, Anna-Niina. 2012. "Prevalence and Socio-demographic Determinants of Infertility, Success of Infertility Treatments and Health of Treated Women." PhD diss., Tampere University.

Part III

Religious Fundamentalism, Humanist Values, and State Dilemmas in an Era of Technological Monsters

10 Reframing Conception, Reproducing Society

Italian Paradoxes

Manuela Perrotta

Introduction

ARTs have developed quickly and broadly over the last few decades, producing a number of new options that have changed the definition of kinship and parenthood, bodies and gender relations, and even culture and life itself. ARTs, in fact, have often questioned the traditional (and taken-for-granted) meaning of kinship, shifting the attention toward the hegemonic medical-technological devices.

Although ARTs are globally accepted as concrete options for overcoming unintended childlessness, the potential "disruptive" power of reproductive technologies has not produced the same social effects all over the world. ARTs have enabled innovative forms of kinship and parenthood in many social and cultural contexts (Thompson 2005; Inhorn and Birenbaum-Carmeli 2008), while participating in the reinforcement of the traditional family model in others.

National regulation of ARTs can be seen as the expression of local, morally oriented answers to globally available biomedical knowledge. When these technologies meet national institutional and political actors, they become situated within a specific social order and set of moral values. This interweaving of elements produces specific procreative interfaces, the loci where the law and reproductive practices meet (Melhuus 2005).

The contribution of this chapter will be to show how ARTs, when embedded in a specific cultural and social order, can be used by more (and even less) powerful actors as instruments for reproducing a traditional model of society. To accomplish this aim, the chapter analyzes the case of Italy, which does not reflect the expectations of changes in family patterns often related to ARTs; rather, it represents a reinforcement of the status quo through the enforcement of a monolithic (and singular) model of family, consisting of a married father and mother with biologically related children, preferably born within marriage. The Italian case is particularly relevant for three main reasons: the restrictive national regulations; the institutional attempt to create a unique (Catholic) moral and ethical view on reproductive issues; and the actual distance between politics and lay people. The case of ARTs in Italy, therefore, will be used as a key lens through which to look at the relationship between science, biopolitics, and citizenship.

The chapter is organized as follows: First, it describes the cultural and religious background of Italian society to situate the procreative interfaces in relation to the main moral and ethical positions. Next, it reconstructs the legislative path and discusses the myth of the Italian test-tube "Wild West." Finally, it presents some ethnographic examples[1] to discuss the paradoxes emerging from reproductive practices and discourses.

The Cultural Background

In order to situate the chapter's arguments, I will start with an introduction to its Catholic cultural matrix. The introduction of the law on assisted reproduction in Italy in 2004 was the result of a long negotiation process performed by numerous political and social actors, who deployed different rationalities and resources to support diverse proposals for change. The debate on the ethical and moral aspects of ARTs was extremely heated, with radically opposed ethical, moral, and religious stances being taken. The Catholic lobby, highly influential in the Italian debate, proposed that restrictions should be imposed on therapeutic treatments by virtue of the moral argument that an embryo is not only a lifeform, it is also a person.

It has to be said, however, that although the Catholic Church had and continues to have a big influence in Italy, Catholicism cannot be taken for granted as a cultural framework. First, even though the number of *declared* Catholics forms a majority, a lack of belief and practice, as well as atheism, agnosticism, and skepticism, are extremely common. A common division (Garelli 1991) is made between the Catholic majority, who accept the generic definition of "Catholic," and the Catholic minority, who are intensely religious and of whom one-tenth belong to groups, movements, or associations. This division is important because it helps to explain the relevant differences in moral and ethical positions.

The public presence of the Church, however, has become much stronger in recent years, especially after the disappearance of the Christian Democratic Party (Democrazia Cristiana) in 1994, whose main ideological sources were found in Catholic social teachings and who had been in power for almost 50 continuous years. As Garelli (2007) pointed out, for an array of reasons, Italian Catholicism is currently experiencing a period of notable vitality and dynamism, which is widely expressed in the public sphere and in the culture. Recently, Diamanti and Ceccarini (2007) spoke about an "influential minority" that is well represented by the Catholic Church, which is deep-rooted in associations of various inspiration and acts as a lobby.

The Catholic hierarchy and religious groups act to influence topics of great public concern that are crucial to the construction of society in the future. ARTs represent just one example of how Catholic morals have retained supremacy in legislative practices (see DiMarco 2009).

The public opposition of the Church to ARTs has a long history. In the 1950s Pope Pius XII declared the use of assisted insemination (ARTs did not exist at that time) an "unnatural act" (referring to masturbation) and, therefore, a sin.

In 1987, the Congregation for the Faith Doctrine, the former Holy Office (Sant'uffizio), published a document entitled "Donum Vitae: Instruction on Respect for Human Life and Its Origin and on the Dignity of Procreation"[2] (see also Just, this volume), which permitted only homologous insemination (i.e., with gametes from the couple) if it did not replace the conjugal act. The focus of this declaration was to preserve the sanctity of marriage and reinforce its link with reproduction. The position of the Catholic Church was elucidated again in 1995 by John Paul II in the evangelical letter "Evangelium Vitae,"[3] in which the Pope argued that biomedical technologies go well beyond a reasonable dominion over nature. At this time, the main criticisms were directed against non-therapeutic research on human embryos and their destruction or cryopreservation, the selection of characteristics or gender of the newborn, heterologous fertilization (i.e., with gametes from donors external to the couple) and all cases of surrogate motherhood.

Notwithstanding this moral and ethical condemnation, the dominant Catholic rhetoric did not seem to correspond to the uses and customs that were actually in place. Referring to the year 2013, the annual report of the Health Ministry to Parliament reported that 71,741 couples had undergone treatments with 12,187 live births (2.4 percent of all children born in Italy in 2013[4]).

The Normative Framework: The Myth of the "Test-Tube Wild West" and Law 40

The first attempt to regulate ARTs in Italy was proposed in 1958 (later revived in 1963, although neither of these Bills led to a debate in Parliament). In the years that followed, there were many attempts to legislate the issue of reproductive technologies, but they did not bring any concrete results. The second half of the 1990s, in particular, was rich in unsuccessful regulatory attempts. In 1996, for the first time, The Democratic Party of the Left (Partito Democratico della Sinistra) intervened on this issue with the intention of regulating these practices rather than prohibiting them. After this Bill, several others followed. The process ended with the enactment of Law 40 in 2004,[5] which included much more restrictive prohibitions than the proposals submitted earlier.

In order for us to understand the emergence of Law 40 and its strict limitations, I believe it is essential to present the cultural climate in which the public discussion was framed. Before the introduction of this law, Italy as a nation was referred to as the "test-tube Wild West" to highlight the absence of rules regulating ARTs. This was particularly fostered by press coverage of the pioneering work of Severino Antinori, a controversial Italian obstetrician and gynecologist, who, in 1989, started to experiment with the in vitro fertilization of women who had experienced non-precocious menopause. In 1994, with Antinori's help, a 63-year-old woman was impregnated and became the oldest child-bearer in the world. The media sensation caused by Antinori's achievements, accompanied by futuristic visions of human cloning, serves as an example of the test-tube Wild West cited in the public debate.

According to the media, the first regulatory norms for ARTs in Italy were enacted in 2004, whereas previously there was a lack of legislation. Although this is true in terms of an overall national law, an agreed regulatory system was already in force long before the enactment of Law 40.

The first public regulation of ARTs was introduced in 1985, when a ministerial circular (known as "Circolare Degan"[6]) forbade the treatment at public clinics of single individuals, unmarried couples, and homosexual couples, as well as banned heterologous fertilization and the creation of embryos for therapeutic purposes or research. Because of the absence of specific legislation concerning private clinics, the need for self-regulation was embraced by the Italian General Medical Council, which approved the final version of the Code of Medical Ethics in 1995 (published as Fineschi 1996). This code prohibited all medical practitioners working in the public or private sector from using four specific fertilization techniques (Art. 41): surrogate motherhood of any kind, insemination of homosexual couples or single women, insemination after the partner's death, and the insemination of women after non-precocious menopause.

Finally, an ordinance issued by the minister of health[7] in 1997 "prohibited the publicizing and sale of human gametes and embryos" in both public and private clinics. A chronological reconstruction of these prohibitions (summarized in Table 10.1) allows for a better understanding of Law 40's path. Although the regulations were not comprehensive national legislation, it can be claimed that all the *subversive* options, in terms of changes in kinship relations or being open to the new family models made possible by ARTs, were not legally available in Italy before 2004: since 1985 in the public clinics and since 1995 in all of them. These restrictions, moreover, were mainly characterized by conservative moral and ethical values.

These regulations, however, were unknown to the public. I argue that the myth of the test-tube Wild West was used in the public debate to achieve consensus in the majority of the population that was not familiar with these techniques and the restrictions already in place. Comprehensive national legislation on ARTs was put forward as necessary to remedy the lack of specific legislation on the matter and to counter the risk that improper use might be made of these technologies. However, this public rhetoric ignored all the rules and regulations that were already active in the field, thus producing a cultural and political context in which the state could intervene to regulate what had previously been within the jurisdiction of the professions. The restrictiveness of Law 40 was generated in this cultural climate, in which the specter of the test-tube Wild West haunted Italy.

Law 40 not only forbade surrogate motherhood of any kind, insemination of homosexual couples and singles, insemination after the partner's death, and treatment for women after non-precocious menopause; it also prohibited heterologous fertilization, the production of more than three embryos per cycle, the cryopreservation of embryos, and the performance of preimplantation genetic diagnosis. Furthermore, the law mandated that all the embryos produced must be transferred to the uterus, even if they were potentially malformed.

Table 10.1 Italian Regulatory Path of ARTs

Year	*Institution*	*Bans*	*Jurisdiction*
1985	Minister of Health	ART treatment of singles, unmarried couples, and homosexual couples; heterologous fertilization (i.e., with gametes from donors external to the couple); producing embryos for therapeutic purposes or research.	Public clinics
1995	Code of Medical Ethics	Surrogate motherhood of any kind; insemination of homosexual couples and singles; insemination after the partner's death; insemination of women in non-precocious menopause.	All medical practitioners
1997	Minister of Health	Publicizing and sale of human gametes and embryos.	All clinics
2004	Parliament	ARTs for anyone except stable heterosexual couples of fertile age; surrogate motherhood of any kind; heterologous fertilization; producing more than three embryos per cycle or using them for purposes other than transferring to the woman's body; cryopreservation of embryos; pre-implantation genetic diagnosis.	All clinics
		Deleted bans for constitutional illegitimacy	
2009	Constitutional Court	Producing more than three embryos per cycle or using them for purposes other than transferring to the woman's body; cryopreservation of embryos.	All clinics
2014	Constitutional Court	Heterologous fertilization.	All clinics

The novelty of Law 40 was to endow the embryo with personhood and to declare that the embryo's rights prevailed over those of the mother. The main effect of the limitation in embryo production and the prohibition on embryo freezing is that female patients now have to undergo all the hormonal treatments and clinical procedures for each IVF cycle. In other countries, more embryos than needed are routinely produced and cryopreserved to avoid repeating all the procedures, which are painful and dangerous for the woman. What is intriguing is that the law gave embryos more rights than a fetus, since Law 194 of 1978[8] on abortion has not been overturned or modified to create further restrictions on abortion.

The law was widely discussed and criticized in terms of both its ethical and clinical aspects (Clarke 2003; Robertson 2004). A broad political movement developed around these criticisms. It mobilized public opinion for some months (open letters written by Italian and international scientists against the restrictions imposed by the law, petitions, newspaper articles, etc.) and led to a referendum to abrogate the law. However, the referendum was not successful because the quorum (50 percent plus one of those entitled to vote) was not reached (just 25.3 percent voted). The reasons for the failure of referenda are multiple. As suggested by Metzler (2011), the Catholic hierarchy did not call for Italians to support the law (voting no) but instead invited them to abstain, with the aim of invalidating the referendum. In addition, in the last few years before this law, abrogative referenda had obtained little success, and this one had less hope than the others because of difficulties with its technical aspects and the perception of the topic as only being relevant to a few people, those with infertility problems.

Despite the failure of the referendum, couples, fertility clinics, and associations appealed to the Italian Constitutional Court to modify some of the restrictions. In March 2009, the Constitutional Court (ruling no. 151/2009) declared the partial constitutional illegitimacy of Law 40, with particular regard to the limitation of only three fertilizable oocytes in each cycle, the compulsory transfer of all the embryos obtained, and the prohibition of embryo cryopreservation. Moreover, some fundamental statements were made by the Court: first, embryo protection is limited by the need to ensure a concrete possibility of achieving a successful pregnancy; and second, the supremacy of physicians' judgment was reaffirmed, recalling that, according to Italian constitutional jurisprudence, gold-standard therapeutic practice is governed by the "autonomous responsibility of the attending physician in selecting, with the full consent of the patient, the best suitable treatment for the case" (Benagiano and Gianaroli 2010).

In April 2014, the Constitutional Court (ruling no. 162/2014) also declared that the prohibition on gamete donation in ART treatments was unconstitutional, as it violated couples' fundamental right to have children. Although, as a result of this, gamete donation is currently legal in Italy, procedures for procuring donor gametes have still to be specified and the debate on the practical application of donor techniques is still ongoing.

Italian Paradoxes: (Unintended) Effects on Reproductive Practices and Discourses

The legal history presented above produced many effects (intentional and otherwise, see Spilker, this volume) on the reproductive practices and discourses of Italy. I will discuss the more controversial effects according to an analytical division, although the phenomena are often overlapping.

The Creation of the Pre-Embryo

In the months before the enactment of Law 40, the Italian public debate turned to the issue of the "beginning of life" as the new primary ethical and moral issue. Moreover, this debate was framed as a controversy promoting two opposing factions: the so-called "pro-life" faction (summarized by the slogan "the embryo is one of us"), which aimed to defend human life from its inception (understood as conception and identified in the union of egg and sperm); and a second faction, which did not construct the embryo as a person and advocated putting the rights of the mother before those of the unborn child. These positions brought different legal ramifications, particularly regarding the possibility of freezing surplus embryos: the first group clearly rejected embryo cryopreservation as a means to defend human life; in contrast, the second was in favor of the freezing process, which was seen as a valuable tool to limit the negative effects of repeated hormonal treatments and surgery for oocyte collection. As we have seen, the position that prevailed in Italy was the first of these.

To avoid these restrictions, during the first months after the enactment of the law, employees at reproductive clinics, and their professional associations, questioned the notion of the *embryo*: when can a fertilized oocyte be considered an embryo and, thus, constitute a life and a person? Some scientists proposed an intrinsic distinction between an embryo and a pre-embryo (that is, an oocyte fertilized less than 36 hours previously in which the appearance of the two pronuclei indicates that fusion between the male and female elements has not taken place yet) on the basis of a medical interpretation of the law, which enabled them to circumvent its provisions. This attempt to negotiate the limitations imposed upon the medical profession by redefining the category of embryo was subsequently blocked by ministerial circulars and guidelines establishing the term; although Italian law made reference only to the "embryo," the restrictions also applied to the pre-embryo because it had clearly been the legislators' intention to protect potential *life* from its beginning, i.e., the moment of encounter between oocyte and spermatozoon.

This strategy (see also Gherardi and Perrotta 2011) shows how, even in the medical community, the moral and ethical concerns of the Catholic Church came to dominate the reproductive discourse. In fact, the term embryo was (and still is) widely used both within and outside the scientific community because it is considered a simpler and more comprehensible term to communicate with personnel external to the laboratory (doctors, nurses, anesthetists, and so on) and with patients. The generic expression "fertilized oocyte" and, especially, the term "embryo" are often used, whereas biological nomenclature (zygote, morula, or blastocyst) is often set aside in reproductive clinics.

Although the term embryo is used by professionals for communication purposes and is often a way to "bond" with prospective parents, the practice of naming zygotes as embryos reinforced the so-called "social life of the embryo" (Franklin and Roberts 2003). While the adoption of the term embryo by the medical community has never been challenged, paradoxically the use of the term pre-embryo was perceived as a manipulative attempt made by the practitioners with the goal of sidestepping regulation with a terminological shift.

Nationalizing Embryos

With the introduction of Law 40 and its prohibition on freezing embryos, which lasted until 2009, it was necessary to take action to resolve some ethically controversial issues: what was to be done with the embryos produced before the law that every clinic had in storage? How could the principle of equating the embryo with a person and, therefore, guaranteeing it the same rights, be applied retrospectively to these already-existing embryos?

When Law 40 was enacted, there were around 30,000 cryopreserved embryos stored in national biobanks in Italy. Some of these embryos were intended for use by aspiring parents in further attempts to begin a pregnancy. However, what would happen to the embryos belonging to couples who had already had children and did not want any more? What would happen if the couple did not intend to procreate further for some reason (separation, adoption, age, etc.)? In that case, the law stated that the embryos produced and frozen before the enactment were to be kept in their current state at the expense of the couple, or must be declared "abandoned" (in legal terms). Couples were, therefore, required to pay for the maintenance of their own embryos (the costs for the cryopreservation of embryos vary from clinic to clinic, but they range from €500 to €1000 per year), or sign an abandonment form, giving up all rights to them.

Instructions have yet to be issued about what is to be done with the abandoned embryos, which were supposed to be transferred to an "orphan embryo bank." This biobank was set up, but the embryos have never been transferred, due to both legal reasons (the possibility of disputes) and economic constraints (the need for additional funds for the transport of the embryos). What is certain is that other options, such as donation to other couples, donation for research purposes, or disposal, which represented the fate of 77 percent of frozen embryos before the enactment of the law (Cattoli *et al.* 2005), are now illegal.

Although expressions like *orphan embryos*, *abandoned embryos*, and *adoption of embryos* recall the principles of the law that equates them to persons, this definition is, in fact, problematic and morally controversial. However, what is most surprising is that, although embryos produced either before or after the introduction of the law cannot be used for research purposes, neither this nor other laws forbid stem-cell research in the country. The prohibition on embryo research envisaged by Law 40 is not a legal preclusion of research on embryonic cell lines created in other countries. This is partly due to EU legislation that stipulates the free circulation of goods and, therefore, makes it impossible to prohibit the importing of stem cells. Therefore, Italian scientists are allowed to do stem-cell research in Italy as long as they do not use Italian embryos (Metzler 2011). Because of the ambiguity of banning research on embryos by virtue of their alleged sacredness, those groups of scientists are tolerated but not publicly supported. Interestingly, one unexpected effect of the ban on embryo freezing has been the promotion of research on gamete cryopreservation (and particularly "egg freezing" – which had a more modest success rate before 2004), of which Italy became a pioneer during the years of prohibition on embryo freezing (2004–2009).

The Invention of "Miracle Moms"

The limitations introduced by Italian legislation have generated a widespread phenomenon of medical travel to countries with more liberal policies. A study conducted between October 2008 and March 2009 by the European Society for Human Reproduction (Shenfield *et al.* 2010) shows that Italians lead the world in seeking cross-border reproductive care (31.8 percent of all foreign patients).

People are willing to cross borders for treatments illegal in their own country, and cross-border reproductive care is not socially stigmatized, although it is not publicly supported either. To explore this paradox, I analyze the cases of many famous women who became mothers at 45 years of age or older and who have appeared in the Italian media over the last few years. Postponing maternity, in fact, is a socially accepted, and often encouraged, phenomenon. Higher levels of education among women, together with a huge increase in female labor-market entry and a lack of care services, have led not only to a drastic reduction in Italy's birthrate (the average number of children per Italian woman was just 1.39 in 2013), but also to women choosing to postpone pregnancy until they are older than 30 years (in 2013, the average age of women giving birth was 31.5 years).[9]

However, in the scientific community, conceiving in a *natural* way after age 45 is considered unusual, if not impossible. Therefore, the pregnancy (among others) of a well-known rock singer at the age of 56 (or 54, according to other commentators) drew much attention in Italian society. The matter of concern, however, was narrowed to the opportunity to become a mother at that age. Moreover, it was framed from a gendered perspective, debating how and if the concept of equal opportunities should be used to justify postponed motherhood and providing another example of how gender and bioethics are often intertwined in reproductive practices (Spilker and Lie 2007). Even the declaration of the singer's gynecologist to an Italian newspaper was passed over in silence: "The baby has not been conceived with egg donation, as some might think, but after a long process of care over the years which has allowed this result." However, Antinori spoke out against this explanation: "A case of homologous insemination after 48 years of age is simply not possible: there is not one example cited in the literature."[10]

However, it is not relevant whether this single pregnancy was due to egg donation in a foreign country or another technical solution (for instance, cryopreservation of her own egg at a young age). What is interesting is the absolute vacuum of knowledge within which this and other "miraculous" pregnancies (a number of well-known women from show business have had late babies in the last few years) are presented. In the public debate, there is no discussion of how these pregnancies are initiated. Nor is the theme of reproductive travel mentioned. The only exceptions are online forums[11] dedicated to this topic (currently, one of the main sources of information for people looking for treatment), where the question of egg donation in these cases is explicitly discussed, supposedly because aspiring mothers have more knowledge than other lay people. Among these users, the discourse is framed in different ways. Some users condemn both the singer and the Italian press for misinformation. Others justify the choice of the women to hide their use of egg donation because it means hiding the lack of biological connection with their children. Many women on such forums share this concern, arguing that it would not be accepted in Italian society.

Conclusions: Reframing Conception, Reproducing Society

In the previous pages, I have tried to narrate an unruly story, unraveling the paradoxes of the Italian situation, in which: (a) embryos have more rights than fetuses and mothers; (b) the term embryo has been naturalized with the participation of the medical community, but the term pre-embryo is perceived as deceitful; (c) certain practices are illegal within the country (such as gamete donation), while neither illegal nor socially stigmatized when performed abroad; (d) the state forbids research on Italian embryos while allowing scientists to import foreign stem cells; and (e) the state openly discriminates against some of its citizens, such as those who are not allowed to undergo treatments in Italy and cannot afford to travel abroad. However, people are still willing to cross borders for treatments illegal in their own country. All of these paradoxes need some final reflections.

First, all of these elements demonstrate the distance between politics and lay people, moral arguments and daily life. If the state was trying to create a new moral order in the country, this attempt failed. Second, the effect of the law has been to build an image of a moral and ethical defense of life, represented by the embryo. Although this cultural image reflects the standpoint of many politicians and members of the Church's hierarchy, it does not seem to be shared by the majority of Italian citizens. Third, the procreative interfaces have produced a reframing of conception that allows for a traditional and conservative reproduction of society based on the traditional family model grounded in blood ties.

What makes Italy a particular, and peculiar, case is that the reproduction of society is cosmetic: a system of double standards allows for concrete changes while retaining formal shapes. I name this the "Italian anomaly," that is, the reproduction of a double standard (in moral and ethical meanings) through the rhetoric of different actors: political, religious, and lay. One example of this double standard is the way in which medical travel is dealt with in the public debate, where the expression "cross-border reproductive care" is unknown and the phenomenon is usually referred to as "reproductive tourism." As observed by Kroløkke (this volume), a terminological and theoretical debate has arisen over how to describe the search for ARTs across national and international borders. Speaking about tourism denies one of the core reasons for travel: the impossibility of gaining access to this kind of care in patients' own countries. Accordingly, as some authors have suggested, it would be more appropriate to talk about "reproductive exile" (Inhorn and Patrizio 2009). In this sense, I argue that the use of the term "tourism" in the Italian debate – willingly or unwillingly – reinforces the idea of individual choice and locates the discussion in the domain of a free market, rather than focusing on access to care and legal restrictions. At the same time, the ambiguity of the term "tourism" also allows users to avoid engaging with the social stigmatization of practices that are illegal in the country and often on the edge of ethical and moral acceptance (as in the example of "miracle moms").

Finally, the social and cultural reconstruction of the Italian reproductive interface and discourse has made the rethinking of what Hanafin (2007) defined as *reproductive citizenship* more urgent. Hanafin developed this concept to differentiate it from the notion of *ethopolitics* proposed by Nikolas Rose (2001). In recent years a form of affirmative biopolitics has been emerging, which does not reflect the traditional distinction between those who exercise power and those who are its subjects. Rose claims that, in advanced liberal democracies, individuals and collectives demand rights, call for recognition and respect, and increasingly define their citizenship in terms of their rights to life, health, and care. The notion of ethopolitics highlights these forms of deliberative participative politics. As Hanafin (2013) notes, in the landscape of reproductive citizenship in Italy, forms of ethopolitics can be seen in the movements of individuals who are attempting to self-style their reproductive choices (for instance, constantly appealing to the Constitutional Court). However, politicians and the Roman Catholic Church vigorously oppose such a policy and constantly attempt to prevent the creation of this right. Hanafin defines this phenomenon as *vitapolitics*, which is "not a politics of empowerment but a politics of entrapment in an imagined natural order" (2007, 5). Defining the rights of an embryo as a proto-citizen, in fact, means establishing a monolithic view of bioethical issues. This bioethical position accommodates the conservative and patriarchal models of gender and familial relations, impeding the pluralist development of multi-ethical frameworks. However, on a practical level, much of civil society chooses personal reproductive options that openly go against this bioethical position. As I have shown in this chapter, this produces a number of paradoxes that bring forth a variety of emerging tensions in Italian society, which will require further exploration.

Notes

1 This chapter is based on ethnographic data collected during and after my PhD research, which include participant observations in three ART clinics, 25 interviews with professionals, 12 interviews with couples, and document analysis (including data

collected via newspapers and websites, data published by the Ministry of Health, and material produced by the Italian Constitutional Court). For reasons of space, however, the chapter will not present in-depth ethnographic data. For more details, see Perrotta 2008, 2010.

2 See www.vatican.va/roman_curia/congregations/cfaith/documents/rc_con_cfaith_doc_19870222_respect-for-human-life_en.html, last accessed November 23, 2015.

3 See http://w2.vatican.va/content/john-paul-ii/en/encyclicals/documents/hf_jp-ii_enc_25031995_evangelium-vitae.html, last accessed November 23, 2015.

4 According to ISTAT there were 514,308 live births in 2013. However, this has to be considered a low estimate because of the non-predictable number of children born in Italy as a result of using these techniques abroad.

5 Law No. 40, February 19, 2004, "Norme in materia di procreazione medicalmente assistita" [Regulations relating to medically assisted procreation] published in the Official Gazette No. 45, February 24, 2004.

6 Ministerial circular n. 100/119657/32.2.14 "Limiti e condizioni di legittimità dei servizi per l'inseminazione artificiale nell'ambito del Servizio Sanitario Nazionale" [Limits and conditions of legitimacy of services for artificial insemination within the National Health Service], issued by the Minister of Health on October 10, 1985.

7 Ordinance "Divieto di commercializzazione e di pubblicità di gameti ed embrioni umani" [Prohibition on marketing and advertising of human gametes and embryos], issued by the Minister of Health and published in the Official Gazette No. 55, March 7, 1997.

8 Law No. 194, May 22, 1978, "Norme per la tutela sociale della maternità e sull'interruzione volontaria della gravidanza" [Rules for the social protection of maternity and on abortion] published in the Official Gazette No. 140, May 22, 1978.

9 Data source: ISTAT, The National Institute of Statistics, available on the website http://demo.istat.it/index.html, last accessed, November 23, 2015.

10 Gianna Nannini madre con la tecnica proibita. Antinori accusa: «Impossibile alla sua età quella omologa». [Gianna Nannini mother using the forbidden technique: Antinori's accusation: "Homologous fertilization impossible at her age"]. La Stampa, November 28, 2010.

11 See discussions on this issue on forums of the websites of the major patient associations: www.madreprovetta.org, last accessed November 23, 2015; www.cercounbimbo.it, last accessed November 23, 2015; www.alfemminile.com, last accessed November 23, 2015; www.fertilita.org, last accessed November 23, 2015.

References

Benagiano, Giuseppe, and Luca Gianaroli. 2010. "The Italian Constitutional Court Modifies Italian Legislation on Assisted Reproduction Technology." *Reproductive Biomedicine Online* 20: 1398–1402.

Cattoli, Monica, Andrea Borini, Luca Dal Prato, Maria A. Bonu, Mirella Patuelli, and Carlo Flamigni. 2005. "Stored Frozen Embryos: The Influence of Italian IVF Law." *Human Reproduction* 20 (suppl. 1): 48i.

Clarke, Hilary. 2003. "Italy Approves Controversial Legislation on Fertility Treatment." *The Lancet* 362 (9401): 2076. Accessed November 23, 2015. doi: http://dx.doi.org/10.1016/S0140-6736(03)15157-4.

Diamanti, Ilvo, and Luigi Ceccarini. 2007. "Catholics and Politics after the Christian Democrats: The Influential Minority." *Journal of Modern Italian Studies* 12 (1): 37–59.

DiMarco, Erica. 2009. "The Tides of Vatican Influence in Italian Reproductive Matters:

From Abortion to Assisted Reproduction." *Rutgers Journal of Law and Religion* 10 (2): 1–31.

Fineschi, Vittorio, ed. 1996. *Codice di deontologia medica* [*Code of Medical Ethics*]. Milano: Giuffre.

Franklin, Sarah, and Celia Roberts. 2003. "Innovative Health Technologies: The Social Life of the Embryo," published by the Department of Sociology, Lancaster University, available at www.lancaster.ac.uk/fass/resources/sociology-online-papers/papers/roberts-franklin-social-life-of-embryo.pdf. Accessed November 23, 2015.

Garelli, Franco. 1991. *Religione e chiesa in Italia* [*Religion and the Church in Italy*]. Bologna: Il Mulino.

Garelli, Franco. 2007. "The Public Relevance of the Church and Catholicism in Italy." *Journal of Modern Italian Studies* 12 (1): 8–36.

Gherardi, Silvia, and Manuela Perrotta. 2011. "Egg Dates Sperm: A Tale of a Practice Change and its Stabilization." *Organization* 18 (5): 595–614.

Hanafin, Patrick. 2007. *Conceiving Life: Reproductive Politics and the Law in Contemporary Italy*. Burlington: Ashgate.

Hanafin, Patrick. 2013. "Law, Biopolitics and Reproductive Citizenship: The Case of Assisted Reproduction in Italy." *TECNOSCIENZA: Italian Journal of Science & Technology Studies* 4 (1): 45–68.

Inhorn, Marcia C., and Daphna Birenbaum-Carmeli. 2008. "Assisted Reproductive Technologies and Culture Change." *Annual Review of Anthropology* 37: 177–196.

Inhorn, Marcia C., and Pasquale Patrizio. 2009. "Rethinking Reproductive 'Tourism' as Reproductive 'Exile.'" *Fertility and Sterility* 92 (3): 904–906.

Melhuus, Marit. 2005. "'Better Safe Than Sorry': Legislating Assisted Conception in Norway." In *State Formation: Anthropological Perspectives*, edited by Christian Krohn-Hansen and Knut G. Nustad, 212–233. London: Pluto.

Metzler, Ingrid. 2011. "Between Church and State: Stem Cells, Embryos, and Citizens in Italian Politics." In *Reframing Rights: Bioconstitutionalism in the Genetic Age*, edited by Sheila Jasanoff, 105–124. Cambridge: MIT Press.

Perrotta, Manuela. 2008. "The Organizational Construction of the Body in the Assisted Reproductive Technologies." In *Women on Biotechnology*, edited by Francesca Molfino and Flavia Zucco, 171–181. Milano: Springer.

Perrotta, Manuela. 2010. "Situated Practices as the Locus of Technological Change." In *Beyond Knowledge Management – Sociomaterial and Sociocultural Perspectives within Management Research*, edited by Silvia Jordan and Hermann Mitterhofer, 147–169. Innsbruck: Innsbruck University Press.

Robertson, John A. 2004. "Protecting Embryos and Burdening Women: Assisted Reproduction in Italy." *Human Reproduction* 19: 1693–1696.

Rose, Nikolas. 2001. "The Politics of Life Itself." *Theory, Culture & Society* 18 (6): 1–30.

Shenfield, Françoise, Jacques de Mouzon, Guido Pennings, Anna P. Ferraretti, Anders Nyboe Andersen, Gau de Wert, and Veerle Goossens. 2010. "Cross Border Reproductive Care in Six European Countries." *Human Reproduction* 25 (6): 1361–1368.

Spilker, Kristin, and Merete Lie. 2007. "Gender and Bioethics Intertwined: Egg Donation within the Context of Equal Opportunities." *European Journal of Women's Studies* 14 (4): 327–340.

Thompson, Charis. 2005. *Making Parents: The Ontological Choreography of Reproductive Technologies*. Cambridge: MIT Press.

11 The Veto of Moral Politics

The Catholic Church and ARTs in Ireland

Orla McDonnell

Introduction

Over the last three decades, the assemblage of techniques associated with In Vitro Fertilization (IVF) has been re-designated from the novel and controversial status of "New Reproductive Technologies" or "Artificial Reproductive Technologies" to legitimate and routine medical practice as "Assisted Reproductive Technologies" (ARTs). This process of normalization involves a confluence of factors, including the medicalization of infertility, the expansion of therapeutic rationales in line with expanding technological capacities and, not least, the expansion of local and global markets providing private fertility services. At the same time, the normalization of ARTs is culturally bound by the institutional contexts of different jurisdictions, as the various chapters in this volume testify. In Ireland, for example, the residual power of the Catholic Church, despite its diminishing institutional authority, has operated as a moral veto against the opening up of a policy debate on the legitimacy of ARTs in the formation of families and broader regulatory issues. The consequence of this has been many years of state passivity with respect to the changing social context surrounding reproductive and sexual politics and family formation, which have altered the normative context in which ARTs have taken hold. There is always a residual novelty in the way that technologies associated with ARTs can disrupt the normative frameworks that render certain practices legitimate, as recent cases in the Irish courts demonstrate. The medicalization of infertility has been a key boundary definer, but this can only go so far in delimiting the radicalizing potential of ARTs, since infertility is not exclusively a biological category and ARTs are not in the proper sense treatments for infertility but rather alternative means of having a child who may or may not be linked genetically to a parent.

While, in Ireland, IVF was first recognized as a legitimate therapeutic practice under Medical Council guidelines in 1989 (Medical Council 1989; McDonnell and Allison 2006), ARTs have until recently operated in a legal vacuum, due to what I will describe as the veto of moral politics – a political impasse associated with the residual power of the Irish Catholic Church institutionalized as national moral norms. Indeed, given the legacy of biopolitics in Ireland, which was shaped in no small way by the moral monopoly of the Catholic Church, one could well have expected the State to have moved toward a restrictive regulatory regime similar to that of Italy in 2004 (Perrota, this volume). Instead, ARTs were left to the self-regulatory domain of the medical profession, which shifted from restrictive codes of practice banning donor gametes and the freezing of embryos in 1989 and limiting IVF to married couples in 1994 to more liberalized codes in subsequent ethical guidelines (Medical Council 2004; 2009). It is over ten years since the government-appointed Commission on Assisted Human Reproduction published its report (2005) recommending a statutory framework for the regulation of ARTs. However, it is only recently that legislative action has been taken with the introduction of the Children and Relationships Act 2015.[1] Part of this Act deals in a partial way with ARTs and, for the first time, legally regulates the relationship between children conceived using donor gametes or donor embryos and their parents.

The development of a private market in infertility treatments and the lacunae opened up by the diminishing power of the Catholic Church, particularly with respect to healthcare and medical ethics (McDonnell and Allison 2006), coupled with the exceedingly slow pace of the State's response to the need for statutory regulation facilitated the normalization of ARTs as a treatment for infertility. An important caveat with respect to this normalization in Ireland is that it has occurred in the context of infertility therapeutics and medical ethics, while the imperative of political decision-making concerns how ARTs contribute to the creation of families. Medical ethics, however, are a wholly inadequate substitute for policy-making given that ART practices are subject to competing claims that challenge the presuppositions of existing laws governing rights and obligations relating to family formation. Given that legal innovation is a key aspect of the network of relations that serve to legitimize and, hence, normalize controversial and novel technologies, this chapter will assess how the veto of moral politics in relation to the traditional institution of the family and the status of the embryo created political inertia with respect to the statutory regulation of ARTs in Ireland for over three decades.

Toward a Liberalized Agenda for ARTs

The task of enrolling public and expert support for a regulatory framework governing ART practices was assigned to an expert commission. The Commission on Assisted Human Reproduction (CAHR) was established in 2000 following the publication of a *Green Paper on Abortion* (Government of Ireland 1999) alerting policy-makers to the implications for ART practices arising from the constitutional ambiguity of the term "unborn." The limited public airing of the Commission's deliberations, the exceedingly long time it took to report on its recommendations, the lack of policy debate following its publication, and the political inertia that continued until recently are indicative of the State's ambivalence about the legal and bioethical complexities arising from ARTs. The most controversial aspect of the Commission's report, which endorsed a liberalized regulatory regime, was the recommendation that the constitutional protection afforded to the embryo/"unborn" should not apply to the IVF embryo prior to implantation. The purpose of this was to remove any uncertainty about the legal basis of embryo freezing and preimplantation genetic diagnosis, as well as providing legal certainty in relation to embryonic stem-cell research under certain regulatory conditions.

Embryo freezing proved a particularly contentious issue for the Medical Council and, as therapeutic rationales came to outweigh moral absolutes on the status of the embryo, the medical profession sought to keep the term "embryo" out of its professional and public deliberations by substituting it with the terms "fertilised ova," "pre-embryo," or "zygote" – technical terms that are used interchangeably as less emotively evocative of and morally charged by abortion politics (McDonnell and Allison 2006). Prior to the publication of the Commission's report, the Medical Council (2004) gave ethical approval to embryo donation (referred to as "fertilised ova"). This de facto lifting of ethical restrictions on embryo freezing meant that the proposed liberal regulatory regime was not politicized vis-à-vis the self-regulatory domain of the medical profession. This facilitated a shift in the emergent regulatory discourse from an ethico-moral to a medico-scientific frame of reference. Subsequently, therapeutic rationales specific to the medical domain have given way to strictly legal concerns arising from a series of high-profile court cases, while a critical moment in terms of the recent turn toward legislative action was the government's decision to hold a referendum on same-sex marriage. Let us now consider the wider institutional dynamics at play in shaping the regulatory politics of ARTs in Ireland.

ARTs and the Familial Nation

Regulatory politics play a decisive role in shaping the meaning of the embryo created through IVF (Bock von Wülfingen 2012; Metzler 2012). Ireland's restrictive abortion regime, which effectively amounted to an outright ban until the Protection of Life during Pregnancy Act 2013, has been zealously defended by the State as a cultural marker of the nation's "pro-life" identity. While the moral and legal status afforded to the embryo is intended to restrict access to abortion, the absence of specific statutory laws governing ARTs should not be taken to imply that the State is either absent from or a benign bystander in these developments. To elucidate this argument, I will briefly examine two decisive court rulings on ART practices to which the State was party.

A landmark High Court case (*Roche v Roche* 2006), which was subsequently upheld by the Supreme Court (*Roche v Roche* 2009) ruled that embryos produced by IVF do not come within the terms of Article 40.3.3 of the Constitution inserted in 1983 to protect "the right to life of the unborn." This case concerned legal action taken by a separated woman who was seeking to have three embryos, frozen after an earlier IVF cycle, implanted in her womb. If the court had ruled that the term "unborn" is defined as applying from the moment of fertilization, the logical corollary of this would be that the "right to life" of embryos created through IVF would be constitutionally protected, effectively strengthening those rights. The case rested on the rights of married couples over their frozen embryos and whether these entailed an assumption of consent for their subsequent implantation; and, furthermore, whether such consent is irrevocable in the event of a couple's separation. The position of the State was that the consent given by the husband to embryo freezing did not require further consent for the implantation of those embryos, irrespective of the changed family circumstances (Carolan 2006). This case served to highlight the State's role as protector of the embryo and of the privileged constitutional status of the family based on marriage, although the latter issue was not central to the ruling of the court. The court drew a legal distinction between the embryo created *in vitro* and the embryo *in vivo*, thus establishing that the protection afforded to the embryo/"unborn" in the Constitution does not apply to the IVF embryo prior to implantation. The courts, however, were reluctant to define the status of embryos created through IVF given the broader public policy issues involved, not just for infertility therapeutics and the legal relationship between prospective parents and children conceived using donated embryos, but also for medical research.

However, the critical turning point in pushing the State to regulate ARTs arose from the legally anomalous situation created by a High Court ruling on surrogacy (*M.R & Anor v An tÁrd Chláraitheoir* [Registrar General] 2013), which is neither prohibited nor regulated in Ireland. This case involved a married couple who were the genetic parents of twins born as the result of a surrogacy arrangement with the wife's sister, and centered on the question of who should be registered as the children's mother. In granting legal status to the genetic mother, the judgment highlighted how biology is contestable and not fixed in terms of normative understandings and cultural codes. The State's case rested on the presumed common law principle of *mater semper certa* – motherhood is always certain, whereas the applicants' case rested on the claim that the blood bonds between the parents and the children were determined by genetics and, in particular, the genetic link between the mother and children. Therefore, the role of biology in defining the natural link between a mother and child was contested. The State, in arguing against the defendants, challenged the notion that motherhood can be defined in terms of genetics alone and put on a legal par with fatherhood. It contended that the laws of nature establish motherhood as different from fatherhood. In recasting the "blood link" as the definer of motherhood and, therefore, placing it on a par with fatherhood in legal, if not in biological terms, the ruling had significant implications for ART practices involving third-party donation. Subsequently, the State won its appeal to the Supreme Court (*MR and DR v An tÁrd Chláraitheoir* [Registrar General] 2014), which re-established the birth mother as the legal mother to be registered on the children's birth certificate. However, the court rejected the State's claim that the principle that motherhood is always certain is firmly established in common law and the core message was that the complexity of the issues raised by surrogacy, particularly with respect to the rights of children, were not a matter for the courts but the legislature. This rebuke by the Supreme Court was reframed by the government as a case of the State being given the green light to govern in the name of protecting those who access ARTs and the welfare of children born as result of those arrangements. Not unlike the "trickster" moment in Spilker's account of family politics and ARTs in Norway (this volume), the term "family" mysteriously disappears from policy discourse as the rationale for legislation is reframed in terms of equality of access and the rights of prospective children born as a result of ARTs.

The Moral Economy of the Family

The discourses of equality and children's rights, particularly the notion of the "best interests of children," have paved the way for a liberalized regulatory agenda with respect to ARTs, which until recently was stymied by the moral politics of the family. In bearing the stamp of national moral-political norms, the sovereignty of the family based on marriage as a moral institution encoded in the Constitution since 1937 was the cornerstone of the pastoral power of the Catholic Church in exercising its moral authority. However, the function performed by the family in shoring up the authority of that Church has been undermined by its declining social power. This is reflected in key cultural and structural changes in family formation and sexual behavior since the 1960s. A parliamentary committee review of family policy (Government of Ireland 2006) formally recognized that policy changes from the 1970s onwards had effectively diluted the constitutional privilege afforded to the family based on marriage, reflecting what it claimed as a radical shift in state support for Catholic social tenets. Yet, the State continued to refuse to endorse a recommendation of the Commission on the Family (Government of Ireland 1998) to broaden constitutional protection to all family types. Let us look more closely at the official rationale that was used to retain the constitutional status quo in the then-government's review of family policy following a public consultation exercise. Retaining the status quo was presented by the parliamentary committee as a pragmatic, political decision given what its report described as a "sharp division" in public opinion between "traditionalist" and "equality" values. Herein lies the dichotomy between public policies that increasingly draw on equality and human rights frameworks as instruments of governance, and the role that natural law derived from Roman Catholic social philosophy historically played *via* the constitutional protection of the traditional family.

In the consultation process, statutory organizations directly involved in implementing family policy in areas such as adoption and social welfare embraced the position that the Constitution should be changed to recognize all family forms in line with equality legislation and human rights protocols. The traditionalist stance was articulated most strongly by the Catholic Church and conservative Catholic lay organizations, including "pro-life" groups. These groups evoked state governance based on equality and human rights discourses as not only a direct threat to the relevance of religion in value-based debates about social change but also as a means of politically diluting the sovereignty of the nation state in defining the public good. For these groups, the politics of abortion is a key stake in any move by the State to endorse change to the constitutional definition of the traditional family, which symbolizes the familial nation and its communal identity as "pro-life." Constitutional recognition of all family types would undermine the principles of natural law and, hence, the symbolic power of religion in the constitutional expression of a national ethos and identity. A crisis of community was a central construct of the moral politics of the family evoked in earlier debates in the 1980s and 1990s on the legalization of contraception, homosexuality, and divorce. This debate has shifted under various social currents and, more recently, the high turnout and support for the marriage equality referendum in May 2015 has been taken as the clearest evidence of an emerging post-Catholic society. For the Catholic Church and Catholic lay organizations, legal recognition of same-sex unions undermines the moral institution of marriage as the site of "procreation" by virtue of its primary function in confirming the natural laws governing the sexes and human sexuality.

The Irish Catholic Bishops' Conference's Committee on the Family disputed claims that state-church relations are the central issue at stake in changes to the value base of the Constitution. Instead, it argued that any such change would only strengthen the hand of the State in undermining the sovereignty of the family. In this sense, it argued that the stakes are highest for the State itself, reminding it of the political risk of undermining the moral economy of the family: "It cannot replace the family without sacrificing its own interest in social cohesion and undertaking responsibilities it has neither the mandate nor the capacity to fulfil" (Government of Ireland 2006, Appendix 1: 118). The family, which is defined in the language of natural laws as the "primary vital cell" (as in the bishops' submission), has considerable symbolic weight for the political positioning of those who wield the veto of moral politics, partly because its traditionalist discourse can be rationalized in line with the longstanding state policy of supplementing and not supplanting the family (Canavan 2011). Hence, in echoing the bishops' forewarning to the State, the status quo was defended on the basis that the traditional family is the primary source of "social solidarity" against the social current of "individualism" that threatens the norms of reciprocity, mutual dependency and caring obligations institutionalized in the normative structures of the traditional family (Government of Ireland 2006, 128).

While the main focus of legislative reform of family policy during the 1980s concerned the discriminatory difference in rights between children born in and out of wedlock, ARTs raise a more complex set of legal problems for the rights of parents and children. However, the implications of ARTs for family policy were not part of the remit of the parliamentary review, although a small number of submissions raised it as an issue to challenge the nomenclature of "natural law," "natural fathers," and "natural mothers" guiding moral and legal discourse on family policy. The National Women's Council of Ireland, in laying out the context of family change in Ireland, drew attention to the normalization of ARTs and the use of gamete donation in disrupting cultural assumptions that equate biological and social parenthood. In challenging the moral discourse surrounding the heteronormative definition of the family, a submission from a gay organization (the Johnny Gay Peer Action Charity Group) pointed out that reproductive potential is not always realized or intended in heterosexual married relationships, while same-sex couples who have children are denied family status. A community-based lesbian organization (LINC) highlighted the precarious legal position of lesbian couples with children. This submission noted that

> if biological parenthood is a legal requirement for birth registration, the issues of donor insemination, egg donation, surrogacy ... will have to be legislated for in all their complexity as they apply to heterosexual couples as well as lesbian and gay couples.
>
> (Government of Ireland 2006, Appendix 1, 179)

The "Familial Nation" and Veto of Moral Politics

Ostensibly, a pragmatic rationale guided the political decision to maintain the status quo. In weighing up the political risk of a constitutional referendum, the Catholic Bishops' Conference's Committee on the Family took the view that any state incursion into the symbolic sovereign domain of the traditional family would fall prey to the kind of intense and divisive politics associated with various constitutional referenda (presumably, it was referring to the referenda on abortion and divorce). The report explained that those who wished to retain the status quo "fear that any change would threaten the position of the family based on marriage [and] would undermine the stability of the traditional family and all the enhancement of the common good that flows from it" (Government of Ireland 2006, 121). The opposing view was described as:

> ... largely people who feel that the basic democratic value of equality should extend to all forms of family life. However they appreciate and respect the contribution made by the traditional family to the common good. While they would like to see the Constitution change they would wish at the same time to maintain support for the traditional family.
>
> (Government of Ireland 2006, 121)

The implication of the semiotics of these statements is clear: all favored support for the traditional family, while *many* did not support giving constitutional recognition to other family forms since this would undermine the family unit that they all recognize and support. Moreover, the few who supported constitutional change argued their case on the basis of a principle of equality, whereas *all* supported the common good emanating from the family based on marriage. The common good that flows from equality was elided here, as were those submissions that questioned unwavering support for the notion that the common good is universally served by traditionalist values in an otherwise pluralist society. The report, therefore, confirmed that the 1937 Constitution, which was directly influenced by the Catholic Church, continued to reflect the desires of the majority. The narrative of the nation state, in which the sovereignty of the traditional family and the self-determination of the State are bound together in their representation of a cohesive, mono-cultural community (Hanafin 2001) remained intact through the symbolic function that the Constitution performs in reproducing the nation state.

The Catholic Church and the Regulatory Politics of ARTs

While the Catholic Church's most recent doctrinal teaching, *Dignitas Personae* (Congregation of the Doctrine of the Faith 2008), is unequivocal in its opposition to ARTs, the Irish Church, in aligning itself with the need for regulation, has not been forceful in calling for a proscriptive regime and has softened its public stance on the immorality of IVF. The Irish Catholic Bishops' Conference (2003) submission to CAHR in 2000 and its subsequent response to CAHR's report in 2005 endorsed the need for the statutory regulation of ARTs on the basis of two key constitutional principles – the right to life of the "unborn" and the privileged status afforded to the family based on marriage. Since doctrinal teaching cannot be the basis of reasoned arguments that others will recognize in a secular state, the substance of its concerns was the emergent liberal regulatory discourse that threatened the core values of the familial (Catholic) nation. While the bishops registered the Church's moral objection to embryo freezing, in contrast to its doctrinal position and a call for a ban on embryo freezing in their 2000 submission, here they conceded that "freezing may well be considered preferable to the wanton destruction of embryos which might otherwise take place and, in so far as the freezing of embryos is allowed by law, it must certainly be regulated" (Irish Catholic Bishops' Conference 2006, 17–18). Again, going against its own doctrinal certainty, it accepted the morally relativist argument supporting embryo donation, stating: "It must be said at the outset that to allow 'surplus' embryos to survive in this way is infinitely preferable to disposing of them or making use of them as objects of research" (ibid., 19). Hence, in terms of regulatory legislation, the position of the Church was aligned with the Medical Council's ethical approval of IVF, embryo freezing, and embryo donation. In other words, the Church has become part of the compromise that in practice has defined the parameters of the normalization of ARTs. However, it was in relation to bioethical governance that the real politics of the Catholic Church were revealed.

The Bishops' Conference vehemently opposed CAHR's recommendation that the constitutional protection afforded to the embryo should not apply to the embryo before implantation and accused the Commission of "never having faced up to the fundamental question of the status of the embryo" (ibid., 29). It was critical of the Commission's presentation of bioethics as a deliberative process involving different values and moral standpoints, arguing that the right to life, dignity, and respect of the human embryo as a human being, and the sovereignty of the family as a moral institution were fundamental (non-negotiable) moral principles. In this respect, the bishops accused the Commission of being disingenuous in claiming that its recommendations on the regulation of ARTs were primarily concerned with the welfare of children. It also charged the

Commission with embedding political bias into its deliberation process by facilitating those with a vested interest in the ART industry, who "either implicitly or explicitly denied the human rights of the embryo" (ibid., 35).

Three less obviously revealing responses by the Bishops' Conference also throw light on how the Church sees the governance of ARTs. The first concerns CAHR's recommendation that national statistics be collated on the outcomes of ARTs. Here the Church, in the name of infertility prevention, could not conceal its own sense of moral authority in recommending that a regulatory authority should exercise biopower by compiling statistics that "indicate the proportion of cases of infertility in which there is evidence of present or previously treated sexually transmitted disease, previous use of chemical contraception and IUCDs or previous abortion" (ibid., 14). The second issue concerned the recommendation that counseling should be integrated into ART services to support client decision-making. Since "non-directive" counseling in medical contexts usurps the pastoral power of the Church and indeed that of health professionals to guide the individual's moral compass in ethical decision-making, the Church sees "…no value in any form of education or counseling which embraces feelings but excludes the essential facts about the nature of the human embryo" (ibid., 21). The third issue concerns the recommendation that "best practice" guidelines on infertility treatment should be developed by the proposed statutory regulatory body for doctors and gynecologists working outside of specialist clinics. The Church was not opposed to such guidelines but argued that these should be developed within the regulatory bodies of the healthcare professionals themselves. This is perhaps revealing of the Church's suspicion of regulatory oversight as a further usurpation of its historical hold over the ethos of the nursing and medical professions through its ownership and control of hospitals.

Conclusion

While a regulatory mandate has been recognized since the mid-1990s, the political strategy adopted by the State until recently has been to allow ART services to self-regulate. The Church in Ireland, as in other European "Catholic countries," has been a key player in shaping biopolitics in relation to the social regulation of sex, sexuality, and reproduction through the institutionalization of a privileged family form. However, since this chapter was first drafted in 2012, governing ARTs at a distance is no longer politically feasible for the Irish State. In the field of reproductive politics, the political risk of legislative inaction was highlighted in November 2012 following extensive media coverage of the death of an Indian woman, living in Ireland, from septicemia associated with a miscarriage after an abortion had been performed at a stage when her health was already dangerously compromised. The controversy centered on her husband's public testimony that his wife's repeated requests for an abortion as her health was deteriorating were ignored because they were told that the pregnancy could not be terminated as long as a fetal heartbeat existed since Ireland was a Catholic country. Following 20 years of legislative inaction on abortion, this case was a critical event in challenging the veto of moral politics. The argument of this chapter is that the State's equivocation in failing to regulate ARTs, inadvertently or otherwise, shored up the veto of moral politics and, hence, the residual power of the Catholic Church as a moral legislature at the expense of its own acknowledged mandate to act. Moreover, in the 2009 and 2014 Supreme Court rulings discussed, the courts stressed that it was the responsibility of the legislature to act with respect to the complex issues that arise from ARTs. Certainly, the symbolic power of the Catholic Church continues to gain traction to the extent that traditional values have purchase in political discourse about the common good, thus lending weight to the veto of the moral (decreasing) minority. While this continues to be the case in terms of the State holding the line that abortion is culturally abhorrent, gay people have been embraced as part of the familial nation through the discourse of equality in expressing the common good. Besides, as the analysis in this chapter shows, the Church had aligned with the shifting ethical position of the Medical Council in pre-empting regulatory action by the State on ARTs, while the Supreme Court (*Roche v Roche* 2009), in determining the status of the embryo *in vitro*, removed a key barrier to future legislatures regulating ARTs in line with changing therapeutic rationales. It now remains open to the State to make the running in determining equality of access to ARTs and broader policy issues with respect to the rights of prospective parents and children.

In the lead-up to the same-sex marriage referendum, the government moved very quickly to introduce the Children and Relationships Bill. Those opposed to same-sex marriage saw this as a cynical political maneuver. They argued that this extension of the constitutional right to marriage would in effect pre-empt the regulation of donor-assisted reproduction and surrogacy by extending the right to natural procreation within marriage to an unconditional right to access ARTs for same-sex married couples. Both the Referendum Commission and the marriage equality campaign argued that there was no link between these issues. While restrictions on access to the domestic market in infertility treatments for single people and gay couples have been imposed through the force of normative conventions in the absence of legislation, the debate opened up by the same-sex marriage referendum made it clear that marriage does not constitute the ultimate legal test in relation to access to ARTs. In the cases discussed in this chapter, neither the right to procreation nor the right to access ARTs were part of the court rulings. Indeed, the legislative vacuum on ARTs has impinged on the rights of married and non-married heterosexual couples in equal measure to those of same-sex couples in terms of lending legal certainty to the rights of parents and children. Under the Children and Relationships Act 2015, equality of access to donor programs is made explicit in allowing for the recognition of single women as sole parents in donor-assisted arrangements, and where couples are involved the other parent is the mother's husband, civil partner, or cohabitant. While surrogacy was originally intended to be part of the Act, this was removed and the then government promised that it would address this and the broader regulatory issues arising from ARTs in the near future. The expectations created about future legislation are also part of the process of enrolling public support for the normalization of ARTs. The discourse driving these expectations centers on equality and the welfare of children, while therapeutic rationales and the expectations created about the future direction of medical science have become part of the background assumptions that paradoxically have never been part of policy or public discourse because of the legacy of the veto of moral politics.[2]

Notes

1 The genesis of this Act, which provides for changes to the laws on adoption, guardianship, parentage, and custody and introduces new legal regulations on donor-assisted reproduction, arose from on-going debates about the status of the family in the Constitution and its implications for policy equality with respect to de facto families. Moreover, the legalization of civil partnership in 2010 had failed to address the legal rights between a child and the non-biological parent in same-sex unions, while changes to adoption law in 2010 had continued to exclude same-sex couples from adoption. Once the government committed to holding a constitutional referendum to allow for same-sex marriage, legislation was required to address parentage and guardianship rights with respect to children in families of same-sex married parents.

2 The expectations created by government pronouncements are that surrogacy will be legalized in tandem with a ban on commercial surrogacy; the creation of embryos for research will be banned, although embryos may be donated for research including embryo stem-cell research; and preimplantation diagnosis will also be regulated to allow for sex-selection where there is a risk of serious genetic disease (Department of Health 2015).

References

Bock von Wülfingen, Bettina. 2012. "The Fruit of Love: The German IVF-Embryo Turning from Abject into Bio-Object." In *Bio-Objects: Life in the 21st Century*, edited by Nicki Vermeulen, Sakari Tamminen and Andrew Webster, 137–150. Farnham: Ashgate.

Canavan, John. 2011. "Family and Family Change in Ireland: An Overview." *Journal of Family Issues* 33 (1): 10–38.

Carolan, Mary. 2006. "Embryos Belong to Mother, Court Told." *Irish Times*, July 5.

Children and Relationships Act. 2015. Irish Statute Books. www.irishstatutebook.ie/ accessed October 8, 2015.

Commission on Assisted Human Reproduction. 2005. *Report of the Commission on Assisted Human Reproduction*. Dublin: CAHR.

Congregation of the Doctrine of the Faith. 2008. *Dignitas Personae*: *Instructions on Certain Bioethical Questions*. www.vatican.va/.../cfaith/documents/rc_con_cfaith_doc_20081208_dignitas-personae_en.html/ accessed April 4, 2012.

Department of Health. 2015. "Government to legislate for Assisted Human Reproduction & Associated Research." Press Release, http://health.gov.ie/blog/press-release/ accessed October 1, 2015.

Government of Ireland. 1998. *Strengthening Families for Life: Final Report of the Commission on the Family*. Dublin: Stationery Office.

Government of Ireland. 1999. *Green Paper on Abortion*. Dublin: Stationery Office.

Government of Ireland. 2006. *All-Party Oireachtas Committee on the Constitution: Tenth Progress Report.* Dublin: Stationery Office.

Hanafin, Patrick. 2001. *Constituting Identity: Political Identity Formation and the Constitution in Post-Independence Ireland.* Aldershot: Ashgate.

Irish Catholic Bishops' Conference. 2003. *Assisted Human Reproduction: Facts and Ethical Issues.* (Veritas Publications 2000). Accessed April 4, 2012. www.catholicbishops.ie/2008/02/07/assisted-human-reproduction/.

Irish Catholic Bishops' Conference. 2006. *Towards a Creative Response to Infertility: A Detailed Response of the Irish Catholics Bishops' Conference to the Report of the Commission on Assisted Human Reproduction.* Dublin: Veritas.

McDonnell, Orla, and Jill Allison. 2006. "From Biopolitics to Bioethics: Church, State, Medicine and Assisted Reproductive Technology in Ireland." *Sociology of Health and Illness* 28 (6): 817–837.

Medical Council. 1989. *A Guide to Professional Conduct and Ethics*, 3rd Edition. Medical Council: Dublin.

Medical Council. 1998. *Constitutions and Functions: A Guide to Professional Conduct and Ethics*, 5th Edition. Medical Council: Dublin.

Medical Council. 2004. *Constitutions and Functions: A Guide to Professional Conduct and Ethics*, 6th Edition. Medical Council: Dublin.

Medical Council. 2009. *Guide to Professional Conduct and Ethics for Registered Medical Practitioners*, 7th Edition. Medical Council: Dublin.

Metzler, Ingrid. 2012. "On Why States Still Matter: In Vitro Fertilization Embryos Between Laboratories and State Authorities in Italy." In *Bio-Objects: Life in the 21st Century*, edited by Niki Vermeulen, Sakari Tamminen and Andrew Webster, 151–170. Farnham: Ashgate.

M.R & Another v An tÁrd Chláraitheoir and Others (2013), IEHC 91 (Irish High Court 2013).

MR and DR and Others v An tÁrd Chláraitheoir and Others (2014), IESC 6 (Irish Supreme Court 2014).

Protection of Life during Pregnancy Act. 2013. Irish Statute Book. www.irishstatutebook.ie/accessed October 8, 2015.

Roche v Roche (2006), IEHC 359 (Irish High Court 2006).

Roche v Roche (2009), IESC 82 (Irish Supreme Court 2009).

12 Desiring Bodies

Problematizing the Matter of ARTs in Poland

Edyta Just

Introduction[1]

For more than 20 years there was inertia within the Polish political parties regarding assisted conception. It could be argued that the inability to set up a law that regulated ARTs at the national level was an outcome of intersecting political and religious factors and the power relations operating behind them. The Polish Catholic Church's reservations about ARTs apparently played a significant role in both the political and public aloofness toward technologically aided reproduction.

For a variety of reasons, the Vatican considers ARTs to be unethical (Congregation for the Doctrine of the Faith 1987, 2008). First of all, they are evaluated as immoral because they bypass the reciprocal encounter, disrupt the bodily connection and expression of love, and as such lead to dehumanization. Second, they are judged as unethical because of the possible donation of sperm and egg cells (the act of treachery occurring within marriage) and the treatment of embryos, which are not approached as human beings (e.g., freezing of embryos), as the Vatican considers them to be. The Polish Catholic Church shares the Vatican's position on ARTs. In countries such as Poland, where the Catholic Church is strong and Catholic doctrine is recognized as important, the Catholic Church itself, along with the practices it recommends, cannot be easily disregarded. By saying this, I am not trying to argue that the strong position of the Polish Catholic Church and its negative assessment of ARTs were the only reasons for the absence of a law concerning ARTs. Yet, even if it was not solely the position of the Polish Church and its doctrine that prevented politicians from proposing and passing ART legislation, still the Church's negative assessment of ARTs could not have been easily bypassed or ignored by Polish politicians.

The breakthrough came about only in 2015, in a year of presidential and parliamentary elections, when the ruling party Civil Platform (*Platforma Obywatelska, PO*) proposed ART legislation known as *Ustawa o Leczeniu Niepłodności* [*The Act on Infertility Treatment*] (Sejm Polski 2015) and then pushed it through both the lower and upper houses of the Polish Parliament. In July 2015, President Bronisław Komorowski signed the Act. However, his decision and the Act itself have been heavily criticized by the Polish Catholic

Church and right-wing politicians from the Law and Justice Party (*Prawo i Sprawiedliwość, PiS*), who are very outspoken about their affinity with the Church. The Act should have come into force three months after it was signed. Yet, *PiS* announced that, once successful in the parliamentary elections, it will immediately block the recently signed Act.

In this chapter, I briefly discuss the inertia around ART legislation in Poland. This discussion is intended to highlight the entanglements between policymaking and religion and the influence the latter may have on the former. By doing so, the text remains in close affinity with those by Perrotta, McDonnell and Mehrabi (this volume), contributing to an understanding of the complex interactions between religion and state policies. Moreover, recognizing the necessity of having ARTs regulated at the national level, I discuss the ways in which ARTs were practiced in Poland and also highlight the problems entailed by the absence of ART legislation. This particular discussion emphasizes the need to introduce national-level legal regulations and is partially based on in-depth, semi-structured and qualitative interviews, which I conducted in 2005 in my mother tongue Polish with Polish doctors and 13 heterosexual Polish couples who had successfully participated in assisted reproduction. Furthermore, I briefly present the content of the Act on Infertility Treatment signed in July 2015. Finally, I argue against one of the Catholic Church's objections to ARTs (i.e., assisted reproduction qualifies as an unethical procedure because conception does not follow a reciprocal encounter) and contend that it is possible to assert bodily connections, expressions of love and lack of dehumanization even when conception is technologically enhanced. In order to argue in favor of ARTs, I refer to the empirical material, the in-depth interviews conducted with the heterosexual Polish couples, and the philosophical concepts of Gilles Deleuze and Félix Guattari (1987, 1994).

ARTs and the Polish Political Agenda

It can be argued that the Catholic Church's ARTs veto significantly weakened politicians' aspirations to enact ART legislation for many years. In 2004, the former Commissioner for Equal Status of Women and Men, Izabela Jaruga-Nowacka, stressed that the Polish Catholic Church's attitude toward assisted reproduction was responsible for the political restraint around ARTs (Tomczak 2004). Interestingly, when broadcasting official statements, members of the liberal and leftist parties never described Catholic doctrine as influential in their decision-making processes. However, as Jaruga-Nowacka made clear, the Polish Church's position and its message could not be easily overlooked or disregarded. In this sense, I shall contend that the Vatican's dismissal of ARTs, as transmitted by the Polish Catholic Church, became binding for many politicians.

In 2005, the probability that assisted reproduction would eventually be seriously debated became even more minuscule. In that year, the parliamentary elections were won by the very conservative and ultra-Catholic parties, for whom obeying Catholic rules and objectives was mandatory. Then, in 2007, the liberals came to power. However, they were equally unwilling to commence a constructive and conclusive debate about ARTs. Some efforts at regulation were undertaken, but the discussions that were initiated lacked solidity and resulted in no concrete resolutions.

The situation changed slightly at the end of 2008 when a proposal for a new law concerning ARTs, known as *Ustawa o Ochronie Genomu Ludzkiego i Embrionu Ludzkiego oraz Polskiej Radzie Bioetycznej i Zmianie Innych Ustaw* [*The Act Regarding the Protection of Human Genome and Embryo, Polish Bioethical Council and Changes to Other Acts*] (Sejm Polski 2008), was presented by the liberals. They hoped that with the introduction of this law Poland would finally meet EU requirements and ratify the Bioethics Convention of the European Council.[2] The content of the law was prepared by the Team for Bioethics, consisting of lawyers, doctors, biologists, philosophers, and ethicists, led by Jarosław Gowin from *PO*. The proposed law was very restrictive and exclusive, e.g., only couples who are married, heterosexual, diagnosed as infertile, and without major illnesses (undefined by the law) can participate in assisted reproduction; egg and sperm donation and sperm banks are forbidden; only one embryo can be produced and if two embryos are formed both of them must be transferred; embryos cannot be cryopreserved (frozen) unless there are medical contraindications or a woman for any reason decides against the transfer.

This proposal resulted in intense debates not only within political circles, but also in society at large. Parties such as Left Democratic Alignment (*Sojusz Lewicy Demokratycznej, SLD*) and New Left from the Parliamentary Team for Population and Development (*Nowa Lewica z Parlamentarnego Zespołu na rzecz Populacji i Rozwoju, SdPl*), and also members of *PO* considered it too restrictive. Politicians from *SLD* emphasized that they would never support such a restrictive and abusive law. The representatives from *SdPl* sent an official objection to the Gowin Team's Bill. There was also opposition to the Bill from *PiS*, but they argued that it was not restrictive enough (Gazeta.pl 2009). Twenty-three deputies belonging to *PiS* announced their determination to propose a law entirely forbidding ARTs in Poland.

Even though the proposed law was very restrictive and perhaps could have been accepted by the Polish Catholic Church (precisely because of its restrictive nature), it still allowed the practice of ARTs, which according to Vatican documents such as "Donum Vitae" (Congregation for the Doctrine of the Faith 1987) and "Dignitas Personae" (Congregation for the Doctrine of the Faith 2008) should be forbidden. The heated discussions lasted for the first three months of 2009. Then suddenly, at the beginning of April 2009, *PO* decided not to commence the parliamentary debate on its proposal. As a result, no resolutions were passed. The former Health Minister, Marek Balicki (*SdPl*), emphasized that *PO* did not want to have a transparent standpoint with regard to ARTs and was troubled by the eventual reaction of the Polish Catholic Church. He suggested that, from the beginning, the *PO* efforts to regulate ARTs were elements of its public relations strategy (*Interia.pl* 2009). It can thus be argued that for *PO* it was better to drop the whole issue instead of either implementing or changing the content of the proposed law. The implementation of the law could have possibly resulted in a decrease in public support for *PO*. By the beginning of 2009, opposition to the Bill from those who wanted a more liberal law was increasing within the public sphere. The official public protest against the debated law was sent to the Prime Minister, Donald Tusk (*PO*),[3] and supported by various non-governmental organizations.[4] Importantly, a survey of public opinion carried out in March 2009 showed that 77 percent of Poles accepted IVF for married couples, 53 percent also for unmarried couples and 51 percent for single women. Yet, 46 percent considered adoption to be a better way of "getting" a child than IVF, while 36 percent chose IVF. Interestingly, 52 percent accepted the production and cryopreservation of embryos (Gazeta Wyborcza 2009a). Yet, modification of the Bill's content would have probably triggered a critique by the Polish Church. Silence fell once more over the whole subject of assisted reproduction.

The situation changed again in 2013 with the introduction of the governmental program known as *Program Leczenia Niepłodności Metodą Zapłodnienia Pozaustrojowego na lata 2013–2016* [*IVF Treatment for Infertility for 2013–2016*] (In Vitro 2013). However, this program regulated the application of ARTs only for medical centers and couples selected to participate in it. Back then, the Polish Prime Minister, Donald Tusk (*PO*), stated that the political climate did not allow a constructive discussion or the passing of ART legislation at the national level (Kazimierczuk 2013).

With this brief overview of the long-standing inertia regarding ART legislation in Poland, I have striven to highlight the interconnection of policymaking and religion and the impact of the latter on the former. Although I am not claiming that the Polish Catholic Church should be held solely responsible for this inertia, there is a credible argument that it played a significant role in political inaction toward regulating ARTs at the national level. Given the influence that religion may have on policymaking, it would be interesting to research and reflect upon the reasons why *PO*, after many years of political apathy, finally managed to introduce ART legislation in Poland. Although time needs to pass before we can assess the practices this law may engender, it seems that its content cannot be evaluated as utterly restrictive. Yet, importantly, given the entanglements between religion and policymaking, it is also important to observe the future of this law in conjunction with the outcomes of future parliamentary elections in Poland.

The Practice of ARTs in Poland

The first Polish IVF child was born at Białystok Medical Academy in 1987. Since then many medical centers have offered ARTs, even though legal arrangements to regulate their application did not exist. The only exception was the above-mentioned governmental program introduced in 2013, regulating the practice of ARTs for those selected to participate in it.

For more than 20 years, it was difficult to precisely estimate the total number of clinics that offered ARTs. Furthermore, clinics were not obliged to present their statistics and, even if they did report them, the given numbers could not be easily verified for credibility. Therefore, it remained a substantial challenge to gather information about the clinics' location and the quality of the medical procedures offered there. People who opted for ARTs must have expended a great deal of energy to find clinics and choose the most appropriate one. Even after a clinic was finally selected, prospective parents could not be really sure whether the assistance offered there was of good quality or not. In this sense, it can be said that the application of ARTs in Poland undeniably lacked transparency. Furthermore, the Polish appliance of assisted reproduction was regulated only by the internal directives of individual medical centers. Those directives were conditioned by the economic situation of the clinic, certain cultural beliefs and ideologies, and also by doctors' approaches and viewpoints with regard to reproductive issues. This indicates that the ways in which prospective parents were admitted and procedures conducted might have varied significantly between medical centers. Usually, only heterosexual couples were accepted for ARTs. Single women, along with lesbian and gay couples, were not considered eligible. It was up to a clinic to suggest how the treatment would proceed, e.g., in making a choice between intracytoplasmic sperm injection (ICSI) and IVF. Since ICSI was said to be more efficient, and since ARTs were not funded through the public budget, prospective parents who were given a choice usually favored ICSI. Clinics also made decisions concerning the number of transferred embryos. The general practice was to transfer two embryos or, if a woman was more than 35 years old, three. Moreover, since the practice of ARTs was only regulated by the medical centers' internal directives, it was up to clinics to supply their patients with enough information and psychological support. However, due to financial reasons and the fact that doctors worked in several different medical institutions, prospective patients could not always count on having the opportunity to discuss their case, clarify ambiguities or express worries whenever they felt the need to do so.

Undoubtedly, the governmental program represented a crucial change in the management of ARTs in Poland. Even though this program regulated the practice of ARTs solely for the medical centers and couples who participated in it, important improvements could still be observed. First of all, the medical centers selected for the program were obliged to meet the set quality standards with regard to both equipment and personnel. Second, the program envisioned the foundation of a registry containing all the important data concerning ART treatments in the clinics which took part. Those clinics had to report the results of the treatments they conducted to the registry as well as to the European Society for Human Reproduction and Embryology (ESHRE). Alongside the registry, there was also a Program Board responsible for the monitoring, assessment, improvement, and development of the program. In this sense, it can be said that the governmental program tried to safeguard the quality, but also the transparency, of the practice of ARTs. In terms of other regulations, access was granted only to heterosexual couples medically diagnosed as infertile,[5] although a given couple did not have to be married. A female participant could not be older than 40 at the time she was admitted to the program. If for a given couple no ova or spermatozoids could be obtained, no ova were produced, recurrent miscarriages occurred, or the uterus was severely damaged or did not exist then the couple could be excluded from or not accepted onto the program. Sperm banks or the possibility of obtaining genetic material from third parties were not addressed or discussed. Every couple who participated in the program was entitled to three cycles.[6] Importantly, the program ensured that ovarian stimulation was adapted to a female patient's needs and it regulated procedures linked to this stimulation and the retrieval of egg cells in a detailed manner. With regard to the methods of fertilization, both IVF and ICSI could be implemented. The latter could only be applied under certain conditions such as endometriosis, idiopathic infertility, male infertility, or unsuccessful fertilization after the implementation of classic IVF. Women under 35 could have six egg cells fertilized. However, if the fertilization was unsuccessful twice or if a woman was older than 35 then all the retrieved egg cells could be inseminated. However, it was recommended that only one embryo be transferred unless it was medically justifiable or if a woman was over 35, when two embryos could be transferred. If, for any reason, embryos could not be transferred, they were cryopreserved. The cryopreserved embryos could not be destroyed but had to be stored until they could be transferred. If the transfer resulted in pregnancy, the couples were obliged to report to the clinic in which IVF had been conducted any complications during the pregnancy, and also the health of the born child and especially any developmental and/or genetic defects.

Although some of the practices that the program engendered might be deemed problematic (e.g., access only for heterosexual couples; lack of ova/sperm donation), it nevertheless ensured the quality and transparency of the ART practices and seemingly took women's interests and well-being into consideration (e.g., regulations regarding egg cell stimulation/retrieval; the transfer and cryopreservation of embryos). However, as mentioned above, the program only regulated ARTs for the clinics and couples who participated in it. Given the impact of the absence of ART legislation on participants, the positive changes introduced by the program (e.g., quality standards, transparency), and that many of those desiring a child fell outside of the program's parameters, the introduction of sensible ART legislation became essential. As mentioned above, it is still too early to evaluate the practices that this law, The Act on Infertility Treatment signed in July 2015, may stimulate, but I must emphasize that this Act is not very restrictive.

Like the governmental program, this Act sets quality standards for equipment and the training of personnel. Only medical centers that can meet all the quality requirements will be able to offer ARTs. The Act also authorizes the existence of ova/sperm/embryo banks. Up to six egg cells can be fertilized or, if the woman is more than 35 years old or her health condition indicates the need, a higher number can be fertilized. Up to two embryos can be transferred and all the non-transferred embryos will be cryopreserved (Newsweek 2015). Importantly, these embryos can be given for adoption. The Act, however, embodies the governmental program's resolution that only heterosexual couples may take advantage of ARTs. Although the fact that unmarried couples may be admitted is important, single women and homosexual couples are still not considered eligible. Furthermore, the Act does not discuss the funding of ARTs from the public budget, which may severely affect those striving for technologically assisted reproduction. There is also some anxiety that the financial support secured by the current governmental program will cease to exist if the parliamentary elections are won by the right-wing party (Steinhagen 2015).

ARTs Becoming Ethical

The Vatican and the Polish Catholic Church have issued many objections to ARTs. Given the limited length of this chapter, I will argue against just one of the objections voiced.

The Vatican's "Donum Vitae: Instruction on Respect for Human Life in its Origin and on the Dignity of Procreation Replies to Certain Questions of the Day," (Congregation for the Doctrine of the Faith 1987) presents the comprehensive position of the Catholic Church on assisted reproduction. According to this document, human conception should result from the reciprocal encounter. This is because the reciprocal encounter allows for the connection of bodies and the expression of love (spirit) while those bodies are connected. As technologically enhanced reproduction deprives prospective parents of the reciprocal encounter, the bodies cannot truly connect. Due to the fact that the connection between bodies is lost and love (spirit) cannot be expressed, the body becomes reduced to its pure physiology: tissues, organs, and cells. The body is reduced and thus objectified and dehumanized. Consequently, the human subject no longer represents a unity. It undergoes a split between the body and the spirit, which results in the objectification and dehumanization of the subject. As such, the human subject is faced with the loss of its dignity.

In my argument, I go beyond Cartesian dualism, which resonates with the discourses of the Church. Instead, I shall refer to the ontology of the human body/subject as proposed by French philosophers Gilles Deleuze and Félix Guattari. According to Deleuze and Guattari (1987, 1994), human subjectivity is embodied and the body is desire driven; it constantly forms linkages and connections with its surroundings, it becomes productively affected and undergoes various becomings, changes, and deterritorializations.[7] I read my empirical data, the interviews with 13 heterosexual Polish couples, with the philosophy of Deleuze and Guattari as my lens. Shifting the ontological perspectives in this way, I argue that, contrary to the viewpoint of the Vatican, bodily connections and expressions of love can take place when conception is technologically enhanced. In ART processes, the prospective parents' bodies cannot remain indifferent toward each other.

For example, when embryo transfer was discussed by my informants, the woman was usually accompanied by her male partner, and the transfer took place while the partner was present so that the couple was in a way "in it" together, even though of course it was the woman whose body was acted upon. By focusing on Ali's story, I shall illustrate how, seen through the lens of Deleuzian and Guattarian philosophy, the transfer process can be seen as a shared process of becoming.

While undergoing embryo transfer, Ali and her partner, both driven by the desire to have a child, were immersed in affects of trust, belief, and love. The doctor came in with a catheter. The procedure started. Ali became the pure affect of hope and happiness. Her partner was seeing-hearing what Ali was experiencing. The partners held hands in indivisible entanglement.

Those moments of acute perception, of seeing-hearing and of holding, were moments of commenced connections that left "no-body" unchanged and unaffected. Those were the moments of becoming deterritorialized. The partners were becoming each other and they were being affected. They were becoming "her partner," "his partner," "warmth," "smile," "her hand," "her-partner-squeezed-hand-body," "his-looking-eyes," "his-warm-comforting-voice-body," "her-squeeze," "his hand" and "his-squeezed-hand-body"; affects of love, hope, happiness, compassion, and empathy that supported Ali as she underwent the procedure and allowed her partner to become constructive and intensively engaged in the assisted conception.

When seen from the perspective of Deleuzian–Guattarian ontology, the prospective parents' bodies do not remain separate and indifferent toward each other during the procedure of assisted reproduction. Interpreted in this context, my informants' stories demonstrated desires in motion and constant connections. They told about many becomings and deterritorializations launched by the technology and the doctors. They spoke of becoming one another, each other's eyes, lips and smiles. Becoming each other's warmth, squeezes, hugs, embraces, hands, audibly comforting voices, and billions of affects of love, empathy, hope, gratitude, expectation or happiness.

In the Deleuzian and Guattarian framework, the desiring bodies connect, become affected and connect again, endlessly. The becomings and deterritorializations, which vary in intensity and speed, occur ceaselessly. The bodies connect with everything that occupies their territories and so they also connect with each other enjoying their own singular deterritorializations. There is not a single moment when the bodies do not connect. To see, to hear, to taste, to smell, and to touch is to connect. To see a smile, tears, pain, sadness, or happiness; to hear somebody's voice, shouts, complaints, grief, or euphoria; to taste somebody's lips, to feel somebody's hug or squeeze means to connect. The bodies not only connect but in fact become each other. One body when seen, heard, or touched enters the spaces of the other's body. There is a specific deterritorialization of the body when it becomes the other body's eyes, hands, tears, smiles or hugs. Thus, from this ontological position, the Vatican's statement that the connections between the prospective parents' bodies are lost when ARTs and couples interact is contradicted. When the human body is conceptualized as becoming deterritorialized/affected, but also sensing, perceiving, psychic and emotional (Deleuze and Guattari 1987, 1994; Grosz 1994; Braidotti 2002), it is possible to say that whenever there is contact between bodies, they do connect, become, and become affected immediately, responding by turning into love, happiness, horror, empathy, sadness, regret or hope. If bodies do connect in this passionate and intense way, no reduction or split occurs, and it seems possible to argue against the Vatican, emphasizing that no objectification or dehumanization takes place and that the human being does not lose its dignity through the use of ARTs.

To recognize the peculiarities of the bodies involved is also to suggest that to a certain extent those are the elements intrinsic to both ARTs and the doctors due to whom the prospective parents' bodies start to connect, become each other, and are affected. In this sense, I want to risk suggesting that ARTs neither result in a lack of connections between the prospective parents' bodies nor prevent love from being expressed; by contrast, ARTs create, support, and fuel connections. Furthermore, ARTs can be conceptualized as stimulators of the prospective parents' bodily connections, which can result in a very creative and affirmative "experience" of life by the couples participating in assisted reproduction. It seems that, instead of blaming ARTs for the disruption of linkages between bodies, they should be seen as amplifiers of those connections. Indeed, when ARTs are employed, the bodies not only connect, but in fact engage more organs in order to do so. Isn't it comforting to realize that one has more organs with which to connect and express love than only a vagina and a penis? Isn't it good to know that when ARTs are involved, the connections are still there, the love is still there, the pleasure is still there, the vagina and penis can have some rest, and yet reproduction still occurs?

Furthermore, to comprehend that desires which "adore" connections govern human subjects is to conclude that nothing can stop "one-body" from creating "shared-spaces," making alliances and reaching out to another body (i.e., the bodies team up with each other and care for each other when going through ARTs, pregnancy and the postpartum period). To recognize the peculiarities of these bodies is to problematize the Vatican's conclusion regarding bodies and the human subject when faced with assisted reproductive technologies. To recognize the abilities/peculiarities of these human bodies is also to be able to propose a different, more positive, ethical assessment of ARTs than the one articulated by the Vatican.

Conclusion

The absence of a legal framework concerning ARTs may possibly jeopardize the well-being of those who wish for a child. Therefore, at least in my opinion, the appliance of ARTs should be accompanied by laws and regulations. There is no law that is ideal, and the Polish Act of 2015 certainly is not. Yet, after more than 20 years, Poland has finally introduced ART regulations at the national level. Importantly, the new law aims to secure the quality and transparency of the practice of ARTs, but it also includes directives concerning donation, fertilization, and embryo transfer and treatment. It is still too early to reasonably assess this new law, but the political apathy and inertia concerning assisted reproductive technologies seem to be over. The law is about to take effect. However, the outcomes of the parliamentary elections in 2015 may change the situation for ARTs in Poland yet again. The Polish Catholic Church does not accept technologically assisted reproduction and neither does the right wing. The entanglements between policymaking and religion are very tangible in Poland. The future of ART legislation and practice remains an open question. Since religion may have an impact on policymaking, and since sensible ART legislation is essential, I have endeavored to problematize the moral standpoint of the Vatican by launching a stream of ethical arguments, based on the philosophy of Deleuze and Guattari. I have proposed a different take on the embodied human subject when immersed in ART procedures. This different sensibility and ontology has led me to altered ethical deliberations and evaluations of ARTs. Yet, as I have just noted, the future of ART legislation and practice remains an open question in Poland.

Notes

1 This chapter is partially based on my PhD Dissertation (Just 2008).
2 The Bioethics Convention of the European Council demands ARTs to be regulated by a law in all EU countries.
3 Donald Tusk was the Polish Prime Minister from November 16, 2007 until September 22, 2014.
4 Thirty-two non-governmental organizations supported the public protest, among them: Federacja na rzecz Kobiet i Planowania Rodziny, Wanda Nowicka (Federation for Women and Family Planning), Stowarzyszenie na rzecz Leczenia Niepłodności i Wspierania Adopcji "Nasz Bocian," Blanka Żukowska, Barbara Szczerba, Michał Damski (Association for the Support of Infertility and Adoption "Our Stork") and Fundacja Centrum Praw Kobiet, Urszula Nowakowska (Women's Rights Center Foundation) (Gazeta Wyborcza 2009b).
5 The program defined the "health impairments" recognized as causes of infertility in detail.
6 One cycle includes hormonal stimulation, retrieval of egg cells, fertilization, and embryo transfer.
7 "Affect is the change or variation that occurs when bodies collide, or come into contact. As a body, affect is the knowable product of an encounter…" (Colman 2005, 11); Becoming is conceptualized in the following way:

> Becoming is neither an imitation nor an experienced sympathy, nor even an imaginary identification. It is not resemblance. Rather becoming is an extreme contiguity within coupling of two sensations without resemblance or, on the contrary in the distance of a light that captures both of them in a single reflection.… It is the zone of indetermination, of indiscernibility, as if things, beasts and persons … endlessly reach that point that immediately precedes their natural differentiation.
>
> (Deleuze and Guattari 1994, 173)

References

Braidotti, Rosi. 2002. *Metamorphoses: Towards a Materialist Theory of Becoming*. Cambridge: Polity Press.

Colman, Felicity J. 2005. "Affect." In *The Deleuze Dictionary*, edited by Adrian. Parr, 11–13. Edinburgh, Edinburgh University Press.

Congregation for the Doctrine of the Faith. 1987. "Donum Vitae: Instruction on Respect for Human Life in its Origin and on the Dignity of Procreation Replies to Certain Questions of the Day," February 22. Accessed November 12, 2015. www.vatican.va/roman_curia/congregations/cfaith/documents/rc_con_cfaith_doc_19870222_respect-for-human-life_en.html.

Congregation for the Doctrine of the Faith. 2008. "Instruction *Dignitas Personae*: On Certain Bioethical Questions," September 8. Accessed November 12, 2015. www.vatican.va/roman_curia/congregations/cfaith/documents/rc_con_cfaith_doc_20081208_dignitas-personae_en.html.

Deleuze, Gilles, and Félix Guattari. 1987. *A Thousand Plateaus, Capitalism and Schizophrenia*. London, New York: Continuum.

Deleuze, Gilles, and Félix Guattari. 1994. *What is Philosophy?* New York: Columbia University Press.

Gazeta.pl. 2009. "PiS Chce Zakazac In Vitro" [PiS Wants to Forbid IVF]. *Gazeta.pl*, April 22. Accessed November 12, 2015. http://wiadomosci.gazeta.pl/Wiadomosci/1,80271,6525146,PiS_chce_zakazac_in_vitro__PO__To_element_kampanii.html?utm_source=Nlt&utm_medium=Nlt&utm_campaign=856991.

Gazeta Wyborcza. 2009a. "Polacy Za In Vitro" [Poles for In Vitro]. *Gazeta Wyborcza*, March 6. Accessed November 12, 2015. http://wyborcza.pl/1,75478,6354394,Polacy_za_in_vitro.html.

Gazeta Wyborcza. 2009b. "Protest w Sprawie 'Ustawy Gowina'" [Protest against "Gowin's Act"]. *Gazeta Wyborcza*, January 5. Accessed November 12, 2015. http://wyborcza.pl/1,75478,6119901,Protest_w_sprawie__ustawy_Gowina_.html.

Grosz, Elisabeth. 1994. *Volatile Bodies: Toward a Corporeal Feminism*. Bloomington, Indianapolis: Indiana University Press.

In Vitro. 2013. "Program Leczenia Niepłodności Metodą Zapłodnienia Pozaustrojowego na lata 2013–2016" [IVF Treatment for Infertility for 2013–2016]. Accessed November 12, 2015. www.invitro.gov.pl.

Interia.pl. 2009. "PO nie zgłosi projektu ustawy w sprawie in vitro" [PO Will Not Report the Act on IVF]. *Interia.pl*, March 18. Accessed November 12, 2015. http://fakty.interia.pl/polska/news/po-nie-zglosi-projektu-ustawy-w-sprawie-in-vitro,1277020.

Just, Edyta M. 2008. "New Reproductive Assemblages: Understanding, Managing and 'Using' Human In Vitro Fertilization (IVF)." PhD diss., Utrecht University.

Kazimierczuk, Agnieszka. 2013. "Premier: Zwłoka ws. Ustawy o In Vitro – Przemyślana" [The Prime Minister: A Delay of the In Vitro Act – Deliberate]. *Rzeczpospolita*, September 26. Accessed November 12, 2015. www.rp.pl/artykul/1051818.html.

Newsweek. 2015. "8 Rzeczy, Które Powinieneś Wiedzieć o Najbardziej Kontrowersyjnej Ustawie Ostatnich Lat" [Eight Things You Should Know about the Most Controversial Act of Recent Years]. *Newsweek*, June 23. Accessed November 12, 2015. http://nauka.newsweek.pl/ustawa-o-in-vitro-co-powinienes-wiedziec-o-ustawie-o-in-vitro-,artykuly,367288,1.html.

Sejm Polski [The Lower House of the Polish Parliament]. 2008. "Ustawa o Ochronie Genomu Ludzkiego i Embrionu Ludzkiego oraz Polskiej Radzie Bioetycznej i Zmianie

Innych Ustaw" [The Act Regarding the Protection of the Human Genome and the Embryo, Polish Bioethical Council and Changes to Other Acts], December 17. Accessed November 12, 2015. http://orka.sejm.gov.pl/Druki7ka.nsf/0/AE4E777E0FBE7940C1257B170039FF7B/$File/1107.pdf.

Sejm Polski. 2015. "Ustawa o Leczeniu Niepłodności" [The Act on Infertility Treatment], June 25. Accessed November 12, 2015. http://orka.sejm.gov.pl/proc7.nsf/ustawy/608_u.htm.

Steinhagen, Dorota, es, groh, kawi. 2015. "In vitro Wchodzi w Życie. Kliniki Leczenia Niepłodności Obawiają się Rządów PiS" [The Act on IVF Comes into Force: Infertility Clinics Fear PiS]. *Gazeta Wyborcza*, June 23. Accessed November 12, 2015. http://wyborcza.pl/1,75478,18407830,in-vitro-wchodzi-w-zycie-kliniki-leczenia-nieplodnosci-obawiaja.html.

Tomczak, Janusz. 2004. "Marzenie o Wlasnym Dziecku" [A Dream of One's Own Child]. *Onet.wiadomości*, March 31. Accessed October 12, 2014. http://kiosk.onet.pl/1156765,1,3,241,druk.html.

13 Germany Goes PGD

The Appeal to Women's and Human Rights Discourse in the Paradigmatic Amendment to the German Embryo Protection Act

Bettina Bock von Wülfingen

Introduction

In January 2009, great media attention was given to the birth of a child at the hospital of the University College of London. Through the use of preimplantation genetic diagnosis (PGD), this child had been picked out from 11 sibling embryos, on the basis that it did not carry the so-called breast cancer gene BRCA1, which often occurred in this family. The diagnosis of this gene is highly disputed due to its merely statistical probability of causing the disease. At that moment, such a selection amongst embryos was impossible in Germany, as *any* manipulation of the embryo was prohibited – until recently. However, as has also been internationally reported, on July 7, 2011 the German Parliament decided to allow PGD in specific cases of severe illnesses genetically detectable in the embryo. Whether this decision signifies a big change for German biopolitics, particularly ARTs, is contested.[1] In any case, manipulation and selection of the embryo is no longer *categorically* excluded. This chapter discusses the broader context of ARTs in Germany and how this new position on PGD is accommodated in the humanist values that have traditionally dominated the ART debate in Germany. It is based on a review study, analyzing past and recent publications by medical representatives, Parliament, and the relevant ministries as well as feminist literature on ARTs in Germany. Additionally, the section on "The recent acceptance of PGD" draws on my previous dissertation study (Bock von Wülfingen 2007), a discourse analysis of hitherto unheard arguments in favor of the combination of biotechnology and ARTs in Germany appearing in public since the late 1990s.

The Embryo Protection Act (EPA) of 1990 bans any manipulation or use of an embryo for any aim other than its transfer into a woman's womb immediately after the stage of fertilization, and IVF itself is also very restricted. A recent amendment (2011) makes an exception for specific, restricted situations in which PGD may be used. There had been a lot of dispute in the Federal Republic of Germany ("West Germany," FRG) during the 1980s to this legal position. During these disputes, in the Bundestag (the German Parliament) feminist arguments joined with those of conservatives in a unanimously critical stance toward

ART methods. In addition, the German intellectual, so-called quality print media followed an agreement that questioning the EPA was perceived as breaking a taboo. In the early years after the millennium, an attempt was made to replace the EPA with a new Reproductive Medicine Law. Although it failed, it nevertheless helped to transform the perception of ARTs in Germany. In 2010 this change became obvious, culminating in the 2011 modification of the EPA. Against this backdrop, it is the aim of this chapter to compare ART discourses before and after 2000.

The first section details the regulation of ARTs in Germany since 1990. In the next section, I describe the specific German cultural and historical background that helps to explain the country's extremely cautious approach to ARTs, which is usually depicted as a consequence of the experience of National Socialism in Germany. This section includes the confrontation with reproductive realities, such as a significantly low birthrate, and pressure from different stakeholders since around the year 2000, who were interested in relaxing the strict regulations. The last section demonstrates that one of the major lines of thought helping to accommodate PGD into the restrictive legislation is the adaptation of the reproductive rights and self-determination discourse from the *in-vivo* to the in-vitro situation, discursively creating – in the German context – what I call an "in-vitro pregnancy."

Regulation of ARTs in Germany

ARTs were around in Germany, as in other countries, long before the advent of IVF and the birth of Louise Brown in 1978. After the period of National Socialism, and in line with a long-standing tradition of privileging the medical profession over, for example, midwifery, German legislation on issues of reproductive medicine concentrated more than that of other countries on the regulation of interference with the female reproductive body, to hinder any unregulated or unwanted sterilization, abortion, or insemination. Therefore, even a simple insemination can only be legally performed by a medical doctor. However, and this is often forgotten, contraceptives and abortion are also a form of ARTs (Clarke 1998; Hofmann 1999). In Germany, such anti-natal reproductive technologies frame the historical background to the discussion of the rights of the embryo as being in conflict with the rights of the woman (as becomes clearer below).

Abortion within the first three months of becoming pregnant was legalized in the German Democratic Republic ("East Germany," GDR) in 1950 on the basis of the "protection of the rights of women" and on medical and eugenic grounds; in 1972, the GDR legalized abortion generally within the first 12 weeks of gestation ("term solution"). By contrast, in the FRG abortion was generally illegal (according to §218 of the Penal Code) and an "indication solution" was enacted according to which, after 1976, exceptions could be made. After the "reunification" of East and West Germany in 1990, the overall German law was changed. Since 1995, abortion has been illegal, but without penalty if performed within the first trimester, although obliging women to attend a professional consultation ("consultation solution"), which in some regions can be difficult to obtain (Hahn 2000; Spieker 2001). Quite apart from its specific political history, Germany is divided into a more Catholic south and a more Protestant north, alongside the rather non-religious former GDR, and therefore it has for a long time been necessary in pragmatic politics to find a balance between those who argue for the liberty of women and society and those defending the life of the embryo as human life.

The relevant legal framework for ARTs and selective reproductive technologies, such as different forms of prenatal diagnosis (PND) and PGD, as well as the storing or cloning of human embryos, is threefold: Its regulation in Germany is mainly divided between the law (Constitutional Law, Criminal Law, and Administrative Law) and the medical "*ärztliche Standesrecht*" (physicians' professional regulations), expressed in the medical guidelines generated by the German Medical Association adapting law to practice. Additionally, social law regulates health insurance payments.

The Embryo Protection Act (EPA) very specifically targets the historically arisen need to accommodate IVF into this framework after its advent in common medical settings in the 1980s. In contrast to Criminal Law (the above-mentioned §218), the EPA does not protect the embryo in the *in-vivo* situation (from the moment of implantation on), but only in the in-vitro situation. Most important are §1, i.e., forbidding the fertilization of an egg cell with any aim other than that of transferring it to the womb of a woman; and §2, which forbids any use of an embryo other than its preservation or for aims other than pregnancy. Clause 8 defines an embryo as a fertilized egg cell with the capacity to develop from the moment of the fusion of the two nuclei on, which occurs after the fusion of egg cell and sperm in the newly formed embryo. Additional clauses prohibit the use of donated (heterologous) egg cells, and surrogate motherhood.

Even after the EPA was enacted, many questions still needed to be resolved, e.g., how could a medical practice make sure that, during IVF, no "extra" embryos were produced? The German Medical Association interpreted the law in such a way as to state in their guidelines that only as many embryos could be produced as would be transferred, resulting in the "rule of three" (Waller 2011): up to three embryos could be produced in one cycle and would all have to be transferred (Bundesärztekammer 2006), leading to the much-discussed rise in triple pregnancies and related early births in Germany (Labahn 2003). Today, it is becoming a more common practice to select upon optical appearance or polar body analysis (an analysis only including information from the fertilized egg cell before fusion of the nuclei, i.e., performed on the so-called pre-embryo) (Kentenich 2015). This has led to a situation of more and more pre-embryos being kept frozen in bio-banks.

It is also the responsibility of the German Medical Association to lay out guidelines regarding who is eligible to access IVF: in Germany, doctors are prevented from providing IVF or donor insemination to lesbians, singles, or queer families, not by law but by the guidelines that limit this service to heterosexual couples living in a long-term relationship. Therefore, only insiders know the names of medical doctors who also deal with lesbian couples.

The social welfare regulation plays a pivotal role in "normalizing" (or not) a medical technology: In Germany, until 2004 statutory health insurance fully covered up to four IVF cycles for couples diagnosed as infertile. However, the rearrangement of the German economy to a more flexible neoliberalism and the subsequent cuts in public spending, along with new prioritization, interfered with this situation, so that, since 2004, only 50 percent of the cost of three attempts is paid. This led to a drop of treatment numbers of about one-third.[2] However, less then ten years later and despite this regulation the treatment numbers were back to those in 2001.[3]

German Embryos in Culture

In order to better understand why Germany is so cautious about the introduction of ARTs and PGD, it is necessary to explain the categorical protection of the embryo, as well as the idea of the protection of the mother. The categorical protection of the embryo that reigned until the decision in favor of PGD in specific cases, and that still holds for most politicians in Parliament, embodies the ethical principle that any human embryo is per se endowed with human dignity. This approach sets no preconditions for its protection and does not therefore distinguish between embryos at different stages. As a result, all human embryos are viewed as equal to one another and to any other form of human life (clause 8 of the EPA).

The categorical EPA therefore contrasts strongly with a more utilitarian approach. In political debates on the EPA and new regulations for reproductive medicine, it was argued that weighing the suffering of adults against any other form of human being, be it only a structure of just one or several cells, did not work well: This kind of prioritizing clashed with the German memory of an oversteered rationalism and the relativized value of human life under Nazism. In this vein, then-president Johannes Rau argued that "the memory of it [eugenic experimentation in Nazi Germany] is a continuous appeal: nothing may be above the dignity of the individual human being" (Rau 2001). Apart from the protection of traditional concepts of the family, the feminist perspective on PGD, which saw it as "medicalizing" women, similar to any technique involving IVF (Augst 2001), was also mobilized to argue against PGD (ibid.).

It is not only the historical German experience with the Nazi regime that accounts for the less pragmatic and more cautious position of regulators in Germany toward ARTs. Jasanoff (2005) stresses that all countries are special in the way they deal with new technology. What counts is the traditional local ways of defining knowledge and risk. Thus the comparatively slow changes in the EPA can in part also be attributed to Germany's rather dogmatic approach to the regulation of knowledge and technology use in general (Jasanoff 2005). In her elaboration of what she calls "civic epistemologies," Jasanoff states: "modern techno-scientific cultures have developed tacit knowledge-ways, through which they assess the rationality and robustness of claims that seek to order their lives" (Jasanoff 2005, 255). According to her research on the regulation of ARTs in the years after 2000 in different countries, the case of the United States contrasts sharply with that of Germany: in the United States, where the state seldom interferes, industry, the sciences, activists, and patient groups negotiate with each other over what should be deemed knowledge – even, if necessary, in court.[4] The lack of intention and the increase in channels of public presentation through television and the internet corroborate the impression of objectivity. In Great Britain, on the other hand, the state plays a more important role. Here, experts generally tend to win public trust in their authority through long service to the common welfare. Similar to the United States, British culture is also oriented toward pragmatism and empiricism. In Germany, it is the state and its institutions that are viewed as essential to the authorization of knowledge. Regulation is mainly carried out through legislation. According to Jasanoff, the law in this case works as a barrier between the public sphere on the one hand and the state and expertise on the other. Thus, the public is only consulted until a situation worthy of a legal change is found. Thereafter, it is assumed that the whole terrain of reason will be sufficiently represented by the relevant (expert) committees. Expertise and objectivity are defined by one's affiliation to relevant institutions. In addition, Germany tends to allow new technologies to be tested in other, more pragmatic and adventurous countries before introducing them (Jasanoff 2005).

Additionally, and in part further explaining the above, the Kantian notion of the human as a being who cannot be sold or enslaved also plays a role in motivating the prohibition of surrogate motherhood and egg-cell donation (i.e., "protecting" women from "selling" their bodies (Augst 2001) as well as protecting traditional concepts of the family). On all these grounds, during the 1980s there was a consistent rejection of reproductive and (genetic) diagnostic technologies within the different strands of feminism.

Moreover, these positions were represented in Parliament during the debates leading up to the enactment of the Embryo Protection Act in 1990. The German Greens in Parliament highlighted the embedding of women within a (problematic) and patriarchal social context and the fear of eugenics. Following this line of argument, the propagation of new reproductive (and genetic) technologies, as well as concerns for infertile women, derived from a "reactionary family concept and both are eugenic projects at all times" (Augst 2001, 141). The critique even referred to global German politics: Opponents of ARTs stressed that the concerns for infertile women were due to a pronatalist stance and in sharp contrast to the population policy of the Federal Ministry for Economic Cooperation and Development in so-called developing countries. Following this discourse, IVF and prenatal diagnostic interventions were "not only hazardous for the users' self-esteem but also represent an attack on the physical integrity of all women" (Bündnis 90/Die Grünen 1990, 4). The politicians argued that women and their bodies were exploited, with contextual references to influential feminist activists such as Maria Mies, Gena Corea, and the international group FINRRAGE (Graumann 1999).

The Social Democratic Party (SPD), while being generally in agreement with the "Green standpoint," argued that IVF should only be allowed when a woman in a stable heterosexual relationship was a victim of accident or illness which led to her infertility.[5]

The debates on the legalization of embryonic stem-cell research around the year 2000 raised similar issues. In contrast to earlier debates, which placed research into genetic diagnosis and human embryos within a discursive framework of patriarchal exploitation, Green feminists were now turning to the problem of commercialization and power relations related to biological material. Meanwhile, a discourse of basic rights, once adopted from the feminist fight for abortion and now referring to a couple's rights to reproductive choice, had entered the debates in favor of PGD, as the following perspective on the time after 2000 will show.

The Recent Acceptance of PGD: Feminist Technology and the Equal Rights of the Parents

Germany not only holds a special position in terms of the restrictive regulation of ARTs, but also regarding its overall rates of reproduction, which in turn back arguments for state support of IVF. Twenty-one percent of German women aged 40–44 are childless, which is more than in any other European country (Statistisches Bundesamt 2009). After falling rates each year, in 2013 Germany's birthrate sank to 8.28 per 1,000 of the total population, the lowest in the world (HWWI 2015).

In the reunified Germany, the age of mothers giving birth has steadily been increasing, reaching 30.9 in 2014 (Statistisches Bundesamt 2015). Earlier interview studies have pinpointed individual reasons of a mostly economic and work-related nature for this trend: women postpone children until they have a more stable job situation with a higher income (Brähler and Ströbel-Richter 2002). Since 2007, the government has tackled the issue of low birthrates by introducing different measures that ultimately break with the model of the mother being the only "real" parent, paving the way for more equity within a parenting couple. Financial support for the parent who reduces paid work to care for their children during the first few months had previously been so low that only the partner with a lower income, in most cases the mother, would stay home (Gutschmidt 1997). In 2007, this financial support was changed in such a way that it became attractive for the, usually male, better earning member of the couple to step up to the parenting responsibilities. This, however, did not make much difference in the later care of the child: It is only recently, since August 2013, that every child from the first birthday on has had the right to daycare (BMFSJ 2015), allowing more parents to combine professional life and parenting and to share parenting more equally.

Meanwhile, alongside the overall rising age at first childbirth, the infertility rate also rose, and, linked to this, the number of women seeking infertility treatment (Kentenich 2015). In 2013, the 130 infertility treatment centers reported a total of 84,051 treatment cycles with 51,242 treated women (representing a continuous increase since 2005) (Deutsches IVF-Register 2014). This increase has, in turn, supported more pressure for a less restrictive ART policy.

The recent change in the law to allow PGD in specific cases, and the accompanying argumentation, is a case in point, highlighting the pressure for a liberalization of ART policies. But it also follows earlier (and still ongoing) (ibid.) attempts to replace the EPA with a general new law on reproductive medicine. Gerhard Schröder, who in 1998 was the new leader of the social-democratic government, aimed to develop Germany into a location for the biotech industry at the turn of the twenty-first century. This change in government policy was accompanied by recurring attempts by different professional organizations and individuals (among others, the pharmaceuticals industry, physicians, and researchers) to replace the Stem Cell Act and the Embryo Protection Act with less restrictive regulations (Deutscher Bundestag 2008a and 2008b). While the German media reflected the urge to view Germany as a location for biotechnologies in their articles, more liberal feminist positions also appeared. Between 1995 and 2003, the so-called quality press frequently invited experts, mostly from the United States and Great Britain, to share their visions of the future use of ARTs and comment on the more advanced applications in other countries (Bock von Wülfingen 2007, 2012). My analysis of these media texts, which in the overall discourse were still exceptional, found that laboratory technologies combining biotechnology and ARTs were presented as a "normal" method of fertilization that should in all cases replace today's still common "do-it-yourself conception" (Bock von Wülfingen, 2007).[6]

In 1999, the most prominent German feminist print magazine, EMMA, was the first journal to dedicate a couple of pages to the US chemist and popular scientific author Carl Djerassi. His article dealt with the supposedly imminent liberation of women by means of extracorporeal procreation and its coupling with genetic technologies (Djerassi 1999). Thus, some of the arguments put forward in public debates since the 1990s in favor of a less restrictive Embryo Protection Act have been reminiscent of Simone de Beauvoir, who argued that it was not the social conditions of reproduction that were mainly responsible for the "oppression" of women, but rather the biological linkage of reproduction to the female body (Hofmann 1999). Arguments from Shulamith Firestone's radical early work "The Dialectic of Sex" (1970) also showed up in popular biomedical articles demanding the liberation of women from their biology through ARTs. Alongside this discourse of "liberation from nature," further elements of the international movement for *reproductive rights* and the right to abortion also appeared (*Women's Voices* 1993; Schultz 1994): "Whether to freeze her egg cells at 30 and have them re-implanted at 40 would be a patient's own decision," suggested Hans van der Ven, a gynecologist from Bonn (cited in Lakotta 2001). This would shift the "power relations between man and woman" (Djerassi, cited in Thimm and Traufetter 2000). And, as the Italian gynecologist Antinori suggested, human cloning should be allowed, "[b]ecause for me, having children is a human right" (Antinori, cited in Keller 2002).[7] Obviously, the now commonplace "*Selbstbestimmungsrecht*" (the basic right to self-determination) was not at all prominent in pro-natal ART discourses before 2000, but instead has its roots in international struggles against sterilization campaigns, and in Germany in fights against the penalization of abortion, for example, around 1995 in the "*Mein Bauch gehört mir*" campaigns ("my womb is mine"). The popular slogan "pro-choice," which was used to promote freedom of choice in the US literature, mainly in the context of defending the right to abortion, had also entered the discourse.[8]

Thus, in the years around 2000 new discursive traits on ARTs entered Germany, mainly from Great Britain and the United States, which had previously been taboo.

Despite all the discursive investment, the 105th Annual German Medical Conference (Deutscher Ärztetag) in 2002 decided against a change in the Embryo Protection Act and in favor of a prohibition on PGD (Bundesärztekammer 2011). According to the delegates, PGD had too little chance of medical success; additionally, its legalization could have severe societal effects (Schmidt 2003). Similarly, in 2003 the German Parliament voted against a change in the EPA, condemning the mere idea in parliamentary debates (Deutscher Bundestag 2003).

On July 6, 2010, however, the German Federal Court had to decide in the case of a gynecologist who, on various occasions in 2005 and 2006, had performed embryo selection at the request of couples who knew that at least one of the partners carried a disease that would severely affect the fetus or child. Although, according to earlier common sense, this was the illegal act of PGD, the German Federal Court now decided in favor of the physician. Additionally, it obliged the German Parliament to adapt the EPA to include PGD.

In June 2011, the German Medical Association, together with other medical and scientific organizations, voted in favor of a change in the law to enable PGD (Bundesärztekammer 2011), and finally, on July 7, 2011, the German Parliament also voted in favor of the legalization of PGD in very specific circumstances for those couples at risk of passing on severe illnesses to their child for which no therapy existed (Deutscher Bundestag 2011).[9]

The court and the German Medical Association argued that the legislators who drew up the EPA in 1990 had not foreseen such a technology as PGD, the ultimate aim of which was to achieve a pregnancy. The doctor thus had not breached Clause 2 of the EPA, which, as described above, forbids any use of an embryo other than its preservation and the establishment of a pregnancy. Additionally, a comparison with abortion played a fundamental role: Part of the argument in favor of PGD from the medical experts' side was the idea that the in-vitro situation of the embryo was to be handled in analogy to the termination of a pregnancy. In the latter case, the status of the *nasciturus* is balanced against the status of the mother; thus, the so-called conflict of interests between the pregnant woman and embryo in the case of abortion. As said before, termination of pregnancy is an issue dealt with by the Criminal Law.[10] It is "retrospectively not considered as a right of women to refuse the birth of an unwanted child, but as a situation comparable to the killing of somebody in an emergency situation when one's own life is in danger" (Krones and Richter 2004, 625). Therefore, until recently abortion was considered incomparable to PGD in the German context. However, this understanding has changed.

In the case of PGD, in 2011 the German Medical Association argued that, if we extended the constitutional protection of human dignity to the in-vitro embryo, we would have to weigh it against the constitutional rights of the involved *couple*. The latter, according to the dominant position in the juridical literature, was to be given higher priority (Bundesärztekammer 2011, 1453f.). Most recent German bioethical publications even suggest that prohibiting PGD would transgress the *constitutional rights of the parents* (Hufen 2010, 140ff.; Weschka 2010). The comparison, according to the current medical discourse, suggests itself as PGD would just prevent a "probational pregnancy" and chronologically forestall a conflict situation after PND (Woopen 1999; Hepp 2000; Loewenich 2008, 408ff.).

The interjection that a distinction had to be drawn between the more problematic situation of a physical relationship between a pregnant mother and the *in-vivo* embryo and the seemingly less problematic situation of (potential) parents of an in-vitro embryo (Graumann 2004) was turned down: The denial of a conflict in an intended but not yet initiated pregnancy was "not convincing and is rather seen as a formalism" (Nentwich 2011, 3).

The legal change in the 1990s regarding the regulation of abortion invites this new comparison with PGD: Prenatal diagnostics had already created a situation in which, in most cases of a "positive" finding, women invoke their right of "late abortion." According to the change to §218 in 1995, which is the paragraph on termination of pregnancy, it is not necessarily the medical condition of the child but the *psychological* condition of the *mother* in terms of her capacity regarding its upbringing that can be invoked for a non-penalized abortion after the twelfth week of gestation. Although not in the legal discourse, in the public realm, the term applied to a situation in which a child will have high caring needs is the "*Selbstbestimmungsrecht*" of the mother.

Conclusion

During the first decade of the twenty-first century, Germany's handling of reproductive issues changed considerably. We observe a shift from the mother as the "real" parent toward a stronger consideration of a (heterosexual) couple as the parenting entity, in both the realm of childcare, especially in the equal treatment of parents, and regarding PGD, where *both* parents together assume a new and stronger position vis-à-vis the embryo. The reference to equality and fundamental rights, such as the right to self-determination, has helped to incorporate PGD into the framework of humanist values that surrounds ARTs in Germany.

As already mentioned, the term "reproductive rights" in the current German PGD discourse has now been extended to *intending* parents with a high probability of passing on "genetic disorders" to their potential child, leading to what, under German conditions, we can call "in-vitro parenting." Obviously, the discourse of human rights as applicable to ARTs that was introduced into the German media discourse around 2000 is now established at the national regulatory level. During the past decade, the "freedom of reproductive choice," along with the right to self-determination and its extension from the mother to the couple, has traveled from struggles over anti-natal techniques to ARTs, and into the arguments of the German Federal Court and medical representatives.

Notes

1 Bettina Bock von Wülfingen, "Contested change: How Germany came to allow PGD" (forthcoming).
2 See the preamble to the Deutsches IVF-Register 2004–2008, e.g., Deutsches IVF-Register 2008.
3 Deutsches IVF-Register 2010.
4 Jasanoff calls this system "muddling through."
5 E.g., Herta Däubler-Gmelin in Augst 2001, 142.
6 From a selection of over 1,000 articles published between 1995 and 2003 that emerged from a database search using terms such as "human reproduction," "cloning," and "IVF," 35 articles – those which presented positive accounts of our future combined with genetic and reproductive technologies – underwent a micro analysis of discursive strands and metaphors.
7 See also Severino Antinori, in Trautfetter and Wüst 2001, 206.
8 See, e.g., Stock 2000, 190–2.
9 Draft by Flach and others in Waller 2011, 755.
10 Bundesverfassungsgericht, "Urteil vom 25.2.1975 (1 BvF 1,2, 3, 4 5, 6/74) zum Schwangerschaftsabbruch," BVerGe 39 (1975), 1–95; Bundesverfassungsgericht, "Urteil vom 28.5.1993 (2 BvF 2/90 und 4, 5/92) zum Schwangerschaftsabbruch," BVerGe 88 (1993), 203–366.

References

Augst, Charlotte. 2001. "Verantwortung für das Denken. Feministischer Umgang mit neuen Reproduktionstechnologien in Großbritannien und der Bundesrepublik." [Responsibility for Thought. Feminist Converse with New Reproduction technology in Great Britain and the GDR]. In *Jahrbuch für Kritische Medizin* (34): 135–156. Hamburg: Argument.

BMFSJ. 2015. "Gute Kinderbetreuung." [Good Childcare]. Online information, 9.9.2015, Bundesministerium für Familie, Senioren, Frauen und Jugend, Berlin. Accessed December 8, 2015. www.bmfsfj.de/BMFSFJ/Kinder-und-Jugend/kinderbetreuung.html.

Bock von Wülfingen, Bettina. 2007. *Genetisierung der Zeugung*. [*Genetisation of conception*]. Bielefeld: Transcript.

Bock von Wülfingen, Bettina. 2012. "The Fruit of Love: The German IVF-Embryo Turning from Abject into Bio-Object." In *Bio-objects: Life in the 21st Century*, edited by Niki Vermeulen, Sakari Tamminen and Andrew Webster, 137–150. Aldershot: Ashgate.

Bock von Wülfingen, Bettina. Forthcoming. "Contested Change: How Germany Came to Allow PGD."

Brähler, Elmar, and Yve Ströbel-Richter. 2002. "Familienfeindlicher Zeitgeist?" [An Anti-family Zeitgeist?]. *Reproduktionsmedizin* 18: 275–282.

Bundesärztekammer. 2006. "(Muster-)Richtlinien zur Durchführung der assistierten Reproduktion, Novelle 2006." [(Exemplar-) Directive for the Implementation of Assisted Reproduction, Novella 2006]. *Deutsches Ärzteblatt* 20: A 1392–1400.

Bundesärztekammer. 2011. "Memorandum zur Präimplantationsdiagnostik (PID)." [Memorandum for Preimplantation Diagnostics]. *Deutsches Ärzteblatt*, 31–32:B 1449–1456.

Bündnis 90/Die Grünen. 1990. *Entschließungsantrag der Fraktion Bündnis 90/Die Grünen. 19. Okt. 1990, Bundestagsdrucksache 11/8179.* [*Motion for a resolution of the Green Party Bündnis90/Die Grünen. October 19, 1990. Official Record 11/8179*]. Bonn: Deutscher Bundestag.

Clarke, Adele. 1998. *Disciplining Reproduction.* Berkeley, Los Angeles: University of California Press.

Deutscher Bundestag. 2003. *Drucksache 15, 15. Wahlperiode, 18.02.2003.* [*Official Record 15, 15th term of election, February 18, 2003*]. Berlin: Deutscher Bundestag.

Deutscher Bundestag. 2008a. *Entwurf eines Gesetzes zur Änderung des Stammzellgesetzes. BT-Drucksache 16/7981, 6.2.2008.* [*Draft Act amending the Stem Cell Act. Official Record 16/7981, February 6, 2008*]. Berlin: Deutscher Bundestag.

Deutscher Bundestag. 2008b. *Keine Änderung des Stichtages im Stammzellgesetz. Adulte Stammzellforschung fördern. BT-Drucksache 16/7985, 8.2.2008.* [*No changes for the record date for the Stem Cell Act. Support for adult stem-cell research. Official Record 16/7985, February 8, 2008*]. Berlin: Deutscher Bundestag.

Deutscher Bundestag. 2011. *Gesetzesentwurf. BT-Drucksache 17/5451, 12.4.2011.* [*Draft law. Official Record 17/5451, April 12, 2011*]. Berlin: Deutscher Bundestag.

Deutsches IVF-Register. 2008. *Jahrbuch 2007.* [*Yearbook 2007*]. Bad Segeberg: Ärztekammer Schleswig-Holstein.

Deutsches IVF-Register. 2010. *Jahrbuch 2009.* [*Yearbook 2009*]. Bad Segeberg: Ärztekammer Schleswig-Holstein.

Deutsches IVF-Register. 2014. *Jahrbuch 2013.* [*Yearbook 2013*]. Bad Segeberg: Ärztekammer Schleswig-Holstein.

Djerassi, Carl. 1999. "Der entmachtete Mann." [The Disempowered Man]. *EMMA*, no. 5.

Graumann, Sigrid. 1999. "Germ Line 'Therapy': Public Opinions with Regards to Eugenics." In *Genetics in Human Reproduction*, edited by Elisabeth Hildt and Sigrid Graumann, 175–184. Aldershot: Ashgate.

Graumann, Sigrid. 2004. "Präimplantationsdiagnostik, embryonale Stammzellforschung und das Regulativ der Menschenwürde." [Preimplantation Diagnostics, Embryonal Stem-cell Research and the Regulative of Human Dignity]. In *Biomedizin und Menschenwürde*, edited by Matthias Kettner, 122–44. Frankfurt am Main: Suhrkamp.

Gutschmidt, Gunhild. 1997. "Die Mütterfalle." [The Mother Trap]. *EMMA*, no. 1.

Hahn, Daphne. 2000. *Modernisierung und Biopolitik: Sterilisation und Schwangerschaftsabbruch in Deutschland nach 1945.* [*Modernization and Biopolitics: Sterilization and Termination of Pregnancy in Germany after 1945*]. Frankfurt am Main: Campus.

Hepp, Herrmann. 2000. "Präimplantationsdiagnostik – medizinische, ethische und rechtliche Aspekte." [Preimplantation Diagnostics – Medical, Ethical and Legal Aspects]. *Deutsches Ärzteblatt* 97: 1213–1221.

Hofmann, Heidi. 1999. *Die feministischen Diskurse über Reproduktionstechnologien.* [*The Feminist Discourses on Reproductive Technologies*]. Frankfurt am Main, New York: Campus.

Hufen, Friedhelm. 2010. "Individuelle Rechte und die Zulassung der Präimplantationsdiagnostik." [Individual Rights and the Admission of Preimplantation Diagnostics].

In *Recht und Ethik in der Präimplantationsdiagnostik*, edited by Carl F. Gethmann and Stefan Huster, 129–153. München: C. H. Beck.

HWWI. 2015. "Niedrigste Geburtenrate weltweit." [Lowest Birth Rate Worldwide]. Hamburg Institute of International Economics: Pressemitteilung May 29, 2015. Accessed December 8, 2015. www.hwwi.org/fileadmin/hwwi/Mediencenter/Pressemitteilungen/2015_Pressemitteilungen/2015–05–29-BDO/20150529_PM_IBC_Geburtenrate_HWWI.pdf.

Jasanoff, Sheila. 2005. *Designs on Nature. Science and Democracy in Europe and the United States.* Princeton: Princeton University Press.

Keller, Christoph. 2002. " 'Ihr Kinderlein kommet.' " [Oh, Come, Little Children]. *Die Zeit*, no. 50.

Kentenich, Heribert. 2015. *Was kann die Fortpflanzungsmedizin – was soll sie nicht sein?* [*What Reproductive Medicine Can Achieve – And What Should It Not Be?*]. Lecture at the conference Ethische Aspekte der Fortpflanzungsmedizin, Alt Rehse, October 2.

Krones, Tanja, and Gerd Richter. 2004. "Preimplantation Genetic Diagnosis (PGD): European Perspective and the German Situation." *Journal of Medicine and Philosophy* 29 (5): 623–640.

Labahn, Rüdiger. 2003. "Pressemitteilung: Lübecker Klinikchef klagt: 'Das Embryonenschutzgesetz hat in weiten Teilen versagt' " [Press Release: Head of Clinic in Lübeck Complains: 'Embryo Protection Law Failed in Large Parts']. Informations- und Pressestelle Universität zu Lübeck. Accessed December 8, 2015. http://idw-online.de/pages/de/news69240.

Lakotta, Beate. 2001. "Nachwuchs in der Warteschleife." [Offspring on Hold]. *Der Spiegel*, July 16.

Loewenich, Volker von. 2008. "Präimplantations-Diagnostik." [Preimplantation Diagnostics]. In *Gegenseitigkeit. Grundfragen medizinischer Ethik* [*Reciprocity. Fundamental Questions of Medical Ethics*], edited by Klaus Gahl, Peter Achilles and Rainer-M. E. Jacobi, 405–13. Würzburg: Könighausen und Neumann.

Nentwich, Hans-Jürgen. 2011. "Präimplantationsdiagnosik (PID) aus pädiatrischer Sicht (aktualisierte Fassung, Juni 2011)." [Preimplantation Diagnostics from a Paediatric Perspective]. *Monatsschrift Kinderheilkunde*, 7: 1–4.

Rau, Johannes. 2001. "Wird alles gut? Für einen Fortschritt nach menschlichem Maß." [Everything Will Be Alright? For Progress on a Human Scale]. Berliner Rede, May 18. Accessed December 8, 2015. www.bundespraesident.de/SharedDocs/Reden/DE/Johannes-Rau/Reden/2001/05/20010518_Rede.html.

Schmidt, Harald Thomas. 2003. *Präimplantationsdiagnostik. Jenseits des Rubikons?* [*Preimplantation Diagnostics. Beyond the Rubicon?*] Münster: LIT Verlag.

Schultz, Susanne. 1994. "Feministische Bevölkerungspolitik?" [Feminist Demographic Policy?]. In *Gender Killer*, edited by Cornelia Eichhorn and Sabine Grimm, 11–23. Berlin, Amsterdam: Edition ID Archiv.

Spieker, Manfred. 2001. *Kirche und Abtreibung in Deutschland.* [*Church and Termination in Germany*]. Paderborn: Ferdinand Schöningh.

Statistisches Bundesamt. 2009. *Pressemitteilung vom 29. Juli 2009, 283/09.* [*Press Release from July 28, 2009, 283/09*]. Wiesbaden: Statistisches Bundesamt, Pressestelle.

Statistisches Bundesamt. 2015. "Durchschnittliches Alter der Mütter bei der Geburt ihrer lebendgeborenen Kinder in Deutschland, 2013." [Average Age of Mothers at the Birth of their Live-born Children in Germany, 2013]. Accessed December 8, 2015. www.destatis.de.

Stock, Gregory. 2000. "'Der Geist aus der Flasche.'" ['Genie Out of the Bottle.']. *Der Spiegel*, April 10.

Thimm, Katja, and Gerald Traufetter. 2000. "Küss die Hand, gnädiges Ei." [Kiss the Hand, Gracious Egg].*Der Spiegel*, November 27.

Traufetter, Gerald and Christian Wüst. 2001. "'Menschenrecht auf Kinder'." ['Human Rights to Have Children.']. *Der Spiegel*, Feburary 5.

Waller, Katharina. 2011. "Ein zeitgemäßes Fortpflanzungsmedizingesetz für Deutschland." [A Contemporary Law on Reproductive Medicine for Germany]. *Gynäkologe* 44: 754–758.

Weschka, Marion. 2010. *Präimplantationsdiagnostik, Stammzellforschung und therapeutisches Klonen. [Preimplantation Diagnostics, Stem-cell Research and Therapeutic Cloning*]. Berlin: Duncker und Humblot.

Women's Voices. 1993. "A Declaration on Population Policies." *Population and Development Review* 19 (3): 637–640.

Woopen, Christiane. 1999. "Präimplantationsdiagnostik und selektiver Schwangerschaftsabbruch." [Preimplantation Diagnostics and Selective Termination of Pregnancy]. *Zeitschrift für Medizinische Ethik* 45: 233–244.

14 Matters of Donation and Preserved Relations

Co-Construction of Egg Donation and Family Structures in Iran

Tara Mehrabi

Introduction

The Islamic Republic of Iran is the first Islamic country in which gamete donation can be practiced legally. It has been legal since 2003. Iran benefits from relative religious freedom concerning ARTs, as well as the medical possibilities of high-tech ART clinics and experts. In fact, more than 50 active specialized medical centers offer infertility treatments across the country, although only to heterosexual married couples; none of the centers accepts single women or non-heterosexual or non-married couples. Not only are many infertile Iranian couples using donor technologies, but Iran is also a major destination for "fertility travelers" (Inhorn 2011) from other Islamic countries. According to Marcia Inhorn (ibid.), ARTs are growing quickly in Iran, which gives it, together with Egypt, a leading position among Muslim countries in the Middle East.

In this chapter, I examine the "naturalization" and "normalization" (Thompson 2005) of egg donation in Iran in conversation with Islamic doctrine and socio-cultural understandings of family structures and relatedness: a process which I refer to as the Islamization of egg donation in Iran. Inspired by feminist technoscience studies and feminist materialisms (see Thompson 2005; Smelik and Lykke 2008), I aim to show that the Islamization of egg donation in Iran is a multilayered process that highlights the entanglement of technologies, bodily materiality, religion, and socio-cultural values on reproduction and biological kinship. It is a process in which Islamic doctrine and the socio-cultural realities of biological relatedness, egg donation technologies, and bodily materiality *co-construct* one another. Islamization is a process that is not only occurring on the macro scale of Islamic discourses but, as I will show, it also takes place as infertile Iranian women interact with egg donation technologies, and renegotiate meaning (such as cultural and religious values around biological motherhood) and materiality (for instance ova and milk).

I draw on the material I collected during two periods of fieldwork in 2010 in Tehran, the capital of Iran. Each period lasted for three weeks in a private infertility clinic, during which I interviewed a total of 18 women who were considering egg donation as a possible treatment. I conducted the interviews in my mother tongue, Farsi, which is the official language of Iran. I have lived most of my life in Iran and I am familiar with the religious and cultural context; yet, I recognize that it is an extremely diverse country in terms of religion, ethnicity, culture, language, and class, to name just a few. Such diversity both limits the scope of my study and affects my position as a researcher as I was both an insider and outsider to my informants during my fieldwork. For instance, my informants and I could (partially[1]) relate to each other in terms of gender, culture, and religion. Yet, we would drift apart as I was not a married woman nor was I a strict believer in Islam, which was brought up on occasion by my informants. I also collected data from the websites of several infertility clinics, and the Ministry of Health and Medical Education's website.

Background to the Study

Before the Islamic Revolution in 1979, Islam was a matter of culture and personal beliefs, but afterwards it became a state/nation affair, the de/legitimization of everyday life, and the politicization of shi'ism (Najmabadi 1994). In other words, as Afsaneh Najmabadi writes, shi'ism became the dominant "new political sociability" (ibid., 365) in contrast to other existing socio-political systems, such as communism and/or Western politics of modernization. The new regime was not only interested in social models, such as the new welfare model or education, but also in revitalizing a culturally pure Islamic nation, one which was not affected by Western cultures; therefore, the regime was also concerned with individuals and their way of life, such as their clothing and behavior.[2] As such, "the question of women," female (reproductive) bodies, women's lives, and their natural role and place in the socio-political and cultural order of the new Islamic society of Iran became crucial to the new regime. Women were defined as the nation's reproductive bodies, as mothers and wives, while the homeland was articulated as mother (earth/homeland), which strongly linked together matters of nation, religion, gender, sexuality, reproduction, and nature. It is thus no wonder that family planning and its technologies, such as contraceptives, abortion, and, most relevant to my chapter, infertility treatments, have been highly debated in post-revolution Iran.

Moreover, Iran is a Shia Muslim country, which makes it different from Sunni Muslim countries in its political understanding and practices of Islam.[3] Unlike Sunni, Shia allows *Ijtihad*, which is an individual interpretation of the Quran by high-ranking religious authorities. As such, Shia Islam is more flexible in relation to social and political changes; for example, when it comes to accommodating controversial techno-scientific innovations such as egg donation. However, despite its receptiveness, such flexibility also has limits. The flexibility of *Ijtihad* allows change as long as it sustains Islamic values based on Islamic doctrine. This is to say that gamete donation in Iran is caught in a paradox: gamete donation has been authorized by Shia Islamic laws, yet it is also highly restricted and governed within Islamic ideals and doctrine of *natural* reproduction, the nuclear family, and Islamic kinship.

There have been many studies on ARTs and gamete donation in Iran, such as anthropological studies of kinship (Tremayne 2009), ethical and religious aspects

(Larijani and Zahedi 2007), law and ethics of gamete donation (Tremayne 2009, 2012), and socio-economic studies of ARTs and their effects on women (Abbasi-Shavazi *et al.* 2008). I am inspired by many of the studies mentioned, yet I situate my study within the field of feminist materialism and feminist techno-science studies and as such I focus on how bodily materiality, socio-cultural aspects, and religious discourse interact with the technology and co-construct one another. In addition, my interpretation of the situation in Iran differs from some of the above-mentioned studies; I will discuss these differences below.

According to Emily Martin (1991), egg and sperm have often been defined in relation to heterosexual reproduction and cultural imaginaries of masculinity and femininity as dichotomous, even when discussed in scientific terms. However, reproduction and the meanings of egg and sperm have changed radically with the arrival of assisted reproductive technologies and stem-cell research. As many scholars, such as Verena Namberger (this volume), show, eggs and embryos have become commodities on a global reproductive market that can move across the borders of bodies, laboratories, and nations. Reproduction, once imagined to be a heterosexual penetrative act, has transmuted to incorporate queer modes of reproduction in the laboratory as well as wider notions of relatedness (Mamo and Alston-Stepnitz 2014). Frozen germ cells and embryos at fertility clinics render a sense of reproductive control while, at the same time, they have become the biological material that is used for purposes other than reproduction, namely bioeconomic research and futuristic therapies (Waldby and Cooper 2010). In this "ontological choreography" of ARTs (Thompson 2005), infertility technologies, kinship, reproduction, body parts, social orders, ethical discourses, and laws become constantly rearranged into new relationships to one another. In other words, while new technologies such as ARTs can potentially offer non-normative and novel modes of kinship or reproduction, they also enact new modes of capitalist consumerism, stratified access, or modes of exploitation that are based on sex/gender, ethnicity, socio-economic status, and more (Rapp 2011). As feminist technoscience studies scholars often have underlined, technologies are not free from power relations and certainly not innocent.

I would like to contribute to the understanding of this kind of dynamic reality of ARTs with a focus on Iran. I also claim that a feminist analysis of these realities should not get stuck in the binary construction of assisted reproduction as either embedded in oppression or giving rise to women's agency (see Thompson 2005). These facets co-exist within the Iranian context and it is therefore important to engage with them simultaneously. In other words, inspired by my informants' stories and life experiences of infertility and ARTs, I understand ARTs as "new ways of embodying reproduction, some of which would disrupt conventional families and gender stereotypes" (ibid., 70). However, depending on the intersectionality of women's identities, their interaction with these technologies differs in ways that simultaneously reflect structural oppression and modes of agency.

In writing about the Islamization of ARTs in Iran, I am inspired by Varley (2012), who studies how family planning organizations have used Islamic doctrine as a device through which a specific form of "biopower" operates to control and govern women's reproduction and sexuality. Her understanding of Islamization interrogates the secular versus Islamized discourses and narratives of family planning in Pakistan, and questions how women internalize this Islamized family planning rhetoric. I, however, understand Islamization as a more dynamic process that occurs simultaneously within the space of family and the larger discourse and *practices* of infertility treatment. It is not only a social and discursive construction of reproduction and family relations that is at stake here, but also bodily materiality, such as when egg and sperm change meaning and function within ART practices. Islamization as such is an organic movement that occurs simultaneously at material and discursive, technological and biological/natural, micro and macro scales. It is a process in which not only do Islam and Islamic ways of life need to be altered in innovative manners to accommodate the technology, but also the technology needs to be molded and practiced in new ways to fit the "local moral word" of Iranian society (Inhorn 2003). As such, Islamization is not essentializing *one true Islam*; rather, it appreciates the situatedness of Islam and its entanglement with technology. This perspective stresses the multiplicity and fluidity not only of the technology but also of Islam.

Last but not least, Islamization is always already a process of (de)naturalization in which nature can be renegotiated. As Thompson argues, within the context of ARTs, biological parenthood has been transformed into a partial phenomenon that highlights the importance of the practices of "doing" kinship rather than "being" a parent (Thompson 2005, 146). This means that many parents apply different strategies, such as receiving an egg donation from a family member, so as to make sense of their relationship to the child as not only social but also natural. Parents make and naturalize their parenthood through reformulating biological relatedness by other means, such as blood.

To sum up, I employ Islamization as an *analytical tool* to write about the negotiation between bodily matters and kinship relations when a Western technology enters the Middle Eastern Islamic context of Iran. I argue that the Islamization of egg donation both destabilizes the "good old orders" of Islamic life and also simultaneously reinforces them.

Islamization of Assisted Reproductive Technologies in Iran

IVF technologies entered Muslim countries in 1980, following the *fatwa*[4] of leading religious authorities of Al-Azhar University in Egypt (Inhorn 2003). Since then, IVF technologies have spread around Islamic countries and become a reality for many Sunni and Shia Muslims. According to the same *fatwa*, IVF is only allowed for legally married couples who cannot conceive otherwise. Any procedure that involves a third-party donor, namely, egg donation, sperm donation, embryo donation, and surrogacy, is prohibited (ibid.). The Shia Islamic approach has taken a different route due to the built-in mechanism, namely, *Ijtihad*, which is the individual interpretation of the Quran by religious authorities, and *Sigheh*, which is a temporary marriage (Tremayne 2009). In Iran, as a theocracy, decisions are mainly made by the religious authorities on the rightfulness of specific acts or life choices (ibid.). Religious people[5] follow the lead of their religious authority of choice and his *fatwa* justifies their choices and actions. However, as Tremayne (2012) argues, ARTs are arriving in the country so fast and so many clinics and infertile couples are already using them that the religious authorities need to catch up with the treatments already being practiced rather than preconditioning the premises of such practices.

During the late 1990s, Iran's supreme leader, Ayatollah Khamenei, issued a *fatwa* permitting donor technologies if practiced in an Islamic manner, implying that no touch or gaze should be exchanged between the donor and the recipient. Moreover, as Tremayne (2009) argues, even though Khamenei did not explicitly underscore the temporary marriage between the donor of the egg and the husband of the infertile couple as a precondition, temporary marriage has been widely understood and practiced as a way to pursue egg donation following from interpretations of Khamenei's statement. However, not all Shia authorities who are entitled to *Ijtihad*, take the same progressive position toward IVF, not to mention third-party donation (see Sadeghi Moghadam 2006; Sistani 2006; Merghati 2007). Less progressive Shia authorities express concern about the possibility of *Zina* (adultery), disruption of the child's blood-line or *nasab*, and the possibility of marriage between siblings/incest. Moreover, a majority of the Shia religious authorities in Iran are generally resistant toward sperm donation, often prohibiting it, while in return being ambivalent about egg donation, carried out on the precondition of temporary marriage (see Sadeghi Moghadam 2006; Merghati 2007). What is problematic according to these authorities is not the technologies themselves but what they can potentially do; namely, disrupt Islamic kinship structures and values around reproductive relations. As Simpson (2013, 87) writes, the problem of gamete donation lies in the "complexity that arises in attempts to name and frame the substances, sentiments, and relationships to which it gives rise." Egg and sperm donation in Iran needs to be Islamized so as to be done in a manner which will sustain the Islamic kinship system and reproductive relations, just as much as Islamic kinship and reproductive relations need to be altered in relation to these technologies.

In the following, I will discuss the way in which, as part of the Islamization process of ARTs, family ties have been renegotiated on novel grounds.

That Which Can Be Donated

The legitimization of third-party donation in Iran, which is mostly discussed in relation to Khamenei's *fatwa*, is referred to in terms of an "Iranian ART revolution" (Abbasi-Shavazi *et al.* 2008), being a "marriage savior" (Inhorn 2006) or entering "the brave new world" of IVF technologies (Inhorn 2011). As Inhorn (2011, 87) writes "Iran is leading the way into this 'brave new world' of high-tech, third-party assisted conception, with Islamic bioethical discourses being used to justify various forms of technological assistance." I think there is a need for a more critical interrogation of that which these technologies enact, though, in terms of exclusions and conservation of normative family structures. In other words, a concern of this chapter and the fieldwork on which it is based, is that, in the process of legitimization, these technologies are being constantly and strongly debated, and appropriated by Islamic doctrine. This means that kinship and bodily materiality are constantly negotiated in ways that are embedded in normatively gendered, heteronormative,[6] and nationalist[7] power relations, encouraged by Islamic ways of reasoning. Therefore, I pursue questions such as: How are Islamic values and discourses about kinship and "proper" reproductive relations and conception mobilized in interaction, and co-constructed, with technologies and bodily matters such as eggs and sperm? How are politics of gender, kinship and reproduction negotiated and mobilized in ART practices and bodily materialities such as eggs and sperm? How does this politics not only "save" families, but also keep Islamic family structures intact?

In the absence of any straightforward laws in Iran, egg and sperm donation rely upon the *fatwas* of religious authorities. In Islam, it is the father who holds the right to the child and it is the father from whom the child gets her/his identity and lineage (Gheblei 2007).[8] As already mentioned, sperm donation is prohibited by a majority of Shia authorities (see Gheblei 2007). The minority who do allow it, argue that the lineage of the child is tied to the biological father indicating that the child can never inherit from the social father (see Nazari Tavakoli 2006). In addition to this, the practicalities of sperm donation (to be carried out in an Islamic manner) have made sperm into a bodily matter that is not as well-tuned to third-party donation as eggs are. As Tremayne (2012) argues, in the case of male infertility, couples are left with two options. One is embryo donation. The second is that the couple could divorce, and the wife could then temporarily marry the donor of the sperm. After embryo transfer she would terminate the temporary marriage contract and remarry her husband. Since divorce and remarrying has proven to be time consuming, such couples often choose embryo donation. In other words, even if the woman is capable of having her own biological child, if the husband is challenged, the woman is systematically, if not discursively, prevented from having genetic ties to the future baby. This was evident in the clinic in which I did my fieldwork. The doctors there refused to offer sperm donation due to the related complications, while they were very open and even enthusiastic about egg and embryo donation.

Another noteworthy issue concerns the ways in which religious authorities approach the relation between sperm and fatherhood differently from that between eggs and motherhood. The majority of Shia authorities link sperm to fatherhood, and as such they understand the sperm donor to be the father of the child, implying that the child shall inherit from him, and not from the social father (Merghati 2007). The relation between eggs and motherhood is considered by the same community to be more dynamic. There are at least three major groups of voices, all of them having different understandings of biological motherhood. One group ties motherhood to the egg and argues that the donor is the rightful mother of the child. The second group argues that carrying a baby and giving birth is that which enacts a woman as a mother, tying motherhood to the womb, gestation and the process of giving birth. The last group considers both the donor of the egg and the surrogate to be mothers to the baby (Sadeghi Moghadam 2006;Merghati 2007).

On the one hand these differences between enactments of eggs and sperm as the locus of parenthood open up space for alternative modes of motherhood while limiting and reducing fatherhood to the provision of sperm. On the other hand the differences speak to the politics of Islamic kinship, which is mobilized differently in eggs and sperm. Biological fatherhood is non-negotiable while motherhood is ambivalent. Motherhood can be imagined as something to be shared between two women while fatherhood has to be singular. Motherhood can be a matter of genetics/eggs, gestation and nurturing or both, while fatherhood is strictly bound to genetics/sperm.

The Islamization of ARTs is more evident in the case of eggs and sperm being enrolled in a heteronormative romance. An embryo has to be donated in an Islamic manner. This means that the egg and sperm involved in the process of conception have to originate from a legally married couple. Moreover, the embryo can only be donated to a legally married couple of Iranian nationality (Roshan 2007). In this scenario the eggs and sperm are strongly linked to bodies and their religious context. Eggs and sperm can only be mixed if they are legally bound through marriage, because any physical contact between an unmarried man and woman (except for close family members) is prohibited by Islam. As such it appears as though the marriage of the couple is automatically passed into the eggs and sperm. It is as though Islamic concerns about the mixing of bodily fluids between two unmarried adults are revitalized and guarded against through the Islamization of the embryo and modes of embryo donation. Not only are eggs and sperm gendered yet again, but also their modes of mixing together are appropriated in a particular manner in which technologies, science and Islamic gender politics meet.

Third-party donation needs to be seen in relation to Islamic understandings of kinship and family structure, gendered bodies and their places/roles in the Islamic order in which female bodies are yet again “raw material” and means of production in an economy of (re)production (Gimenez 1991). On the one hand, Islam acknowledges that eggs and the sperm are of equal biological importance in conception, and as such the child is always related to both mother and father. Yet within the politics of Islamic kinship and the Islamization of third-party donation I suggest that the egg is considered to perform only as a means of (re) production, rather than embodying a value in and of itself as the sperm does. The egg does not symbolize lineage or the child’s identity as the sperm does. This means that eggs are not as controversial and political as sperm. All in all, Islamic values, gender politics, kinship and reproductive relations are mobilized in and through bodily matters such as eggs, sperm and embryos.

However, when it comes to practice, as Tremayne (2009) argues, not every clinic or couple perform such Islamic rituals when receiving donated gametes. Indeed, in practice, many of the above-mentioned Islamic reasoning processes and conditions are challenged in different ways. For instance, in one case, one of my informants even changed her religious authority of choice (*Marja*) because this *Marja* was prohibiting egg donation. This does not contradict my argument, though, because politics is not a one-way street, nor is the Islamization of ARTs. As I further discuss in this chapter, my informants were also negotiating the premises of egg donation and motherhood inspired by their Islamic heritage. Even though my informants were relying on the religious interpretation of their authority of choice, and even though they were relating to Islam, they had their own novel models of doing kinship. These processes of navigation and finding one's way are also part of what I understand as the Islamization of ARTs.

Family Relations

Marriage and parenthood are strongly encouraged within Islamic doctrine. In order to save the marriage of a couple suffering involuntary childlessness, some religious authorities allow egg donation via temporary marriage. A married man can temporarily marry a single woman for a specified amount of time, from one hour to 99 years, based on the couple's mutual agreement. This means that the husband and the egg donor can be bound together via temporary marriage when fertilization occurs in order to avoid adultery.[9] The husband and the donor end the temporary marriage after the embryo has been transferred. The donor has to be a single, previously married woman, either a widow or a divorcee. Many of my informants told me that they were choosing egg donation because they feared their husbands' polygamy. These women said that they have been facing such a threat to their marriages for a long time. In some cases, the husbands had not mentioned polygamy themselves, my informants told me, but the husbands' families were constantly bringing up the subject, and introducing possible future brides to the husbands. In two cases, my informants themselves were considering the possibility of polygamy for their husbands because they were feeling guilty about their infertility. Based on my material, I agree with Inhorn (2006) that third-party gamete donation can be a marriage savior, when enacted through a temporary marriage. However, I also want to highlight that temporary marriage itself, and most importantly as a *precondition* for gamete donation, is a two-sided coin. I believe that the act of polygamy, sometimes celebrated as a form of flexibility which allows for third-party donation, is, indeed, a very power-laden and normatively gendered way of life. The existence of polygamy was one of the main reasons for my informants to consider egg donation, in order to prevent their husbands from remarrying. Many of my informants were upset not only because of their infertility, but also due to the fact that their husbands could and would engage in polygamy. Ironically these informants, who were choosing egg donation to prevent their husbands' polygamy, would agree to such polygamy as a precondition for treatment. Some of the informants actually understood it to be necessary because they did not want to sin, and because they were concerned about practicing ARTs in a properly Islamic way. Some of my informants, however, were not happy about the situation, and had many concerns. One even told me that she was concerned that her husband may develop loving feelings for the egg donor and try to establish a relationship with her after the procedure in order to hold on to the temporary marriage, or to marry her.

In many parts of the world, ARTs are no longer considered new technologies but mundane practices. In Iran, ARTs are trapped in a paradox in which they are both a mundane practice and also new in terms of the religious and legal complexities. While Islamization allows unconventional modes of reproduction, it is also concerned about preserving bodily materiality (such as sperm and eggs) and familial relations within an Islamic order which is strongly situated within the ideals of the nuclear family and biological kinship. As such, egg and embryo donation is a means by which the nuclear Islamic family can be achieved and sustained in the case of infertility. Even though Iran is an emerging pioneer in terms of gamete donation, the politics of family and reproduction remain strictly within a patriarchally gendered and heteronormative dynamic. Against this background, I will look into the complexities that make both questions of agency and oppressive power relations relevant for Iranian women when it comes to decisions about egg donation. As Thompson (2005) argues, there are no straightforward answers to such questions, because the realities of ARTs are complicated and often move between these apparently dichotomous positions of agency versus oppression.

In the following, I will recount stories of my interviewees' encounters with egg donation in a clinic in Tehran, in which they were actively engaging with the technology in order to redefine biological relatedness, yet were also affected by the existing power structures.

Doing Kinship: On Becoming a Biological Mother

My informants dealt with their anxieties about egg donation through the renegotiation of biological motherhood by other means. Since my aim was to study the intersection of Shia Islam and ARTs in Iran, my stories do not include the heterogeneous group of women who do not relate to Islam or self-identify as believers. This limits the scope of my study and I do not want to present an overarching generalization, but rather situated samples of what it *can* look like when Western technology meets Shia Islam in Iran. To an Iranian woman, reproduction potentially involves further dimensions aside from fulfilling her identity, such as financial security, social respect, and security, care, and financial support in old age (Abbasi-Shavazi *et al.* 2008). While having children is highly valued both socially and religiously and is expected from a married couple, the child is also expected to be a biologically related offspring.

Family Relations

The biological relatedness of a baby to its parents is not only about the structures of the nuclear family but also the arrangement of relations within the extended family. Within Islamic doctrine, the concept of *mahram* and *na-mahram* is well known. To be *mahram* to someone means that they are close family members, and therefore marriage is not allowed between them. In other words, being *mahram* embodies the closeness and relatedness of a family (namely: sister-brother, aunt-uncle, grandparents, but not cousins). Islam has particular orders and codes on how to behave in the presence of *na-mahram* (those who can marry each other) and *mahram* (those who cannot marry each other). Some of my informants were concerned about whether their child would be *mahram* to the future aunts/uncles in the absence of genetic ties. So gamete donation not only disturbs the traditional relations between mother and child but also affects the whole family and their modes of relating. Therefore, my informants were trying to renegotiate their biological relatedness to the child not only in order to redefine their motherhood but also to establish familial relatedness between the future child and her/his family members.

As a way of naturalizing their relatedness to the baby as biological, that which is not purely genetic, my informants established novel modes of biological motherhood that relied on the entanglement of bodies and matter, such as egg, sperm, blood, and milk. In other words, they were *doing kinship* as partial biological relatedness (Thompson 2005), stressing nurturing practices and bodily fluids, and calling upon their cultural and religious heritage.

Milk, Blood, and Womb

Within Islamic cultures, one becomes a mother not only through giving birth but also by breastfeeding. "Motherhood by milk," or a relationship created by lactation between a nurse and her biologically unrelated nursling, is a phenomenon that stretches the notion of family (Clarke 2007). In Islam, if a woman breastfeeds a child, that woman and the child become *mahram* to each other and enter a relation of kinship by milk. Therefore, the recipient of a donor egg would always already become a mother by breastfeeding the infant even in the absence of genetic ties. So, natural relatedness and motherhood have been enacted as nurturing rather than genetics, which brings me to my second point, blood and womb.

Within the Islamic ideals and cultural values of Iran, motherhood is understood and practiced predominantly, if not entirely, in terms of rearing and caring. Most of my informants tried to redefine their biological ties in terms of nurturing and stressed the importance of "nurturing matters." The fact that the baby was "growing" inside their bodies, feeding off their "blood" or their "being" was what mattered to them. As Heather Paxson (2006) argues, many women redefine motherhood in terms of gestation and birth rather than genetic relatedness. Nurturing the baby (with practices such as changing diapers and caring) on the one hand and nurturing matter (such as blood and milk) during or after the pregnancy were considered by my informants to be a powerful natural force and a natural bond to the infant. As such, my informants related themselves to the baby "biologically" rather than genetically.

Sperm

Many of my informants defined their biological relatedness to the child through their husbands and the fact that the child is biologically related to the father. In fact, sperm was the genetic container that mattered to them. My informants highlighted the social importance of a child being of the father's sperm. They mentioned that sperm donation is not acceptable in Iranian society because socio-culturally and religiously a child needs to be genetically related to the father to be kin. In such a context, they told me that egg donation seemed to them a better option than childlessness or adoption. As Parvin said, "The sperm is my husband's. At the end of the day it is better than adoption. It is better than having somebody else's child." Although the child is being conceived from her husband's sperm and somebody else's egg, she still feels connected to it because the baby is created out of her husband's sperm.

According to Thompson (2005), one of the strategies of doing partial parenthood was to search for relatedness within social, cultural, or familial relations. This means that many women seek relatedness to their child through a "cultural or personal relationship" to the donor or the surrogate mother, who was someone close, such as a friend or a family member (ibid., 167). The family lineage can be achieved through membership of the same ethnicity, family, religion etc. My informants could feel partially related to their future child because they had been living with their partners for many years. Not only had they shared and established common social grounds, histories, and stories but they had also materially influenced each other, living in the same place, eating the same food, breathing the same air, and exchanging bodily fluids over time. Therefore, if the child was related to the father it was as though it was also related to the mother.

Good Egg

Some of my informants were hesitant about egg donation because they did not want any surprises, any "deviancy" that might come along with a donated egg. Therefore, they were negotiating motherhood and relatedness thorough finding a "good egg" that would not only lead to a child who resembled them physically but also embodied qualities and characteristics that mattered to them the most. It was as though they were transferring their selves (material qualities and characteristics) into the future baby even if they were not genetically linked. However, unlike Tremayne's findings (2009) in which her informants were more attuned to the idea of receiving a donated gamete from a relative, none of my informants communicated their treatments to their families but instead were strictly keeping it a secret between the couple.

My informants were well aware that they were not genetically related to the baby, but they sought relatedness through searching for common ground between themselves and the donor, such as skin color and facial appearance, so that the baby would look like them. Harrington, Becker, and Nachtigall (2008) underline that the informants in their study made an effort to read similar facial gestures or behaviors between the baby and the social parents to establish relatedness. Similarly, it was important to my informants to find such similarities with their future baby: similarities that they were searching for in the donor so that they would be passed on to the baby. They were looking for a "good egg" that resembled their characteristics as a "reasonably good person" or a "good Muslim" as well.

I have to mention that women of different socio-economic statuses made different decisions about egg donation. Those identified as working class would go to great lengths to have a baby in order to save their marriage, even if it meant foregoing genetic relatedness. This was often because they feared the failure of their marriage, which could lead to financial problems and socio-cultural stigmatization. They told me that they have invested their youth, beauty, and life in their marriage and they would not wish it to fail due their infertility. Those who had the benefit of financial and socio-cultural resources (such as their family's support) were more skeptical about egg donation. Two of them were even considering leaving the treatment should they have to receive a donated egg to become pregnant.

Conclusion

In this chapter, I have analyzed Iranian women's interactions with egg donation, arguing that egg donation technologies, religion, family structures, and biological relatedness co-construct each other. I discussed the proposition that, within the existing asymmetrical power relations in Iran, a context in which one of the strongest possible subject positions for women is motherhood, ARTs are both providing hope for involuntarily childless women and at the same time keeping them within the Islamic social order and family relations. Although my informants were active agents during the treatment, they were also facing multidimensional constraints. On the one hand, they were interacting with egg donation in order to fit in within the existing Islamic and cultural system and its norms. On the other hand, the informants in my study were strongly interacting with the technology in order to reconstruct kinship and their relatedness to the future baby.

I have shown that my informants redefined their relation to the baby as not only social but also biological through conceptualizing and interacting with the flow of matter and substances between their bodies and the future baby's body. As such, they highlighted the importance of "good eggs" which potentially embody the physical and moral characteristics of the donor. Through searching for similar physical and moral connections between themselves and the donor, my informants were trying to transfer themselves into the baby. They discussed sperm as an important matter that embodies familial relations. They also discussed blood, milk, and womb in relation to rearing and nurturing. These were strategies of naturalizing through which my informants were making sense of their technologically assisted relatedness to their future baby as partial kinship. In other words, they were engaged in a process of doing kinship rather than being kin. In doing kinship, they would naturalize their pregnancy by uniting their social and biological parenthood, through recalling not only their cultural, religious, social, and historical resources but also a variety of material components, namely: egg, sperm, milk, blood, and womb. They were establishing a physical connection between their bodies and the baby's body through *flows of matters* and *relations that mattered.*

Notes

1 Being an Iranian woman means different things to different women; so does being a Muslim woman.
2 For instance, veiling became mandatory. Physical contact such as holding hands with the opposite gender became problematic unless legally related. Eating in public during Ramadan became forbidden. Laughing in public is frowned upon for women.
3 The differences between Shia and Sunni are not about the fundamentals of Islam but historically related to a political difference in terms of leadership after the passing of Prophet Mohammad. After Prophet Mohammad's passing, a divide occurred between a majority of Sunni Muslims who followed Abu-Bakr, the former advisor of the Prophet, and a minority of Shia Muslims following his cousin Imam Ali, as the rightful person to follow the Prophet's line. The latter led to a line of Imams who carried further the legacy of Islam, while the former, Sunni Islam, takes Quran and the Prophet's life lessons as the source for Islamic laws and way of life. Shia is more flexible because it takes inspiration from the life stories and ways of life of Imams who came after the Prophet as well. This difference has major consequences in day-to-day practice, among others in the case of ARTs which I discuss in this chapter.
4 *Fatwa* is the outcome of *Ijtihad* by the religious authorities. It is non-legally binding yet authoritative.
5 Not everyone is a believer or practices Islam even if they are born a Muslim.
6 Single women and non-heterosexual couples are not acknowledged as legitimate recipients. Moreover, when a couple is undergoing treatment, if the husband dies during the procedure, the wife cannot continue with it.
7 For instance, as stated in the Embryo Donation Act, the recipients have to be of Iranian nationality.
8 For instance, a mother is neither entitled to the full custody of the child (she holds it only until the child reaches the age of seven), nor is she considered to be vali, which is a person who holds the right and responsibility to make medical decisions or administer the financial properties of the child (Vasmaghi 2008). A Muslim woman who is married to a foreigner can never pass on her nationality to the child, unless the child is born in Iran and then only after the child reaches 18 years of age (Nikou 2015).
9 This only applies to female infertility. As I discussed earlier, in male infertility embryo donation is often offered to the couple.

References

Abbasi-Shavazi, Mohammad Jalal, Marcia C. Inhorn, Hajiieh Bibi Razeghi-Nasrabad, and Ghasem Toloo. 2008. "The 'Iranian ART Revolution': Infertility, Assisted Reproductive Technology, and Third-Party Donation in the Islamic Republic of Iran." *Journal of Middle East Women's Studies* 4 (2): 1–28.

Clarke, Morgan. 2007. "The Modernity of Milk Kinship." *Social Anthropology* 15 (3): 287–304.

Gheblei, K. Khalil. 2007. "Ahkam-e Vazeei-e Koodakan Nashi az Ehdaye Gamet Dar Rabeteh ba Tavaros" [A Study on the Inheritance of Children Born through Donor Gamete]. *Payesh Health Monitor, Journal of The Iranian Institute for Health Sciences Research* 6 (4): 365–371.

Gimenez, Martha E. 1991. "The Mode of Reproduction in Transition: A Marxist-Feminist Analysis of the Effects of Reproductive Technologies." *Gender and Society* 5 (3): 334–350.

Harrington, Jennifer, Gay Becker, and Robert Nachtigall. 2008. "Nonreproductive Technologies: Remediating Kin Structure with Donor Gametes." *Science, Technology and Human Values* 33 (3): 393–418.

Inhorn, Marcia C. 2003. *Local Babies, Global Science: Gender, Religion, and In Vitro Fertilization in Egypt*. New York, London: Routledge.

Inhorn, Marcia C. 2006. "Making Muslim Babies: IVF and Gamete Donation in Sunni versus Shi'a Islam." *Culture, Medicine and Psychiatry* 30 (4): 427–450.

Inhorn, Marcia C. 2011. "Globalization and Gametes: Reproductive 'Tourism,' Islamic Bioethics, and Middle Eastern Modernity." *Anthropology and Medicine* 18 (1): 87–103.

Inhorn, Marcia C., Pasquale Patrizio, and Gamal I. Serour. 2010. "Third-party Reproductive Assistance around the Mediterranean: Comparing Sunni Egypt, Catholic Italy and Multisectarian Lebanon." *Reproductive Biomedicine Online* 21 (7): 848–853.

Larijani, Bagher, and Farzaneh Zahedi. 2007. "Ethical and Religious Aspects of Gamete and Embryo Donation and Legislation in Iran." *Journal of Religion and Health* 46 (3): 399–408.

Mamo, Laura, and Eli Alston-Stepnitz. 2014. "Queer Intimacies and Structural Inequalities New Directions in Stratified Reproduction." *Journal of Family Issues* 36(4): 519–540. Accessed February, 2012. DOI: 10.1177/0192513X14563796.

Martin, Emily. 1991. "The Egg and the Sperm: How Science Has Constructed a Romance Based on Stereotypical Male-Female Roles." *Signs* 16(3): 485–450.

Merghati, S. Taha. 2007. "Hoghoog-e Koodakan dar Ehdaye Gamet" [Children's Right in Gamete Donation]. *Payesh Health Monitor, Journal of The Iranian Institute for Health Sciences Research* 6 (4): 347–354.

Naef, Garmaroudi. 2015. "Modern Reproductive Technologies in the Light of Traditional Ontologies: An Anthropological Reflection on Assisted Reproduction in Iran." In *Selbstgestaltung des Menschen durch Biotechniken* edited by Robert Ranisch, Sebastian Schuol and Marcus Rockoff, 157–172. Tübingen.

Najmabadi, Afsaneh. 1994. "Power, Morality, and the New Muslim Womanhood." In *The Politics of Social Transformation in Afghanistan, Iran, and Pakistan*, edited by AvMyron Weiner and Ali Banuazizi, 366–89. New York: Syracuse University Press.

Nazari Tavakoli, Saeed. 2006. "Raveshhaye Komaki-e Tolid-e Mesl dar Hoghogh Islam" [Assistant Reproductive Technologies in Islamic Laws]. In *Ehdaye Gamet va Janin dar Darman Nabarvary* [Essays on Gamete and Embryo Donation in Infertility Treatment], 259–318 . Markaz e Tahghigh va Toseeye Oloom-e Ensani, Samt publication: Tehran.

Nikou, Semira. 2015. "Iran's Discriminatory National Law." Last accessed June 19, 2016. http://iranprimer.usip.org/blog/2015/feb/04/iran%E2%80%99s-discriminatory-nationality-law.

Paxson, Heather. 2006. "Reproduction as Spiritual Kin Work: Orthodoxy, IVF, and the Moral Economy of Motherhood in Greece." *Culture, Medicine and Psychiatry* 30 (4): 481–505.

Rapp, Rayna. 2011. "Reproductive Entanglements: Body, State, and Culture in the Dis/Regulation of Child-Bearing." *Social Research* 78(3): 693–718.

Roshan, Mohammad. 2007. "Barressi Hoghoghi Ehdaye Gamet va Janin" [Embryo and Gamete Donation: A Legal Analysis]. *Payesh, Faslnameye pajooheshkadeh oloom e behdashti, Jahad e daneshgahi, sal sheshom, shomareye cheharom, safheh* [*Payesh Health Monitor, Journal of The Iranian Institute for Health Sciences Research*] 6 (4): 407–414.

Sadeghi Moghadam, Mohammad H. 2006. "Mabani Feghhi va Bayestehaye Ghanoon (Nahveye Ehdaye Janin be Zojeine Nabarvar)" [Islamic Considerations and Legal Needs in Modes of Embryo Donation to Infertile Couples]. In *Ehdaye Gamet va Janin dar Darman Nabarvary* [*Essays on Gamete and Embryo Donation in Infertility Treatment*], 144–170 Markaz-e Tahghigh va Toseeye Oloom-e Ensani, Samt publication: Tehran.

Simpson, Bob. 2013. "Managing Potential in Assisted Reproductive Technologies." *Current Anthropology* 54 (S7): S87–S96.

Sistani, Mohammad Reza. 2006. "Tazrigh-e Esperm-e Mard-e Ajnabi dar Rahem-e Zan" [Injecting a Stranger's Sperm in a Woman's Uterus]. In *Ehdaye Gamet va Janin dar Darman Nabarvary* [*Essays on Gamete and Embryo Donation in Infertility Treatment*], 131–144. Markaz-e Tahghigh va Toseeye Oloom-e Ensani, Samt publication: Tehran.

Smelik, Anneke, and Nina Lykke, eds. 2008. *Bits of Life: Feminism at the Intersections of Media, Bioscience, and Technology*. Seattle: University of Washington Press.

Thompson, Charis. 2005. *Making Parents: The Ontological Choreography of Reproductive Technologies*. Cambridge, Massachusetts: MIT Press.

Tremayne, Soraya. 2009. *Law, Ethics and Donor Technologies in Shia Iran*. New York: Berghahn Books.

Tremayne, Soraya. 2012. "The Dilemma of Assisted Reproduction in Iran." FVV in *ObGyn Monograph* 70–74. Accessed January, 2014. URL: www.fvvo.be/monographs/biomedical-infertility-care-in-poor-resource-countries-barriers-access-and-ethics/the-dilemma-of-assisted-reproduction-in-iran/.

Varley, Emma. 2012. "Islamic Logics, Reproductive Rationalities: Family Planning in Northern Pakistan." *Anthropology and Medicine* 19 (2): 189–206.

Vasmaghi, Sedigheh. 2008. "Zan dar Fegh-e Islam" [Women and Islam]. Samadiyeh publication: Tehran.

Waldby, Catherine, and Melinda Cooper. 2010. "From Reproductive Work to Regenerative Labour: The Female Body and the Stem Cell Industries." *Feminist Theory* 11 (1): 3–22.

Part IV

ARTs as Entangled in Demographic Agendas and Biopolitics

15 Babies from Behind Bars

Stratified Assisted Reproduction in Palestine/Israel

Sigrid Vertommen

Congratulate Mommy and Daddy, Majd Has Arrived!

On July 31, 2013, Lydia Al-Rimawi gave birth to a healthy baby boy named Majd Abdul Kareem Al-Rimawi at the Razan Medical Center in Nablus, a city in the northwest of Palestine. As I entered Lydia's hospital room, which was abundantly filled with flowers, family and journalists, her eldest daughter Rand offered me a small gift designed for the baby's visitors: a mini-sized nursing bottle with a chocolate bonbon inside, tagged with the note:

> I came from prison, despite the wardens and the bars. Mention God when you see me. Mention God when you pick me up in your arms. Oh sweet people, Majd has arrived. So congratulate mommy and daddy for what has happened.

It was easy to congratulate the mother, who was sitting on the hospital bed, beaming with pride. Majd's father, however, was only present through his absence. Twelve years ago, Abdul Kareem Al-Rimawi was sentenced to 25 years in prison for shooting at Israeli soldiers. Being denied conjugal visits, the only contact he and his wife have had over the last 12 years has been through a glass window. Although the Holy Land is famous for its miraculous conceptions, Majd's case was particularly astounding. He was conceived through IVF after his father successfully smuggled his sperm out of the Israeli prison where he is being detained. The Rimawis are not the first couple to undertake this spectacular reproductive endeavor. In 2006, Yigal Amir, the convicted murderer of Prime Minister Yitzhak Rabin, was caught smuggling his sperm out of jail before being officially granted the right by the Israeli Supreme Court to conjugal visits with his wife Larissa Trembovler, which resulted in the birth of their son in 2007.

This rather sensational story raises fundamental questions about the right to give birth and the right to be born in Palestine/Israel. Drawing on Shellee Colen's (1995) concept of *stratified reproduction* to indicate that the capacity to control one's reproductive abilities is stratified along gendered, sexualized, racialized, and classed fault lines, Michelle Murphy (2011) introduced the term *distributed reproduction* as a way to upscale the analysis of reproduction beyond the strict microbiological space of the female body to more extensive macro-infrastructures such as state, military, agricultural, and economic infrastructures, which are often unevenly distributed in time and space and accordingly assist, rearrange, foreclose, or harm one's reproductive capacities. This is particularly true for hyper-divided settler colonial societies such as Palestine/Israel, which was founded on the structural removal and replacement of the Palestinian population through the arrival of a new Jewish settler body (Wolfe 2007). My main argument is that Israel's (in)famously pronatalist assisted reproductive policies have been co-produced within a Zionist demographic logic of elimination which aims to create and consolidate a "Jewish majority in a Jewish state" by containing Palestinian fertility. This argument will be gradually developed. First, I will contextualize Yigal Amir's right to father a child within Israel's pronatalist reproductive-demographic climate. Second, I will elucidate the stratified character of Israel's pronatalism by illustrating how its ART policies have been imagined and deployed to promote Jewish fertility, while simultaneously attempting to control Palestinian fertility. In the final part, I argue that assisted reproduction has not only emerged as a biopolitical site for settler colonial control, but has also been appropriated as a tool of contestation by Palestinians. Drawing on Begoñia Artexaga's work on the embodied resistance of Irish political prisoners, I will compare Yigal Amir's quest for parenthood with that of Palestinian political prisoners.

Be Fruitful and Multiply in Splendid Isolation: The Case of Yigal Amir

Yigal Amir became the most despised Jew in Israel after assassinating Prime Minister Rabin during a peace rally in Tel Aviv in 1995. He is serving a life sentence in Ramon Prison in southern Israel, where he has been kept in solitary confinement and under round-the-clock camera surveillance. In 2007, Yigal Amir and his wife Larissa Trembovler, whom he married by proxy while incarcerated, gave birth to a son called Yinon. The marriage and the birth of their child both evoked heated public debates in Israeli society (Steinfeld 2011). The general persuasion of Israelis was that, as a convicted murderer, Amir had lost the moral right to start a family (Smajdor 2009). However, shortly after their controversial marriage in 2004, the Amirs started filing requests with the Israeli Prison Service and with several courts and eventually succeeded in gaining conjugal visits. In her research on fertility politics in Israel, Rebecca Steinfeld (2011) pointed out the remarkable contrast between permitting Amir to have conjugal visits while denying his request to be moved out of solitary confinement. Steinfeld argued that this seeming paradox of procreation despite isolation could only make sense in the context of Israel's exceptionally pronatalist reproductive policies.

Fertility indeed plays a prominent role in Israeli society (Kahn 2000; Weiss 2002; Birenbaum-Carmeli 2004; Nahman 2013). Ever since its creation in 1948, the State of Israel has institutionalized its pronatalist vision through multiple funds and committees that provided social and monetary incentives to establish large families, such as the 1949 Heroine Award for mothers with at least ten children, the 1962 Committee for Natality Problems, the 1968 Demographic Centre with its Fund for Encouraging Birth and the 2002 Israel Council on Demography (Birenbaum-Carmeli 2007, 25). Moreover, Israel has more fertility clinics per capita than any other country in the world and Israelis are by far the world's biggest consumers of IVF (Shalev and Werner-Felmayer 2012; ICMART 2013). Assisted reproductive technologies such as IVF, ICSI, donor insemination, surrogacy, egg donation, egg freezing, and prenatal genetic diagnosis are extremely popular in Israel and most are generously sponsored by the state. For instance, the Israeli government funds every citizen for an unlimited number of IVF cycles until the live births of two children within the current relationship (Birenbaum-Carmeli 2004). In contrast, treatments that restrict family size remain largely unsubsidized in Israel and abortion is still illegal, except for therapeutic reasons (Balabanova and Simonstein 2010). While Vlasenko (this volume) explores the different kinds of subjectivities and governmentalities that Ukraine's pronatalist state rhetoric has generated, my chapter will examine the settler colonial stratification of Israel's reproductive politics.

The Israeli reproductive impulse (Kahn 2000) has often been explained through what Mahmood Mamdani (2000) has dubbed "culture talk," i.e., a myopic focus on the centrality of reproduction in Judaism, Jewish culture and tradition. Some scholars refer to the first commandment in the Torah prescribing Jews to "be fruitful and multiply," the special status of the barren Matriarchs in Jewish tradition, and the compatibility of Jewish law (Halakha) with the scientific grounds of assisted reproduction often resulting in a permissive attitude by the Jewish religious establishment toward ARTs (Nahman 2013). Others refer to the Holocaust and the virulent anti-Semitism prevailing in Europe and Tsarist Russia, which led Jews to equate individual procreation with collective survival (Kahn 2000). Without intending to downgrade the cultural significance of reproduction, I argue that Israel's pronatalist stance on ARTs has been shaped not only by Judaism, but also by ongoing histories of Zionist settler colonialism in Palestine/Israel.

Zionism and Population Management: "Jewish Society Must Be Defended"

Framing the Zionist project in Palestine/Israel as a settler colonial practice rather than a "mere" nationalist ideology, as is often the case, fundamentally affects the analysis of the role, function, and goals of population management. A settler colonial analysis presumes a demographic "zero sum game" in which the settler population can only be enlarged *at the expense* of the natives. As Patrick Wolfe (2006, 2007) has pointed out, the governing logic in a settler colony supports the elimination or replacement rather than incorporation of indigenous peoples. In the case of Zionism, this was reflected in the project of "creative destruction" in Palestine that began at the end of the nineteenth century when Jewish pioneers

– evading horrendous forms of anti-Semitism and invigorated by Zionist ideology and institutions – started immigrating to Palestine and accumulating indigenous lands. This process of territorial maximization coincided with the structural dispossession of Palestinians from their lands.

As feminist scholars on (settler) colonialism have argued, indigenous removal not only materializes through mass killings or expulsions, it can also proceed through settler regulation of sexual and reproductive relations (e.g., Povinelli 2006; Morgenson 2011, 2012). The regulatory management of the reproductive practices of both settlers and natives has been foundational to the *settler colonial* order of things (Stoler 1995). Within this formulation, settlers are destined to "reproduce the nation" while the mere existence, let alone reproduction, of the indigenous population is perceived as an existential threat to the colonial project (Landertinger 2011).

The Zionist population project revolved around defining and developing Israel as a Jewish state, implying that at least the majority of the population should be Jewish. In this sense, the presence of Palestinians, within and outside the borders of what became Israel in 1948, has continued to pose an existential threat to the Jewish collective body. This demographic anxiety is further fueled by the fertility differential between the two groups. Historically, Palestinians had higher birth rates than Jewish Israelis, a trend which is often framed as a *velvet holocaust* or a *demographic intifada* in Israeli discourse.[1] Concordantly, Palestinian women are often depicted as hyper-fertile, premodern, and irresponsible breeders. During a conference in 1995, the renowned Israeli geographer Arnon Soffer claimed that "the most serious threat that Israel faces is the wombs of Arab women in Israel" (quoted in Kanaaneh 2002, 74). In 2008, after the military attack on the Gaza Strip, Israeli soldiers designed t-shirts portraying a pregnant Palestinian woman in the crosshairs of a gun, accompanied by the slogan: "One shot, two kills" (Waghorn 2009). Similarly, in her research on the sexual colonization of Native American women, Andrea Smith (2002) argued that the bodies of native women were particularly targeted in settler colonial states because of their threatening ability to reproduce the next generation and to assure the continuance of the indigenous peoples.

Israel has attempted to create a Jewish majority in two significant ways. First and foremost, by attracting Jews from the Diaspora (preferably Ashkenazi Jews from Europe or Russia) through the Law of Return, which automatically grants every Jew in the world the right to Israeli citizenship and nationality, and by simultaneously denying Palestinian refugees their Right to Return. Second, by issuing pronatalist reproductive health policies that stimulate Israelis to reproduce *their* nation. As Roberto Bachi, the first director of Israel's Central Bureau of Statistics and an advisor to the Council for Demographic Problems summarized it, already in 1944:

> The demographical competition between the Arabs and Jews in Israel will be decided not only by the number of immigrants we manage to bring to Israel, but first of all by the reproduction of Arabs and of Jews. Therefore,

> we must aspire to a bigger increase in the birth rate and in order to achieve it we must create a comfortable environment and appropriate conditions for a multitude of children.
>
> (Quoted in Steinfeld 2011, n.p.)

This intimate connection between reproductive and demographic policies remains reflected in Israel's standpoint on more advanced ARTs. When commenting on Israel's exceptionally generous IVF policy, Mordechai Gur, former Minister of Health, stated that "IVF is still cheaper than a newcomer" as a means of increasing the population (quoted in Birenbaum-Carmeli 2004, 900).

Distributed Assisted Reproduction Within the Jewish and Demographic State

Analyzing the history of Israel's fertility policy, Portugese (1998) concluded that Israel has been as concerned with reducing the Palestinian birth rate as it has with increasing the Jewish one. A famous example was the Heroine Mother Award, a birth prize initiated by Ben Gurion in 1949 to grant all mothers financial compensation on the birth of their tenth child. The award was dropped after ten years when it turned out that mostly Palestinian-Israeli mothers were claiming it. In 1968, Israel established the Fund for Encouraging Fertility, which offered cheap housing loans for large families on the condition that at least one family member had served in the Israeli army, clearly excluding Palestinian citizens of Israel since they usually do not serve in the army. Similarly, the 1970 Veteran's Child Allowance Scheme offered extra child allowances to large families in which at least one member had served in the army (Kanaaneh 2002). In 1992, when discussing a Bill in the Knesset that would end this discriminatory practice by equalizing child allowances for all families, the founder of the right-wing Moledet Party, Rehavam Ze'evi, remarked: "This proposal is an incentive for making more Arab children. They will live off us forever. They will give birth to 50, 60, 70 children and we will pay them discharged soldiers grants" (quoted in Portugese 1998, 108).

This *selective pronatalism* (Kanaaneh 2002) can also be detected in Israel's policies on more recent ARTs, although in more nuanced and subtle ways. Legally speaking, Palestinian citizens of Israel are entitled to the same fertility treatments as Jewish Israelis, but the colonial reality often prevents them from enjoying these equal reproductive rights.[2] In 2010 for example, the Israeli Knesset voted in a controversial law that both allowed Israeli women aged between 21 and 35 to sell their egg cells to the Israeli state in return for substantial financial compensation and offered Israeli women aged between 18 and 54 the opportunity to request egg donation covered by their National Health Insurance. One of the amendments to the Egg Donation Bill stipulated that the donor and the recipient of the egg cell are required to share the same religion, which makes it impossible for a Jewish woman to donate an egg cell to a Muslim, Christian or Druze couple or vice versa without the approval of an Exceptions

Committee. Since, in practice, Palestinian women rarely donate egg cells in Israel, this amendment ensured that they will also never benefit from egg cell donation (Nahman 2013; Vertommen 2016).

Palestinian Israelis' access to IVF is mostly limited because of the deplorable condition of the healthcare and public transport infrastructure in those areas of Israel that are densely populated by Palestinians, such as the North, the Triangle and the Naqab. The distributed character of Israel's architecture of ARTs becomes very visible when mapping out the country's existing fertility clinics (Murphy 2011). Of the 25 IVF units in Israel, none are located in Arab hospitals. Nazareth, for example, the biggest Palestinian city inside Israel, has no IVF unit. The majority of Israeli IVF units are based in areas that are predominantly Jewish. This, in combination with a systematic lack of adequate public transport services to/from Palestinian-Israeli localities, has curtailed the access of Palestinian-Israeli woman to assisted reproductive services (Zu'bi 2011).

According to Mira Hibner Harel, the Legal Advisor of the Ministry of Health (MOH), "Arab-Israeli women are equally represented in the use of assisted reproductive services in Israel" (interview Mira Hibner Harel, West-Jerusalem, February 20, 2012). Unfortunately, there are no official figures to support this claim. Despite the government funds that are being poured into ARTs, there is a surprising lack of official data concerning ARTs in Israel. In this sense, Israel's 25 public IVF clinics enjoy a substantial degree of self-government. The Ministry of Health offers very few professional guidelines concerning the screening of IVF candidates, potentially leaving space for individual fertility doctors to arbitrarily refuse patients. However, after conducting a survey with Israeli fertility doctors on their attitudes regarding access to fertility care, Daniel Sperling and Yael Simon (2010) concluded that only a minority of doctors requested information from IVF candidates concerning their nationality, religion, or military service. Moreover, many of the Jewish and Palestinian-Israeli fertility doctors I interviewed confirmed that Palestinian-Israeli couples had little trouble in finding their way to fertility clinics. They repeatedly stated that (reproductive) health is one of the few sectors in Israel where ethnic discrimination between Jewish and Palestinian Israelis is limited. In her research on attitudes among Jewish and Arab-Israeli women toward assisted reproductive technologies, Larissa Remennick (2011) argued that "Arab-Israeli" women perceived no discrimination between themselves and Jewish women concerning free access to ARTs. She quoted Tarika, a Palestinian-Israeli teacher from Jaffa: "I am glad that at least in this respect there is no sheer discrimination against Arab citizens. The Jewish doctors may not like facilitating higher Arab birthrates, but they are polite enough not to show it" (quoted in Remennick 2011, 328). Some of the Jewish-Israeli respondents Remennick interviewed did state their reservations about equal access to costly IVF treatments for Arab-Israeli women.

> I know it's very politically incorrect to say, but I think there should be limits to our generosity towards Arab citizens. They don't serve in the army, they pay lower taxes, only a minority of their women work – why should they

> get the same costly services for free? Do we want to pay thousands of dollars for yet another Arab baby who will grow to hate us and maybe will turn his weapon against my son?
>
> (Quoted in Remennick 2011, 330)

The prevailing attitudes, practices, and policies concerning ARTs in Palestine/Israel remain anchored in a demographic logic that closely governs the reproductive capacities of both the indigenous Palestinians and the Israeli settlers. However, ARTs have not only emerged as an important site and technology of biopolitical control, but they have also been appropriated as a biopolitical tool to defy Israel's settler colonial rule, not only by Palestinians inside Israel, who are increasingly making use of these technologies, but also by Palestinians in the West Bank and Gaza. The case of Palestinian prisoners who are smuggling their sperm out of Israeli prisons in an attempt to impregnate their wives through IVF serves as a good example to underpin this claim.

Biopolitical Control and the Resistance of Palestinian Prisoners: "Every Sperm is Sacred"

There are approximately 5,000 Palestinian political prisoners in Israeli jails, serving sentences for offences ranging from stone throwing to killing Israeli soldiers (Addameer 2010). They are classified by the Israeli Prison Service as security prisoners, which a priori excludes them from certain fundamental rights. Family visits, for example, are only allowed for first-degree family members and are restricted to 45 minutes. No physical contact is allowed between husbands and wives. Prisoners are separated from their visitors by a glass partition and only children up to the age of eight are allowed to touch their fathers for a few brief minutes (Baker and Matar 2011). Conjugal visits are strictly forbidden. Obviously, these restrictions have far-reaching consequences for the desires of Palestinian prisoners. The importance of family and reproduction for prisoners became apparent with the case of Walid Daka, a Palestinian security prisoner who has been sentenced to life and incarcerated since he was 25 years old. Since 2008, Daka has been demanding conjugal rights from the Israeli Prison Service, which would allow him the opportunity to father a child, but until now all his requests have been in vain.

In July 2008, Adalah, the Legal Center for Arab Minority Rights in Israel, filed a petition to the Nazareth District Court on behalf of Walid Daka, repeating his request for conjugal rights. The petition clearly made reference to the ethnic discrimination that is visible in the different treatment of Palestinian and Jewish prisoners with respect to conjugal visits. The petition argued:

> Israeli-Jewish prisoners classified as security prisoners are permitted to exercise numerous rights, including conjugal visits, despite their security classification in prison. This is true, for example, in regard to the prisoner Yigal Amir, who was convicted of murdering Prime Minister Yitzhak Rabin

> for ideological reasons and has since fathered a son. Similarly, the Jewish-Israeli prisoner Ami Popper, who was convicted in 1990 of murdering seven Palestinian labourers and wounding 11 others, got married in prison in 1993, and fathered his first child who was born in 1995. Since then, he has fathered another two children.
>
> (Adalah 2008)

Prisons have always been an intensified microcosm of biopolitics in which the body, and especially the reproductive body, of the prisoner constitutes an important site of disciplinary control in the production of a submissive subject (Aretxaga 1997). Palestinian political prisoners are increasingly using their reproductive bodies and *bare lives* to thwart settler colonial policies by smuggling their sperm out of Israeli prisons in an attempt to "artificially" reproduce. According to the Ahrar Center for Prisoners' Studies, this sperm smuggling from inside the jails constitutes a serious challenge to the Israeli jailers (Akram 2014). Allegedly, so far more than 65 Palestinian prisoners have succeeded in sneaking their semen out of prison and into the Razan Medical Center for Infertility in Ramallah and Nablus, where it is stored in freezers awaiting fertility procedures. According to Salem Abu al-Khaizaran, the leading doctor and spokesperson for the prisoners' project in the Razan Medical Center, this has resulted in 18 pregnancies and six live births, with more deliveries expected in the near future (interview August 3, 2013 Nablus). The sperm-smuggling strategy has also started to achieve success in Gaza. In January 2014, IVF babies were born from Gazan political prisoners Tamer al-Zaanin and Fahmi Abu Salah (Sherwood 2013; Akram 2014).

Because of the high cost of IVF in the West Bank – between US$2,500 and US$3,000 per IVF cycle – the Razan Medical Center decided to provide IVF treatments free of cost to the wives of long-term prisoners as part of their community services. Dr. Abu al-Khaizaran claimed that it would be "unreasonable and unethical to charge these poor women whose husbands have been in prison for 15 years or more" (interview August 3, 2013 Nablus). Despite the fact that Islamic law allows the wives of prisoners who have been incarcerated for more than three years to divorce, none of the spouses actually do this. Because of the heroic reputation of political prisoners in Palestine, women feel it is their duty to stand by their husbands and support them. This means that they are often too old to conceive in a "natural" way by the time their husbands are released from prison. "Because we like to have children in our society," Dr. Abu al-Khaizaran continued, "the family of the released prisoner will start pushing him to get married to another woman, and often they do." Hana al-Za'anin, the wife of Gazan prisoner Tamer al-Za'anin, stressed the societal importance of the initiative: "I need to be a mother. Every woman needs to be married and have children. In our society, this is the role of women" (quoted in Sherwood 2013).

Downplaying the political tensions behind his services, Dr. Abu al-Khaizaran emphasized the "humanitarian" importance of the prisoners' initiative. "It's a fundamental human right of everyone, including Palestinian prisoners, to start a family. I look at it from a humanitarian perspective. Neither the Palestinian Authority nor the Palestinian Prisoners' Organization are involved in this project" (interview August 3, 2013 Nablus). Yet, the matter became highly politicized when both the families of the political prisoners and the Israeli authorities made repeated references to the political tension surrounding this issue in the media. Beyond the socio-cultural imperatives, motherhood can also be perceived as a political act in Palestine/Israel. The wives and families of the prisoners made strategic use of the abundant media attention not only to promote the issue of the prisoners to a broader public, but also to inform their own local communities, who might otherwise suspect the wives of adultery when seeing them pregnant while their husbands are in prison. This is why the Razan Medical Center sought the approval and support of religious authorities before continuing with the prisoner's initiative. In April 2013, the Palestinian Supreme Fatwa Council issued an official *fatwa* allowing artificial insemination for the wives of Palestinians in Israeli jails under certain conditions.[3]

Suspicious about the impact of this story on the reputation of Israel's security apparatus and fearful about every event in which Palestinian reproduction is lauded, the Israeli authorities publicly questioned the ability of the prisoners and the Razan Medical Center to accomplish such a reproductive mission. Sivan Weizman, spokesperson for the Israeli Prison Service, doubted whether the sperm could be smuggled out of prison considering the existing security conditions and the tools at the disposal of the prisoners. This question has remained unanswered since neither the Razan Medical Center nor the wives of prisoners have been willing to reveal how the sperm gets smuggled out, in order to ensure the continuation of this reproductive practice. Apart from these logistical considerations, the Israeli Prison Service also questioned the biological viability of the endeavor.

> Sperm expires after a few minutes or hours when it's not kept frozen. The prisoners are taken out of their cells many hours before the visit and it takes the family many hours to reach the fertility clinic, so we don't see how they could do it.
>
> (Interview Sivan Weizman, July 28, 2013)

What followed was a public media quarrel between embryologists, biologists, and government officials about the life expectancy of semen in which Palestinians claimed that sperm – depending on its quality – could survive for between 24 and 48 hours, while the Israelis were claiming a far shorter maximum lifespan. In an ultimate display of colonial biopolitics, the Israeli Prison Service challenged the Razan Medical Center to conduct paternity tests on newborns in order to genetically prove the father–child kinship.

Conclusion

Being refused the right to conjugal visits, Palestinian prisoners who wish to start a family fall back on smuggling out semen and using ART treatments as their last resort. In an interview, the brother of Abdul Kareem Al-Rimawi, stated (quoted in Levy and Levac 2013): "Yigal Amir was allowed conjugal visits with his wife, but Palestinian prisoners are not. That's why we were forced to operate this way." This quote summarizes many of the arguments made in this chapter. First of all, it emphasizes the stratified character of Israel's reproductive policies, which are still embedded in a Zionist demographic logic designed to promote Jewish fertility and "defend Jewish society" against the internal danger posed by native Palestinians (Foucault 2003). Second, it exemplifies that Palestinians are increasingly mimicking the power configurations they are resisting (Kanaaneh 2002). Palestinians on both sides of the Green Line are appropriating ARTs as a biopolitical tool of resilience against oppressive policies. While the Zionist regime has co-produced ARTs as a site of settler colonial control over both its Jewish and Palestinians subjects, Palestinian prisoners are increasingly using these same technologies to defy Zionist policies. This illustrates that the Zionist demographic rationale not only diffuses through the social body, where it co-produces particular reproductive subjectivities, but it is in turn challenged by the same subjectivities it has enabled (Aretxaga 1997). In a final remark during our interview, Lydia Al-Rimawi mentioned that she hopes her son Majd will grow up to be "just like his father," despite his father being labeled as a dangerous criminal by Israel. When asked if she wanted to have more children like this, Lydia answered "*inshallah*" while encouraging other prisoner couples to start using the same reproductive tactic. In this sense, ARTs not only serve as a last resort for Palestinian women to abide by their socio-cultural imperative of motherhood in what is still a patriarchal society, but they also become a site through which Palestinians are negotiating and claiming their reproductive rights in an act of embodied resistance.

Notes

1 According to Israel's Central Bureau of Statistics (CBS) (2013), in the early 1960s the total fertility rate of non-Jews was more than double that of Jews: 7.13 versus 3.39. In 2013 the CBS published a document concluding that Jewish women are now giving birth to an average of three children, compared to 2.53 in 1995 while Muslim women's fertility decreased from 4.74 in 1995 to 3.51 in 2011. (www1.cbs.gov.il/shnaton64/st03_13.pdf).

2 Due to Israel's politics of fragmentation, Palestinians are subjected to different, graduated health regimes. Palestinian Israelis and East Jerusalemites are entitled to the same healthcare provisions as Jewish-Israeli citizens.

3 There are some conditions that must be met for the procedure to be in line with Islamic law. The couple must be married and the pregnancy must be agreed by both partners and preferably their families. Several of the couple's next-of-kin relatives must witness the insemination, and the process must be made public (*Ma'an News* 2013).

References

Adalah. 2008. "Baker's Prisoners' Petition 609/08, Walid Daka v. the Israel Prison Service Nazareth District Court." Accessed June 19, 2014. http://adalah.org/newsletter/eng/jul08/7.php.

Addameer Prisoner Support and Human Rights Organization. 2010. "Palestinian Political Prisoners, November 2010." Accessed July 28, 2014. www.addameer.org/index.php.

Akram, Fares. 2014. "Sperm smugglers score a victory in Gaza." *Al Jazeera*, January 20. Accessed August 22, 2014. www.aljazeera.com/indepth/features/2014/01/sperm-smugglers-score-victory-gaza-201411912315567823.html.

Aretxaga, Begoña. 1997. *Shattering Silence: Women, Nationalism, and Political Subjectivity in Northern Ireland*. Princeton: Princeton University Press.

Baker, Abeer and Anat Matar. 2011. *Threat: Palestinian Political Prisoners in Israel*. London: Pluto Press.

Balabanova, Ekaterina and Frida Simonstein. 2010. "Assisted Reproduction: A Comparative Review of IVF Policies in Two Pronatalist Countries." *Health Care Analysis* 18: 188–202.

Birenbaum-Carmeli, Daphna. 2004. "Cheaper than a Newcomer: On the Social Production of IVF Policy in Israel." *Sociology of Health and Illness* 26 (7): 897–924.

Birenbaum-Carmeli, Daphna. 2007. "Contested Surrogacy and the Gender Order: An Israeli Case Study." *Journal of Middle East Women Studies* 3 (3): 21–44.

Colen, Shellee. 1995. "Like a Mother to Them: Stratified Reproduction and West Indian Childcare Workers and Employers in New York." In *Conceiving the New World Order: The Global Politics of Reproduction*, edited by Faye Ginsburg and Rayna Rapp, 78–102. Berkeley: University of California Press.

Foucault, Michel. 2003. *Society Must be Defended: Lectures at the Collège de France 1975–1976*. New York: Picador.

ICMART (International Committee for Monitoring Assisted Reporduction Technologies). 2013. "World Report on Assisted Reproductive Technologies 2004." *Human Reproduction* 28(5): 1375–1390.

Israel Central Bureau of Statistics (CBS). 2013. "Fertility rates by age and religion 1960–2012." Accessed July 22, 2014. www1.cbs.gov.il/shnaton64/st03_13.pdf.

Kahn, Susan M. 2000. *Reproducing Jews: A Cultural Account of Assisted Conception in Israel*. Durham: Duke University Press.

Kanaaneh, Rhoda. 2002. *Birthing the Nation: Strategies of Palestinian Women in Israel*. Berkeley: University of California Press.

Landertinger, Laura Christine Luise. 2011. *The Biopolitics of Indigenous Reproduction: Colonial Discourse and the Overrepresentation of Indigenous Children in the Canadian Welfare System*. Unpublished thesis, Queen's University.

Levy, Gideon and Alex Levac. 2013. "How Did a Palestinian Prisoner Father a Child Without Seeing His Wife?" *Haaretz*, August 9. Accessed July 18, 2014. www.haaretz.com/weekend/twlight-zone/.premium-1.540642.

Ma'an News. 2013. "Fatwa Council Approves Artificial Insemination for Prisoner's Wives." March 24. Accessed July 25, 2014. www.maannews.net/eng/ViewDetails.aspx?ID=589018.

Mamdani, Mahmoud. 2000. *Beyond Rights Talk and Culture Talk: Comparative Essays on the Politics of Rights and Culture*. New York: St. Martin's Press.

Morgenson, Scott L. 2011. "The Biopolitics of Settler Colonialism: Right Here, Right Now." *Settler Colonial Studies* 1: 52–76.

Morgenson, Scott Lauria. 2012. "Theorizing Gender, Sexuality and Settler Colonialism: An Introduction." *Settler Colonial Studies* 2: 2–22.

Murphy, Michelle. 2011. "Distributed Reproduction." In *Corpus, An Inter-Disciplinary Reader on Bodies and Knowledge*, edited by M. Casper and P. Currah, 21–38. New York: Palgrave Macmillan.

Nahman, Michal. 2013. *Extractions: An Ethnography of Reproductive Tourism*. Hampshire: Palgrave Macmillan.

Portugese, Jacqueline. 1998. *Fertility Policy in Israel: The Politics of Religion, Gender and Nation*. Westport: Praeger.

Povinelli, Elisabeth. 2006. *The Empire of Love: Toward a Theory of Intimacy, Genealogy, and Carnality*. Duke University Press.

Remennick, Larissa. 2011. "Between Reproductive Citizenship and Consumerism: Attitudes towards Assisted Reproductive Technologies among Jewish and Arab Israeli Women." In *Kin, Gene, Community: Reproductive Technologies among Jewish Israelis*, edited by Daphna Birenbaum-Carmeli and Yoram S. Carmeli, 318–339. New York: Berghahn Press.

Shalev, Carmel and Gabriele Werner-Felmayer. 2012. "Patterns of Globalized Reproduction: Egg Cell Regulation in Israel and Austria." *Israel Journal of Health Policy Research* 1(15): 1–35.

Sherwood, Harriet. 2013. "Gaza's First 'Prison Baby' on Way After Jailed Palestinian Smuggles Out Sperm." *Guardian*, October 13. Accessed July 25, 2014. www.theguardian.com/world/2013/oct/13/gaza-first-prison-baby-palestinian-smuggles-sperm.

Smajdor, Anna. 2009. "Incarceration and infertility: do prisoners have the right to access IVF?" *BioNews*. January 19. Accessed June 25, 2016. www.bionews.org.uk/page_38046.asp.

Smith, Andrea. 2002. "Not an Indian Tradition: The Sexual Colonization of Native Peoples." *Hypatia* 18(2): 70–85.

Sperling, Daniel, and Yael Simon. 2010. "Attitudes and Policies Regarding Access to Fertility Care and Assisted Reproductive Technologies in Israel." *Reproductive BioMedicine Online* 21: 854–886.

Steinfeld Rebecca. 2011. "Fruitful." *Tablet*, June 20. Accessed July 20, 2014. www.tabletmag.com/jewish-news-and-politics/70286/fruitful.

Stoler, Ann L. 1995. *Race and the Education of Desire*. Durham: Duke University Press.

Vertommen, Sigrid. 2016. "Towards a Political Economy of Egg Donations: Doing It the Israel Way." In *Critical Kinship Studies: Kinship (Trans)formed*, edited by Charlotte Kroløkke, Lene Myong, Stine Willum Adrian, and Tine Tjørnhøj-Thomsen, 169–184. Rowman and Littlefield International.

Waghorn, Dominic. 2009. "Israeli Army T-Shirts Mock Gaza Killings." *Sky News*, March 20. Accessed June 16, 2014. http://news.sky.com/story/678761/israeli-army-t-shirts-mock-gaza-killings.

Weiss, Meira. 2002. *The Chosen Body: The Politics of the Body in Israeli Society*. Stanford: Stanford University Press.

Wolfe, Patrick. 2006. "Settler Colonialism and the Elimination of the Native." *Journal of Genocide Research* 8(4): 387–409.

Wolfe, Patrick. 2007. "Palestine, Project Europe and the (Un-)Making of the New Jew: In Memory of Edward Said." In *Edward Said: The Legacy of a Public Intellectual*, edited by Ned Curthoys and Debjani Ganguly, 313–337. Carlton: Melbourne University Press.

Zu'bi, Himmat. 2011. *The Experiences of Palestinian Women in Israel Undergoing In Vitro Fertilization Treatments*. Unpublished master's thesis, Bar-Ilan University.

16 From Precarity to Self-Governance

Performing Motherhood through IVF Treatment in Ukraine

Polina Vlasenko

Introduction

On February 22, 2011, 66-year-old Valentyna Pidverbna from Chernihiv, Ukraine, gave birth for the first time in her life. She immediately became famous in Ukraine as the oldest woman to become a mother. Her husband had divorced her because she was diagnosed as infertile. Nevertheless, she decided to undergo IVF treatment and earned the necessary money by selling goods on a market stall for seven years. She conceived a child during her third attempt at IVF using donor eggs and sperm at a fertility clinic in Kyiv.

One month after the birth, medical professionals started to raise concerns that Valentyna was unable to independently take care of her child: she did not listen to their recommendations regarding healthy diet and daily routine, forbade them to examine the baby, did not buy diapers or baby formula, and in general demonstrated an "inadequate worldview." They argued that the life of the newborn girl was in danger and requested her temporary removal from the mother to an orphanage on the basis of child neglect (Department of Healthcare of the Chernihiv Regional State Administration 2011).

Despite the fact that this appeal was unsuccessful, the safety and wellbeing of Valentyna's child remained a focus of media attention for the next four years. The news constantly reported the girl having serious health problems and Valentyna failing to provide her with good living conditions and medical care. The powerful position occupied by these media discourses demonstrates how Ukrainian society is pervaded by perceptions of "good" and "bad" mothering practices, according to which the only people who have the right to become parents are those who align with social norms of marital status, sexuality, reproductive age, and social class, and who comply with medical and social surveillance. The story of Valentyna shows that, despite the ways in which ARTs undermine discourses of the "naturalness" of human reproduction and heterosexual genetic parenthood (Franklin 1997, 10), their use still remains "embedded in a naturalized and normalized logic of kinship" (Franklin 2013, 4). By restricting who can have access to infertility treatments, those who police ARTs often help to achieve gender normalization and exercise control over "the physically or socially deviant, pathological, and dangerous" (Thompson 2005, 81).

In this chapter, I analyze the power mechanisms that allow ARTs in Ukraine to reinscribe normative ideas about motherhood on the bodies of infertile women, through reinforcing the precarity of these women and encouraging them to exercise "freedom" and "autonomy" in taking care of their bodies. In particular, I examine the discourses about ARTs articulated within the framework of the state, medical professionals in fertility clinics, and infertile women who have undergone IVF treatment. The aim is to discuss the political rationalities in ART discourses in Ukraine that shape the subjectivities of infertile women by rendering certain subjectivities un/livable.

The chapter is based on ten interviews with infertile women who successfully underwent IVF, four interviews with medical professionals in fertility clinics, and six with experts in reproductive politics, conducted in Ukrainian and Russian[1] in Ukraine during a six-month period in 2013. Additionally, in order to interrogate the discourse of the state and medical professionals, I analyze national laws and decrees, and articles by obstetricians and gynecologists. To find informants from the group of medical professionals and experts, I contacted the directors of fertility clinics and experts directly by email and telephone. I recruited informants with experience of going through IVF procedures via an IVF online forum,[2] using the snowballing method; this gave me access to members of a particular social network, but it should be noted that my sample is not intended to be representative of Ukrainian society as a whole. All the women I interviewed for the project had IVF treatment between 2003 and 2010 and were between 22 and 38 years old at the time of the procedure. All my respondents were heterosexual. Nine were married and one was divorced. Five of my respondents worked as lawyers, university professors, and managers at international companies, while the other five were housewives. They shared class, sexuality, and marital status, as infertility treatment in Ukraine mainly targets middle-class, married, heterosexual couples.

Biopolitics: Normalization of Motherhood and Precarization of Infertility in ART Discourses in Ukraine

In Ukraine, the realm of biological life, reproductive health and sexuality is both an object and a tool of political strategies concerned with the stimulation of population growth and reproduction of the nation. I refer to this political rationality of population control as "biopolitics" and examine how it shapes and governs the subjectivities of infertile women seeking IVF treatment. At the state level, biopolitics, as conceptualized by Foucault, is exercised through the apparatus (dispositif) of security, which is based on the maintenance of an overall homeostasis, protecting society as a whole, as well as its individual members, from any internal dangers (Foucault 2003, 249; 2007). The Ukrainian state has identified a "demographic crisis", a major "threat to the national interests and national security of Ukraine" (Verkhovna Rada of Ukraine 2003, Ar.7), while the task of "preserving and strengthening the demographic potential of the country and overcoming the demographic crisis" is seen as a major priority for

Ukraine's national security policy (Verkhovna Rada of Ukraine 2003, Ar.8). The population of Ukraine has been steadily decreasing, from 51.8 million in 1990 to 45.4 million in 2014, with deaths consistently outnumbering births each year since 1991 (State Statistics Service of Ukraine 2014). The total fertility rate has also been decreasing, from 1.9 children per woman in 1989 to 1.0 in 2001. Although it has been increasing since then, it remained low in 2013, at 1.5 children per woman (State Statistics Service of Ukraine 2014).

In this context, the Ukrainian authorities and medical professionals see a high level of infertility as contributing to this demographic crisis. In 2010, the prevalence of primary infertility among "child-seeking women exposed to the risk of pregnancy"[3] in Ukraine was 3.3 percent and the prevalence of secondary infertility among women with a prior live birth was 22.1 percent, which is almost twice the global average (Mascarenhas *et al.* 2012, Dataset S1 and S2). Moreover, according to data from the Ministry of Healthcare of Ukraine, female infertility accounted for 78.2 percent of all 58 277 cases of infertility registered in 2013 (Ministry of Healthcare of Ukraine, letter to the author, 2014). As a result, infertility is seen almost solely as a problem connected to the reproductive health and choices of women.

In 2006, the Cabinet of Ministers of Ukraine introduced the state program "Reproductive Health of the Nation until 2015," which declared reproductive health to have strategic importance for the sustainable development of the nation, and aimed at expanding the network of services for reproductive health and family planning (Cabinet of Ministers of Ukraine 2007). Furthermore, one of the aims of the national strategy for demographic development, approved for the period 2005–2015, was to improve female reproductive health, in particular by introducing new methods of infertility treatment (Cabinet of Ministers of Ukraine 2006). Thus, it can be argued that ARTs, in their quest to produce biogenetically related offspring, became discursively framed as a solution to the demographic crisis, allowing the state to maximize the reproductive life of its citizens by alleviating childlessness in infertile women.

The operation of biopolitics is ensured through the accumulation of knowledge and the generation of discourses that configure the habits of its subjects to comply with the norm. In other words, biopolitics produces citizens who, by actively governing themselves, render their bodies useful and obedient (Foucault 1991). Along such biopolitical lines, the state discourses in Ukraine impose norms of motherhood and traditional family values on women. The creation of a family is often presented in state documents as women's natural and primary mission in life, while the failure to preserve "family values," the "moral health of the family," and "conscious parenting" are defined as key causes of the decreasing birth rate and the problems with reproductive health (Cabinet of Ministers of Ukraine 2006). The "reduction of the demographic potential of the family" is seen as being caused by the postponement of marriage and childbearing, single motherhood, a fall in the number of registered marriages, an increase in divorces, childlessness, and having only one child (Cabinet of Ministers of Ukraine 2006). The "spiritual revival of the Ukrainian nation and national "a solution to the demographic crisis," which presupposes encouraging in men and women "the desire to have and raise children" and restoring "the traditions of large families" (Cabinet of Ministers of Ukraine 2006). Moreover, childlessness and parental practices that differ from the conventional model of a full heterosexual family are deemed not "conscious," meaning irresponsible (Cabinet of Ministers of Ukraine 2006).

Additionally, we can observe the way in which the biopolitical demand for motherhood, as well as ARTs as a helping hand in achieving pregnancy, become naturalized at the level of medical professionals. Within the medical discourse about ARTs in Ukraine, the necessity to reproduce is articulated as a matter of "the health of the nation," "national security," and "the sustainable development of society" and as a matter of female biology, natural function, and even "preservation of the species" (Anon. 2007), which leads to a construction of motherhood as a natural desire situated above politics. Medical discourse also uses the tropes of demographics and family values to attach ARTs to conventional reproductive practices (Yuzko and Rudenko 2012, 46). In particular, within this discourse, reproductive medicine is associated with safe motherhood, sexual health, family planning, and population growth (Anon. 2007) and is opposed to infertility, which is identified as a "nationwide medical and social problem" (Mozgova 2005, 102), a demographic crisis, a tragedy, and a "problem of humanity" (Anon. 2007).

Medical interventions into the reproductive process are also naturalized through representations of the female body as having a "natural" need for assistance and not being complete without the interference of doctors. ARTs become a self-evident "natural" solution to the problems, while medical professionals see women wanting to become pregnant with the help of IVF as patients with "sick" mothering bodies, as opposed to "normal" patients experiencing a "spontaneous" or "physiological" pregnancy (Mozgova 2005, 102). IVF patients can be described as having "poor ovarian response" (Sudoma 2005a, 92), "inadequate immune response to pregnancy" (Mozgova 2005, 103), "ectopic pregnancy" (Sudoma 2005b, 99), "high risk of miscarriage," and other "complications during pregnancy and labor" (Mozgova 2005, 102), who are doomed to premature birth (Mozgova 2005, 108) and multiple pregnancies that "create problems for obstetrics" (Anon. 2007).

However, Ukrainian ART discourses not only educate women into desiring to become mothers; they also determine who has the right to reproduce and reflect a stratified reproduction in terms of class, gender, sexuality, and age. As the case of Valentyna demonstrates, ART discourses construct the ideal mother in such a way that she fits traditional gender, sexual, and kinship configurations, while making other subjectivities and practices precarious by not recognizing them. On the one hand, since the basis for ART treatments in Ukraine is defined only through medical indications, in particular diagnosed female and/or male infertility, there are no explicit prohibitions or legal regulations regarding the use of IVF by women above a certain age, singles, lesbian and gay couples, or unmarried heterosexual couples (Ministry of Healthcare of Ukraine 2013). On the other hand, it is strongly implied in the language of state documents that ARTs should be used primarily by heterosexual, married, middle-class couples, who are the only actors mentioned as patients in infertility treatments (Verkhovna Rada of Ukraine 2002, Ar.123).

The conjunction of discourses about the reproduction of the nation and traditional family values articulates the subject position of "mother" as the only intelligible mode of subjectivity available to women. My infertile female informants all admitted having a feeling of unfulfilled femininity because of their inability to give birth:

> I flagellated myself. All this self-hatred. I regret that I did not notice whether it was fall or winter – all that I thought about was children. That's how it is in our country: you have to get married and necessarily have children.
>
> (Patient 2)

Since childlessness and infertility do not provide legitimate subject positions for women within this discourse, even after having a baby as a result of IVF, Patient 2 had to seek psychological counseling to help her accept the fact that she could not get pregnant "naturally." Patient 3 had similar feelings:

> The feeling that you don't have a baby, that you can't get pregnant like everyone else, leaves an imprint on your whole life. If the family doesn't have children the one to blame is always the woman. Psychologically this was eating me from the inside.
>
> (Patient 3)

My informants also reported that they were pressured by their surroundings to combat infertility and undergo IVF.

> Our people aren't considerate enough. Going through all of it and being asked, as a woman in her thirties, why don't you have kids? The opinion of strangers. Still unpleasant, still hurts.
>
> (Patient 2)

A powerful way to link women to a desire to have children is to condemn and stigmatize infertility. For example, Patient 3 admitted that she "couldn't talk to anyone" about her infertility, because most of her close friends and relatives thought it was a result of her "leading life in the wrong way," being "alcoholic" and "psycho." Thus, biopolitics enacts frames of recognition, which render the lives of infertile women unlivable. In this context, the identity of being an infertile woman becomes impossible, since it is not recognized in discourses where the only way for a woman to fulfill herself is to become a mother.

I use the concept of precarity to show how infertile women are shaped as a precarious population, since they do not fit "the norms that govern the intelligibility of the body in space and time" and are not recognizable as subjects (Butler 2009b, x).

Butler argues that any life is vulnerable, since it is completely dependent on the power structures that are necessary to sustain it. However, some lives are made more precarious than others in their dependencies because they do not conform to the norms that determine what counts as a recognizable life. As a result, precarity can be defined as "that politically induced condition in which certain populations suffer from failing social and economic networks of support and become differentially exposed to injury, violence, and death" (Butler 2009a, 25).

Since infertile women are pressured to take up the subject position of "mother" and fit into the power structures that promise them secure and sustainable lives, they seek technological assistance to give birth and to reposition themselves as "normal," acting out the traditional roles of responsible mothers and caring wives. Like those medical professionals who accused Valentyna of child neglect, my informants assume that only women exhibiting certain socially approved behavior, marital status (heterosexual marriage), stable employment, housing, and financial standing should undergo IVF and become mothers. They expect their exhausting struggle for pregnancy, as well as their middle-class social position that enabled them to access infertility treatment, to prove that they are perfect candidates for motherhood. Another strategy that helps to normalize IVF is the emphasis placed by my respondents on the importance of genetic relatedness as the only "normal" grounds for kinship, implicitly marginalizing all other parenting practices. Moreover, they emphasized the role of technology in producing children of a "higher genetic quality":

> I wanted only my children, I didn't want other people's children. Even if I failed at IVF, I wouldn't go to the orphanage anyway. I think there is nothing to be ashamed about. On the contrary, taking into account how these "artificial" children are made, the best sperm and best eggs are selected … genetically they are healthier than those conceived in a drunken fling.
>
> (Patient 4)

Despite the fact that the ART discourse further stabilizes the subject position of "mother," it still does not allow infertile women to fully live out gender norms. Both inside and outside medical institutions, their pregnant bodies are made precarious. Against this background, some of my informants see their treatment as a source of "shame and embarrassment" and feel that "prejudice and incomprehension" are attached to the label "artificial children."

> We hide it from everyone, from all our relatives and friends. If you go to an ordinary hospital, people start to talk. Some nurses can say that it's better to get a dog than a child like that. Our society is not grown-up enough to accept it. Some people hide even from the doctors.
>
> (Patient 3)

Their pregnancies are perceived by obstetricians as more uncertain than "natural" ones, since as women in their thirties and often with multiple pregnancies, they are expected to be more likely to have "complications during pregnancy" and end up with miscarriages. As a result, IVF mothers are regularly put under increased medical surveillance and persuaded into hospitalization in state institutions such as prenatal care/maternity hospitals. Moreover, Patient 2 described how the age of future mothers, the number of children, and means of conception played an important role in articulating herself and her IVF offspring as not normal:

> Since we have this attitude that you are like an outcast, it's very scary. IVF is everything at once: you have a caesarean, you are too old for pregnancy, and you have twins. Some people say that these children are not normal.
>
> (Patient 2)

Neoliberal Governmentality: The Individualization of Responsibility for ARTs in Ukraine

Despite the fact that the discourse of state reproductive policy demonstrates a strategy of biopolitical management of the population through the normalization of motherhood, it also shifts the responsibility for reproductive health onto private clinics and individual women. Thus, power is also exercised through the individualization of responsibility for human life and health, which becomes detached from the state and ascribed to quasi-autonomous non-governmental entities, including private fertility clinics and individuals, who are supposed "to govern their own conduct freely" (Miller and Rose 2008, 215), "to manage their own affairs, to secure their own security with a prudential eye on the future" (Rose 2007, 4).

For example, the reality behind the pronatalist declarations in the state program "Reproductive Health of the Nation until 2015" is a lack of equipment and financial support, insufficient attention to preventive direction and primary care, limited access to services, a low level of awareness about women's reproductive health, and a lack of involvement by men in family planning. Likewise, from 2005 until 2015, the involvement of the state in the provision of medical treatment for infertility was limited to minimal state regulation and very small subsidies that covered around 500–700 IVF cycles a year in only four state fertility centers; for example, in 2013 there were 608 cycles planned for 45 573 registered infertile women (Ministry of Healthcare of Ukraine, letter to the author, 2014). Moreover, it only assisted the first attempt to use ARTs for those women aged between 19 and 40 who lack or have obstructed fallopian tubes, while male infertility was excluded altogether (Ministry of Healthcare of Ukraine 2005).

Furthermore, despite the fact that Ukraine has a national public healthcare system, the provision of ART services by public medical institutions is almost non-existent. Out of 34 fertility clinics in Ukraine, only six are state owned. However, even those do not provide the full range of ART services and have to cooperate with private fertility clinics to fulfill procedures. As a result, the number of IVF cycles conducted annually in Ukraine remains very low – 12511 cycles were conducted in 2012 for 11.3 million women of fertile age (Ministry of Healthcare of Ukraine, letter to the author, 2014).

One expert interviewed for this research argued that the field of ARTs is almost entirely governed by private fertility clinics, while the state system is characterized by corruption, limited accessibility to state medical institutions, and poor expert knowledge (Expert 1). At the same time, all my infertile female informants argued that they needed state support, since they all struggled to afford IVF and had to borrow money or take out bank loans. Patient 5 felt that there is a discrepancy between the pronatalist state discourse and the lack of actual state-supported measures to combat infertility:

> Everyone here talks about our falling birth rate, trumpets it with great force. At the same time, there are people who don't have the possibility to have children although they want to. And nobody helps them since this is seen as only their private problem.
>
> (Patient 5)

Moreover, access to ARTs is largely unregulated by the state, with very few actual restrictions, and a wide spectrum of treatments, including gestational surrogacy and donation of gametes and embryos, are legal and commodified. Against this backdrop, professionals in private fertility clinics promote their autonomy and explain the success of ARTs in the Ukraine primarily by the fact that the field is commercialized and exists independently of the public healthcare system. They view themselves as self-governing organizations and take the lead in decision-making about the implementation of ARTs and the management of infertility.

> We are trying to take the initiative, because if our politicians wrote the laws and instructions on the use of ARTs, this would mean the end of the whole field.
>
> (Doctor 1)

All my infertile female informants claimed that, regardless of the actual reason for infertility, they felt that society blamed them for it, and held them responsible for working upon their bodies to make them fertile. The state discourse reinforces this responsibility by articulating infertility as being associated with "women's diseases" and, ultimately, with the "demographic crisis." For example, the Strategy for Demographic Development mentions only the female factors of infertility and claims that one of the causes of the demographic crisis and low fertility rate in Ukraine is "poor reproductive health, especially of women" (Cabinet of Ministers of Ukraine 2006). They also claim that another cause of this crisis is the improvement in women's social status, in particular "the expansion of their interests outside the family," higher education, employment (Cabinet of Ministers of Ukraine 2006), and "the necessity to satisfy their educational, professional, and civil interests" (Cabinet of Ministers of Ukraine 2004).

Medical professionals also see women as mainly responsible for overcoming infertility. However, instead of employing arguments that draw upon the overarching biopolitical rationality of demographic crisis, they often make women responsible with the help of the discursive techniques of advanced neoliberal governmentality, in particular by articulating the treatment of infertility as a matter of individual consumer choice. Doctors construct women undergoing IVF as independent, active, and responsible customers, capable of making independent decisions regarding their own health:

> Our relationships with the patient are contractual. She is informed about the efficacy or inefficacy of the program. The patient understands what she is paying for and what she is going to get as a result. Therefore, this is her choice.
>
> (Doctor 2)

In contrast to more traditional biopolitical techniques, advanced neoliberal governmentality does not see the population as such as its target; rather, it shapes the will of autonomous bodies and regulates the choices of individual citizens (Miller and Rose 2008, 216). The primary mechanism of these neoliberal technologies is the production of self-sufficient biological citizens (Petryna 2002; Rose and Novas 2005; Heath, Rapp and Taussig 2007). In this vein, medical discourse on ARTs in Ukraine educates infertile women to take care of their health and adopt a knowledgeable relationship to their bodies.

At the same time, the majority of my infertile female informants were going into IVF treatment without a clear understanding of what to expect from their bodies. Because they lacked medical knowledge, they often felt helplessly exposed to medical staff. When Patient 1 describes her experience of the first IVF cycle, she mentions that she was behaving like an "idiot." She laughs at herself now when she explains that she did not even know how to do a pregnancy test back then. However, over the next 11 cycles she learned perfectly well how to decipher what was going on with her body in medical terms and how to control her own tests, medicine prescriptions, drug doses etc.:

> I was controlling my estrogen, progesterone. I was going to the laboratory as if I worked there. Everyone knew me there, I was coming to control my hCG every two days.
>
> (Patient 1)

My interviews with infertile female informants also reveal that another factor contributing to their taking of responsibility is the distrust they feel toward medical professionals. For example, they reported that in private fertility clinics, doctors could prescribe treatment, medicine, or tests not out of necessity, but to satisfy the profit motive. The women often felt neglected and as though they were "on a conveyor belt." Moreover, when seeking care during pregnancy in public medical institutions, they found these to be "indifferent towards patients" and exhibiting "prejudice towards IVF patients."

> I went to the ordinary women's medical consultation and they told me: "IVF? I'm not going to take you, I don't know what to do with you." I went to the head of the department: "You go there, where you got pregnant. Who knows whether the child is going to live?"
>
> (Patient 3)

When left without support from either the state or medical professionals, infertile women are encouraged to handle their infertility treatment and subsequent pregnancy independently by becoming responsible and self-governing biological citizens and conscious consumers, educating themselves about their bodies by seeking information on the Internet, acquainting themselves with the details of medical treatment, evaluating the expert opinions of doctors, and resisting the knowledge monopoly of the medical authorities (Rose 2007, 22).

> I have learned a lot during these protocols. I come sometimes to the physician, she asks me if I have a medical education, I answer: "With our medicine, even if you don't want to, you will become a physician anyway."
>
> (Patient 3)

The women were also sharing information and giving advice to each other in an online forum, which helped them to check and change prescriptions and choose between doctors and clinics. My informants also decided independently of medical staff which medicine and treatments were more appropriate. Patient 1, for example, treated herself independently according to information she found on the web:

> I prescribed myself a treatment. I found it somewhere on the Internet. When I showed the list of drugs to my doctor, she looked at me and asked: "Oh, my God, how do you handle it all?"
>
> (Patient 1)

Attached to "imperfect" bodies while being made fully responsible for their own treatment, infertile women find themselves in a precarious position. They are recognized as intelligible subjects only if they constantly seek to optimize their bodies and govern themselves with aspirations of self-actualization and self-fulfillment in motherhood. Therefore, they manage the precarity of their non-recognition through obtaining medical knowledge and educating themselves in how to care for their infertile bodies. In this way, the precarious standing of infertile women facilitates the work of power in shaping their subjectivities. Instead of being seen as an "exception," their precarity becomes a norm itself, through which power governs. Thus, "precarization in neoliberalism is currently in a process of normalization, which enables governing through insecurity" (Lorey 2015, 11).

Conclusion

This chapter has investigated how, by encouraging women to engineer their bodies and behavior according to the norm of motherhood, the discourses about ARTs in Ukraine tap into the pronatalist rhetoric of the state, which is governed by biopolitical rationality based on the normalization of motherhood. ART discourses are also informed by practices of advanced neoliberal governmentality that rely on the individualization of responsibility. I argue that the success of this biopower is facilitated by the precarious position of infertile women in the Ukrainian context. Biopolitics and advanced liberal governmentality offer frames of recognition in which all subjectivities become impossible apart from those struggling to achieve the ideal of motherhood, including the subjectivity of infertile women who are not living out gender norms in a recognizable way. Since biopower fails to sustain or protect lives that it doesn't recognize, infertile women are exposed to all sorts of insecurity, and the social conditions on which they depend become extremely uncertain. In order to manage this precarity, infertile women adapt themselves to the available subjectivities of mother and responsible, self-governed biological citizen who will optimize her body independently in order to achieve pregnancy through the practices of IVF treatment.

Notes

1 All quotes from the interviews that appear in this chapter were translated from Ukrainian and Russian into English by me.
2 Available at: http://ovulation.org.ua/forum/index.php.
3 Women were seen as exposed to the risk of pregnancy if they "were in a union, were not using contraceptives, and had a child or wished to have one" (Mascarenhas *et al.* 2012, 2).

References

Anon. 2007. "Bezpliddia – Odvichna Problema Liudstva." [Infertility – Eternal Problem of Humanity]. *Zhinochyi Likar* [*Women's Doctor*] 4. Accessed August 28, 2015. http://z-l.com.ua/ru/article/62.

Butler, Judith. 2009a. *Frames of War: When is Life Grievable?* London, New York: Verso.

Butler, Judith. 2009b. "Performativity, Precarity and Sexual Politics: Lecture Given at Universidad Complutense de Madrid." *Revista de Antropología Iberoamericana* 4/3: i–xiii. Accessed August 28, 2015. www.aibr.org/antropologia/04v03/criticos/040301b.pdf.

Cabinet of Ministers of Ukraine. 2004. "The Concept of Demographic Development for 2005–2015." Resolution from October 8, 2004 of No. 724. *Ofitsiinyi Visnyk Ukrainy* [*The Official Bulletin of Ukraine*] 41. Accessed August 28, 2015. http://zakon3.rada.gov.ua/laws/show/724–2004-p.

Cabinet of Ministers of Ukraine. 2006. "The Strategy of Demographic Development for 2005–2015." Resolution from June 24, 2006 of No. 879. *Ofitsiinyi Visnyk Ukrainy* [*The Official Bulletin of Ukraine*] 26. Accessed August 28, 2015. http://zakon3.rada.gov.ua/laws/show/879–2006-п.

Cabinet of Ministers of Ukraine. 2007. "Reproductive Health of the Nation until 2015." Resolution from December 27, 2006 of No. 1849. *Ofitsiinyi Visnyk Ukrainy* [*The Official Bulletin of Ukraine*] 1. Accessed August 28, 2015. http://zakon4.rada.gov.ua/laws/show/1849–2006-п.

Department of Healthcare of the Chernihiv Regional State Administration. 2011. "News." Accessed August 28, 2015. http://uoz.cn.ua/news135.htm.

Foucault, Michel. 1991. "Governmentality." In *The Foucault Effect: Studies in Governmentality*, edited by Graham Burchell, Colin Gordon, and Peter Miller, 87–104. Chicago: University of Chicago Press.

Foucault, Michel. 2003. *Society Must Be Defended: Lectures at the Collège de France, 1975–1976.* New York: Picador.

Foucault, Michel. 2007. *Security, Territory, Population: Lectures at the Collège de France, 1977–1978.* Basingstoke: Palgrave Macmillan.

Franklin, Sarah. 1997. *Embodied Progress: A Cultural Account of Assisted Conception.* London: Routledge.

Franklin, Sarah. 2013. *Biological Relatives: IVF, Stem Cells, and the Future of Kinship.* Durham, London: Duke University Press.

Heath, Deborah, Rayna Rapp and Karen-Sue Taussig. 2007. "Genetic Citizenship." In *A Companion to the Anthropology of Politics*, edited by David Nugent and Joan Vincent, 152–167. Oxford: Blackwell Publishing.

Lorey, Isabell. 2015. *State of Insecurity: Government of the Precarious.* London: Verso.

Mascarenhas, Maya N., Seth R. Flaxman, Ties Boerma, Sheryl Vanderpoel, and Gretchen A. Stevens. 2012. "National, Regional, and Global Trends in Infertility Prevalence since 1990: A Systematic Analysis of 277 Health Surveys." *PLoS Med* 9 (12): 1–12. Accessed August 28, 2015. doi: 10.1371/journal.pmed.1001356.

Miller, Peter, and Nikolas Rose. 2008. *Governing the Present: Administering Economic, Social and Personal Life.* Cambridge, Malden: Polity Press.

Ministry of Healthcare of Ukraine. 2005. "Procedure for Referral of Women with Absolute Indications for the First Course of Infertility Treatment with the Methods of Assisted Reproductive Technology for Budgetary Funds." Decree from November 29, 2004 of No. 579. *Ofitsiinyi Visnyk Ukrainy* [*The Official Bulletin of Ukraine*] 7. Accessed August 28, 2015. http://zakon2.rada.gov.ua/laws/show/z0224–05.

Ministry of Healthcare of Ukraine. 2013. "Guidelines of the Use of Reproductive Technologies in Ukraine." Order from September 9, 2013 of No. 787. *Ofitsiinyi Visnyk Ukrainy* [*The Official Bulletin of Ukraine*] 82. Accessed August 28, 2015. http://zakon2.rada.gov.ua/laws/show/z1697–13.

Ministry of Healthcare of Ukraine. 2014. Letter to the Author.

Mozgova, Olena. 2005. "Kompleksna Diahnostyka Ryzyku ta Poperedzhennia Zahrozy Pereryvannia Vahitnosti u Zhinok pislia Ekstrakorporalnoho Zaplidnennia." [Complex Diagnostics of the Risk and Prevention of the Threat of Miscarriage in Women after In Vitro Fertilization]. *Ukrainskyi Medychnyi Chasopys* [*Ukrainian Medical Journal*] 2 (46): 102–109. Accessed August 28, 2015. www.umj.com.ua/article/697/kompleksna-diagnostika-riziku-ta-poperedzhennya-zagrozi-pererivannya-vagitnosti-u-zhinok-pislya-ekstrakorporalnogo-zaplidnennya.

Petryna, Adriana. 2002. *Life Exposed: Biological Citizens After Chernobyl.* Princeton: Princeton University Press.

Rose, Nikolas, and Carlos Novas. 2005. "Biological Citizenship." In *Global Assemblages: Technology, Politics, and Ethics as Anthropological Problems*, edited by Aihwa Ong and Stephen. J. Collier, 439–463. Oxford, UK: Blackwell.

Rose, Nikolas. 2007. *The Politics of Life Itself: Biomedicine, Power, and Subjectivity in the Twenty-First Century*. Princeton, Oxford: Princeton University Press.

State Statistics Service of Ukraine. 2014. *Population of Ukraine in 2013: Demographic Yearbook*. Accessed August 28, 2015. www.ukrstat.gov.ua.

Sudoma, Iryna. 2005a. "Syndrom Slabkoi Vidpovidi Yaiechnykiv u Tsyklakh Ekstrakorporalnoho Zaplidnennia u Patsiientok iz Adenomiozom." [Poor Ovarian Response Syndrome in In Vitro Fertilization Cycles in Patients with Adenomyosis]. *Ukrainskyi Medychnyi Chasopys* [*Ukrainian Medical Journal*] 2 (46): 92–101. Accessed August 28, 2015. www.umj.com.ua/article/699/sindrom-slabkoi-vidpovidi-yayechnikiv-u-ciklax-ekstrakorporalnogo-zaplidnennya.

Sudoma, Iryna. 2005b. "Chastota ta Etiolohichni Faktory Ektopichnoi ta Heterotopichnoi Vahitnosti Pislia Prohram Ekstrakorporalnoho Zaplidnennia." [Frequency and Etiological Factors of Ectopic and Heterotopic Pregnancies after Extracorporeal Fertilization Programs]. *Ukrainskyi Medychnyi Chasopys* [*Ukrainian Medical Journal*] 4 (48): 99–104. Accessed August 28, 2015. www.umj.com.ua/article/641/chastota-ta-etiologichni-faktori-ektopichnoi-ta-geterotopichnoi-vagitnosti-pislya-program-ekstrakorporalnogo-zaplidnennya.

Thompson, Charis. 2005. *Making Parents: The Ontological Choreography of Reproductive Technologies*. Cambridge, London: MIT Press.

Verkhovna Rada of Ukraine. 2002. The Family Code of Ukraine. *Vidomosti Verkhovnoi Rady Ukrainy* [*The Official Bulletin of the Verkhovna Rada of Ukraine*] 21. Accessed August 28, 2015. http://zakon2.rada.gov.ua/laws/show/2947–14.

Verkhovna Rada of Ukraine. 2003. Law Of Ukraine "On the Foundations of the National Security of Ukraine." *Vidomosti Verkhovnoi Rady Ukrainy* [*The Official Bulletin of the Verkhovna Rada of Ukraine*] 39. Accessed August 28, 2015. http://zakon4.rada.gov.ua/laws/show/964–15.

Yuzko, Oleksandr, and N. Rudenko. 2012. "Stan ta Perspektyvy Rozvytku Dopomizhnykh Reproduktyvnykh Tekhnolohii Likuvannia Bezpliddia v Ukraini." [Status and Prospects of Assisted Reproductive Technologies as Infertility Treatment in Ukraine]. *Zhinochyi Likar* [*Women's Doctor*] 2: 46–49. Accessed August 28, 2015. http://z-l.com.ua/upload/journals/40/block40site9.pdf.

17 Russian Legislative Practices and Debates on the Restriction of Wide Access to ARTs

Maria Kirpichenko

In 2014 there was a Round Table in Russia on the legal regulation of surrogacy organized by the Committee on Family, Women, and Children[1] – a committee of the Russian Parliament (Duma) (Round Table in the State Duma 2014). Its purpose was to make recommendations to Parliament regarding amendments to the existing legal regulation of ARTs in Russia. As a part of the Russian Parliament, the Committee is entitled to initiate legislative work within its jurisdiction, which covers questions related to the Family Code of the Russian Federation, issues relating to the social support of orphans, material benefits to parents of minors, rights of minors, and other matters concerning minors and family support (*Reglament komiteta* n.d.). The Round Table was chaired by Elena Mizulina, a deputy of the Russian Parliament, Doctor of Law, Professor, and a well-known member of the social democratic political party "A Just Russia" (Spravedlivaya Rossiya n.d.) which occupies 64 seats in Parliament (out of 450). Mizulina is a member of the State Parliament, a chairman of the Committee on Family, Women, and Children, and a member of multiple interdepartmental work groups aimed at implementing national priority projects in the sphere of demographic policy, health care, and the rights of minors.

The aim of this chapter is to investigate how the need to limit access to ARTs is argued for, how the "problem" is located and the legislative interventions justified, and what kind of practices are rendered normative within the framework of contemporary legislative initiatives in the sphere of ARTs in Russia.

My engagement with this issue was provoked by an article on a web forum devoted to ARTs in Russia (Lebedev 2014). The article reported on the Round Table, in which the author had participated. It seemed that the Round Table resonated all too well with current family policy-making in Russia, which has been heavily criticized by (feminist) researchers.[2] This triggered my interest and I sought out more material on the issue. I decided to explore the productive and representative short-cuts and silences (un)consciously employed by many Round Table participants in order to reduce the complexity of the social world to a state of reductive and simplistic clarity.

According to Foucault (2007), the law is highly normative. It codifies norms and leaves no space for alternatives, it prescribes and prohibits. The law produces discursive, subjectifying, and lived effects on bodies and subjects (Bacchi

2009). Any transgression of the law is punishable. Legal incentives are generated as a response to social problems, but what is "a social problem"? In line with feminist researcher Carol Bacchi (2009), it is the discursive construction of "social problems" that attracts my analytical gaze in this chapter. From this analytical perspective, borrowed from Bacchi, policy-making is a process of framing and constructing representations of social problems and transporting them into the legal code (Bacchi 2009). Therefore, it is of crucial importance to critically interrogate the way in which a "problem" is shaped within the logics of a legislative initiative.

The main object of my analysis in this chapter is the *Recommendations of the Round Table "Legal regulation of surrogacy: a family-legal aspect"* (*Recommendations* 2014), presented to the Parliament of the Russian Federation, and two verbatim reports of the debate at the Round Table (*Verbatim Report of the Round Table* 2014 and a *Report from the Round Table of the Russian Association of Human Reproduction Members* 2014). Apart from addressing the rights and responsibilities of the people involved in surrogacy arrangements, the Recommendations suggest limiting access to ARTs to married heterosexual couples in need of infertility treatment. One of the verbatim reports, written by a Round Table participant, can be publicly accessed on his blog (*Verbatim Report of the Round Table* 2014; Moskovkin 2014). The text provides a useful insight into the debate at the Round Table meeting, even though it only represents the specific perspective of its author. Another source is a report from the Russian Association of Human Reproduction (*Kruglyi stol v Gosudarstvennoi Dume. Vpechatlenia chlenov RARCh. "Pravovoe regulirovanie surrogatnogo materinstva: semeino-pravovoi aspekt 2014*)[3] which also participated in the meeting.[4] This report provides an account of the event, including a detailed description of procedures.

Legal Regulation of ARTs in Russia

The first IVF baby in the Soviet Union was born in 1986. Nevertheless, it is hard to find legislative traces of ARTs before 1993 when the law "Fundamentals of Legislation on Health Care"[5] was adopted. This law was superseded by a new Federal Law,[6] passed in 2011, which is still in force. The new law defines ARTs as "methods of infertility treatment when some or all stages of conception and early embryo development take place outside the maternal organism (including use of donor and/or cryopreserved germ cells, tissues of reproductive organs, and embryos as well as surrogacy)."[7] This law is the main legal document regulating the use of ARTs in Russia.[8]

The Federal Law currently in force uses the following categories when specifying who is eligible for ART treatments: married/unmarried couples and single women.[9] The category of single men does not appear in the text. However, according to several adjudications, single men have managed to claim their right to parental custody of children born as a result of surrogacy arrangements (Svitnev 2012; Konnov and Gracheva 2013). Several courts have ruled that single men should be granted parental rights in analogy with single mothers

(Svitnev 2012). At a formal level, the law permits rather wide access to ARTs. However, accessibility is in reality very restricted due to the high cost of treatments compared to average salaries (Brednikova, Nartova, and Tkach 2009).

According to V. Korsak, President of the Russian Association of Human Reproduction, about 360,000 treatment cycles performed between 1995 and 2011 resulted in about 80,000 children born in Russia (Rossiiskoe Informacionnoe Agentstvo 2013). In 2011, about 120 private centers provided 65 percent of the overall ART treatments in the country (ibid.).

A number of researchers within the field of medical legislation have criticized the current regulation of ARTs in Russia. They stress inconsistency in the use of medical terms, lack of clarity about the embryo's legal status, lack of clarity regarding the rights and duties of the parties involved in the use of ARTs, and an absence of restrictions on germ cell cryopreservation, usage, and storage (Sergeev and Pavlova 2006; Pavlova 2007; Chikin 2008; Samoilova 2012; Sokolova and Mulenko 2013). Some legal researchers argue for the restriction and regulation of ARTs in line with current, "traditionalist" family policies (Romanovsky 2010), while others describe contemporary Russian legislation in the field as progressive, in terms of protecting the individual's "reproductive rights" (Pavlova 2007), compared with that of many Western countries (Svitnev 2010; Konnov and Gracheva 2013). However, whether wishing for more restrictions or celebrating the progressiveness of Russian legislation in terms of protecting reproductive rights, these researchers all agree that the legal regulation of ARTs in Russia has multiple inconsistencies and "blind spots." This leads to it giving the impression of being simultaneously a rather permissive policy with wide access and imposing quotas for citizens to obtain economic support for infertility treatment.

At the Round Table, the "problem" to be dealt with regarding ARTs in general and surrogacy in particular was constructed as "lack of regulation." Invited participants were parliamentary speakers, experts in the sphere of children's and family rights, medical experts, and Russian Orthodox Church assignees. The meeting resulted in *Recommendations* to Parliament to introduce changes in the Law regulating ARTs. These cover issues of access, the rights and responsibilities of intended parents and surrogates, and, moreover, the question of "informational propaganda" about surrogacy and germ cell donation. The Round Table was declaratively focused upon surrogacy, and it is surrogacy that the preamble of the *Recommendations* addresses directly. However, the document also proposes, more generally, that Parliament should limit access to all kinds of ARTs.

The Round Table had no legislative power as such. But since the *Recommendations* to Parliament were generated by a Parliamentary committee (the aforementioned Committee on Family, Women, and Children), they have the status of a legal initiative and have the potential to trigger (or to legitimize) legislative work.

Theoretical Foundations and Analytical Material

This chapter is inspired by the analytical framework of "What is the problem represented to be?" approach developed by Carol Bacchi (2009). Bacchi's approach is intended to demystify the process of policy-making. It creates a distance to the problem representations of policy-makers, opening them up for critical interrogation and strategic interventions (Bacchi 2009). It provides an analytical instrument to tease out the "problem" as it was shaped at the Round Table and embedded in the *Recommendations.*

The *Recommendations* of the Round Table, which make up one part of my data material, had at least two editions. In the latest version, some points were excluded[10] (see Lebedev 2014). The most recent version, which was re-written by a working group of the Committee and sent to the Round Table participants about a month after the meeting, consists of a preamble and 17 points. Apart from addressing the rights and responsibilities of those who are involved in surrogacy arrangements, the *Recommendations* propose limiting access to ARTs to married couples in need of infertility treatment.

Another part of my data material, the *Verbatim Reports* of the Round Table,[11] will provide a rhetorical context for my analysis of the *Recommendations*, and my discussion of the ways in which the "problem" to be solved was constructed. I will undertake a cross-cutting analysis of the *Recommendations*, the *Verbatim Report*, and a corpus of legislative documents regulating family policy in Russia. The latter consists of the *Concept of Family Policy until 2025*, the *Concept of Demographic Policy until 2025* and the so-called "*Propaganda Law*," forbidding the "promotion" of homosexuality.

The *Concept of Family Policy until 2025*[12] was initiated by the Committee on Family, Women, and Children. The text of the document suggests and justifies a strategy for family policy in Russia until 2025 based on "traditional values." The *Concept of Demographic Policy until 2025*[13] is an official document signed by the President. It elaborates strategies for overcoming demographic decline and proclaims this to be an issue of national priority. Elena Mizulina is one of the main proponents of the "Propaganda Law"[14] passed in 2013. This law subjects "propaganda of untraditional sexual relations" to administrative liability. The law created a stir at both national and international levels, bringing the issue of "homosexualism"[15] to the forefront of public debates in Russia. The law's text and the Parliamentary readings of it demonstrate that contemporary family policy is embedded in homophobic discourses, channeled by the Committee on Family, Women, and Children and by Elena Mizulina herself.

Biopolitics of the Russian State

Achieving replacement level and then growth of the population are priorities for current social policy in Russia, and the issue of demography has, indeed, been on the political agenda of the Russian state since the Second World War. In the 1990s (after the collapse of the Soviet Union) the mortality rate outpaced the birthrate, and average longevity declined (*Concept of Demographic Policy until 2025*, part 2). It is against this background that concerns about underpopulation are articulated in the *Concept of Demographic Policy until 2025*. Consequently, the document highlights the importance of providing wide access to health care, especially in the sphere of reproductive medicine and ARTs.

Legally, wide access to ARTs is coupled with medical insurance quotas for those who undergo infertility treatment. According to the law,[16] IVF is part of "the highly technological medical care supply" covered by the medical insurance scheme. Quotas are allocated regionally and provide an average amount for the cost of treatment. However, quotas are available only on medical indications, which excludes the so-called social infertility of, among others, single women and men who, nevertheless, still constitute an eligible category for ARTs according to Federal Law.

In order to be placed on a quota waiting list one has to undergo multiple medical check-ups, submit a set of documents and get approval from the special Commission of the Ministry of Health and the Russian Academy of Medical Sciences (Brednikova *et al.* 2009). Formally, the number of attempts is not limited; however, to make a second try one has to collect the documents again from the outset and await one's turn (on the waiting list) for a long time, which might exceed a year.

Access to ARTs is mentioned in the *Concept of Demographic Policy until 2025* as a means to solve Russia's demographic problems; in this document, wide access to ARTs is presented as an issue of national importance. However, along with providing access to healthcare facilities and designing other strategies for improving the demographic situation, the *Concept* also endorses the propagation of "traditional family values" and, as I shall discuss, this endorsement has been picked up by the government as the most promising direction for family policy.

Even though measures to increase the birthrate are seen as only one of many strategies to overcome the demographic decline, alongside improving the average life expectancy and living standards, fertility – or more precisely, women's reproductive capacity – has become the main target of social policy (Gurko 2008; Rivkin-Fish 2010; Jarskaya-Smirnova 2010; Shpakovskaya and Chernova 2010; Leykin 2011; Rozenholm and Savkina 2011; Sperling 2015).

Both D. Medvedev and V. Putin (both in the capacity of Prime Minister and President of Russia between 2000 and today) have publicly linked the demographic crisis to the low birthrate (*Restriction of Reproductive Rights in Russia* 2012). They have constructed a public rhetoric of "women's obligations to solve the demographic issue," which poses a threat to the nation (ibid.; Rozenholm and Savkina 2009; Shpakovskaya and Chernova 2010; Leykin 2011; Sperling 2015). The causal link between survival of the nation and women's reproductive capacity serves to legitimize the pronatalist, neotraditionalist (Zhurzhenko 2004; Rivkin-Fish 2010), and neofamilial (Teplova 2007) character of social policy.

The gradual restriction of abortion legislation is a case in point. After Putin's ascent to power, the list of social indications for second-trimester pregnancy termination (within the medical insurance scheme) was reduced to: deprivation of parental rights, the woman's imprisonment, the husband's disability or death, and rape.[17] Since 2012, the list has included only rape.[18] In May 2015, Mizulina submitted two legal incentives to the Russian Parliament. One of them bans the retail sale of abortion medicines. The other aims to withdraw abortion from the medical insurance scheme altogether and from the domain of private clinics. As Denisov, Sakevich, and Jasilioniene (2012) critically point out, since 2000, the policy regarding reproduction has mainly been aimed at preventing abortions by, for example, introducing psychologists and social workers to abortion clinics to persuade women to go through with the pregnancy. As also documented in a written statement from The Henrich Böll Foundation (*Restrictions of Reproductive Rights in Russia* 2012), the Health Ministry's officials refer explicitly to their collaboration with orthodox conservative organizations such as the Socio-Cultural Initiatives Foundation[19] (chaired by Medvedev's wife Svetlana Medvedeva) and the National Glory Center.[20] The latter launched two programs: "Give me Life!" and "Sanctity of Motherhood" with the purpose of "saving the lives of unborn children" (ibid.) and intending "to promote an image of the full family with three or more children as a social norm, and to contribute to steady demographic growth in the country." (Vserossiiskaya Programma "Svyatost Materinstva" n.d.)

It should be mentioned that "marriage" and "family" in the legal context of the Russian Federation refer to a heterosexual union only. However, neither the Constitution of the Russian Federation nor the Family Code directly prohibit same-sex marriages. Nevertheless, other forms of state recognition are not practiced, and cohabitation of heterosexual couples has no legal status either. A few attempts have been made to litigate the refusal of The Civil Registry Office[21] to register same-sex couples. But all these attempts have so far failed. According to the Supreme Constitutional Court Order, marriage is a biological union between a man and a woman and:

> According to the Constitution of the Russian Federation, as well as to the international legal obligations observed by the Russian Federation, the state is not responsible for propaganda, support, or recognition of same-sex unions. Meanwhile, the absence of such formal acknowledgement [of same-sex unions] does not influence the level of recognition or guarantees of rights and freedoms of a citizen of the Russian Federation.[22]

In addition to the *Concept of Demographic Policy until 2025*, which ensures wide access to ARTs as a means of solving the demographic crisis, ARTs are also discussed in the *Concept of Family Policy until 2025*. Here, the approach to ARTs is rather different. The *Concept of Family Policy until 2025* suggests reducing the number of divorces (by, for example, higher divorce taxation); reducing extra-marital births and abortions; increasing the birthrate per family; financially stimulating large families; and regulating ARTs and surrogacy by limiting access.

Taken together, these two documents offer an insight into the contradictory strategies and ambiguities involved in contemporary Russian demographic policies.

ARTs vs "Traditional Family": What Is the Problem?

Both the *Recommendations* and the *Concept of Family Policy until 2025* propose that access to ARTs should be limited to married couples who are in need of infertility treatment. This indicates that the two documents represent wide access to ARTs as a major "problem." With a point of departure in Bacchi's aforementioned "What is the problem represented to be?" approach (Bacchi 2009), I shall now discuss how this particular "problem" representation is made to cohere. First of all, the *Recommendations* make it clear that it is the institution of marriage that makes some individuals eligible for ARTs. It is the civil registration of the couple, implying the state's recognition of their union, that forms the family. Second, in the *Concept of Family Policy until 2025*, the family is defined as the fundamental basis of Russian society and a stronghold of traditional values, which the state's family policy protects and strengthens:

> It is through the family that new generations develop the spiritual qualities intrinsic to their nature. The family acquires immortality in the memory and faith of the generations.... The family reflects a specific worldview and the idea of societal development in the national consciousness of an ancient Russian individual. The Russian Orthodox Church strengthens the spiritual meaning of kinship and family. Thus the family stands not only for a social union of spouses and children, but it is also a spiritual cell and a "small church."
>
> (*Concept of Family Policy until 2025*, 1.1)

This passage establishes a link between the family, the Russian Orthodox Church, and the state. As Butler (2014) points out with reference to the Orthodox Church, it is the Church that embodies the spirit of the nation, proclaiming nationalism a sacred passion. In this way, the separation of Church and State fails (Butler 2014). It is through the family that the Church makes the state vigilant and ubiquitous.

The icon of "the family," as articulated in the *Recommendations*, draws its meaning from the general ideological context provided by the *Concept of Family Policy until 2025*, and is presented as a key factor in the execution of legislative power. The concepts "traditional" and "the family" are at the core of meaning-making. In the Russian context, "traditional" connotes values proclaimed by the Orthodox Church (even though, according to the Constitution, Russia is a multi-ethnic and multi-religious secular state[23]). However, it remains obscure what kind of "traditionalism" is desired by the policy-makers and what its relation to spirituality and the Orthodox Church actually is.

The growing influence of the Church on political decision-making must be understood in the context of its restoration in the wake of the Soviet period, when it was persecuted and almost destroyed. During Soviet times, the Russian

Orthodox Church was more likely to be presented as an antagonist of the national idea, seen from the point of view of the official rhetoric of the government. In this respect, the *Concept of Family Policy* refers negatively to the Soviet era when "the Bolsheviks were deliberately destroying the family … [and] breaking the connection between marriage, religion and the Church" (*Concept of Family Policy until 2025*, 2.12).

In addition, Russian monarchism, which is inseparable from the Church, is also being idealized as a contrast to the Soviet past. Moreover, an idealized version of the "traditional" pre-Soviet past is contributing to a brand of nationalism which implies opposition to the West: "[as a result of the Soviet period] Russia is actively involved in the system of relationships inherent to Western civilization, which idolizes human rights and freedoms, including the rights of sexual minorities" (*Concept of Family Policy until 2025*, 2.12). So the "West," "civil rights," and "sexual minorities" are opposed to monarchic Russia, national authenticity, orthodoxy, and "the family."

The "family," hailed as the "happy object" of the state (Ahmed 2010), and which, against this background, performs as a self-evident concept for policymakers to promote, refers in this context to the conjugal heterosexual couple valorized as an ideal for parenting and as the only possible place where (only procreative) sex should take place (Cutas and Chan 2012, 2). According to the implied norms, the family union has to be composed of two able-bodied, heterosexual, *sui juris*, non-kindred adults who are romantically and sexually involved with each other and who procreate genetically related and "naturally" conceived children. The "family ideal," to which the Russian family policy refers, thus has a (hetero)normalizing effect, deeming other family constellations to fall outside the norm and outside happiness.

In these discourses, ARTs are constructed as capable of producing outcomes that might potentially change the imaginary content of the given state-sustained "family" ideal and provoke uncertainties for the biopolitics of the state. Framed as "an exceptional measure of infertility treatment," ARTs raise the question of whether or not these technologies are to be seen as a medical issue, since medical conditions are, as a rule, not cured by ARTs. These technologies are used as an alternative means of conception/childbearing. ARTs are rather an issue of a social character, used instrumentally in the context of the *Recommendations* to determine who is eligible for parenting and for building "the family." It is directly pointed out in the *Concept of Family Policy*: "Traditional family values include the value of marriage, which is understood only as a union of a man and a woman … with the intent to give birth to and bring up three or more children" (*Concept of Family Policy until 2025*, 1.4).

Hence, the dichotomy of fertility–infertility leans toward hierarchical relationships, in which infertility is seen as a deviation from the norm (Brednikova and Nartova 2007), which is powered by "the family" icon, including the associated expectations of procreation. This results in the stigmatization of infertile people, since ARTs are not only a way of "making" children, but also a way of "making" parents (Thompson 2005; Spilker 2008).

"The Problem" Is Not a Problem: Abjecting Homosexuals

Wide access to ARTs is represented as a "problem" because it threatens the traditional family icon. But what is it that makes wide access to ARTs a threat to "the family"?

Access to ARTs is understood as an opportunity for "homosexuals to get children because they want to be a full-value family."[24] This point of view is also supported by the "problem" identified by the Round Table: "Christian morality condemns child trading and homosexualism" and "When ART is for same-sex couples it is a threat to the nation" (Verbatim Report of the Round Table 2014; Moskovkin 2014).

This is a typical biopolitical representation that is associated with what Foucault calls "state racism," referring to the permanent need for purification of the state from internal threats to the norm and obedience to maintain itself as homogeneous and monist (Foucault 2003, 61–62). Via parenting, same-sex couples might enter into family-building that falls outside the iconic orthodox path and therefore threatens the vigilantism and ubiquity of the state. Then the language of morality is employed as an instrument of repressive power that outlaws some bodies from citizenship (Butler 2014). However, there is not a word about same-sex couples in the *Recommendations*. This aspect of the "problem" is silenced. Gays are rendered invisible and thus ignored. Queer lifestyles are not called into existence by naming them – as an abject they are positioned outside the intelligible, deemed to have no agency at all, to be non-existent.

This ignorance allows policy-makers to deny any kind of discrimination against gays in Russia – a stance demonstrated clearly when, for example, during parliamentary readings of the "Propaganda Law," Mizulina implied that the law is exclusively aimed at the protection of minors,[25] where "propaganda" is defined as:

> distribution of information, directed to shape untraditional sexual guidelines for minors, views on the attractiveness of untraditional sexual relations, distorted perceptions about the social equivalence of traditional and untraditional sexual relations ... imposing information about untraditional sexual relations which provokes interest...
>
> (*Verbatim Report of the Parliamentary Readings* 2013)

The Round Table's way of legitimizing the position that access to ARTs should be limited is embedded in homophobic discourses which resonate with the general discursive universe of the Committee on Family, Women, and Children. But the *Recommendations* never present same-sex family-building and relationships as part of the "problem."

Playing the National Card

During the Round Table (Round Table in the State Duma 2014), and in more general public media addresses,[26] "the nation" was forcefully mobilized to explain why legislative interventions were needed to limit wide access to ARTs. "The nation" in these discourses appeared as: (1) the link between the Orthodox Church, the state, and the individual; (2) an opposition to the "West"; and, at the same time, (3) the follower of an alleged "general Western trend" toward limiting access to surrogacy and ARTs. The Round Table primarily focused on surrogacy, and it was surrogacy regulation that was mainly discussed. However, somewhat contradictorily, the "general trend" toward limiting access to surrogacy and "artificial conception" was constructed through references to several countries where policy designs regarding ARTs, de facto, range from permissive to restrictive (in terms of the classification by Engeli and Rothmayr Allison, this volume).

Furthermore, some problem constructions of the Round Table played the national card in terms of setting up a moral hierarchy between Russia and other countries: "What do you think about surrogacy agencies in Italy arranging surrogacy tourism to Russia?" and "Only 15 countries out of 200 have permitted surrogacy, and half of them because of morality collapse!" (*Verbatim Report of the Round Table* 2014). The first statement suggests that the Russian state is being exploited by Western capitalism via access to surrogacy; the other that surrogacy is immoral, and, as a nation, Russia has a mission to preserve traditional family values.

The construction of a moral hierarchy corresponds to the idea of "Moscow as the Third Rome" (after Rome and Byzantium) originating from the end of the fifteenth – beginning of sixteenth century and still promoted by the Orthodox Church in Russia, implying that the Russian state has a mission to stand as the last bastion of faith and morality.[27] Hence, a reason for limiting access to ARTs is found in the opposition between Russia and the "West" (where the latter is constructed, for example, with reference to gay marriages or feminism). At the same time it is stated in the motivational part of the *Preamble of the Recommendations* that "It is no coincidence that the legislation of the countries that allow surrogacy contains considerable limitations as to the application of this method" (*Recommendations* 2014). This statement is followed by a list of countries (some European countries, some states of the USA, Israel) where the use of *surrogacy* (not ARTs) is limited by law. However, the logic of the *Recommendations* is disrupted. The document suggests limiting access to ARTs on the grounds of legal restrictions on surrogacy in other countries. In the overall discursive framework of the Round Table, these countries were constructed as representing "immoral" conditions, but, at the same time, they appeared to be role-models of restrictive regulation of ARTs. In this way, the Round Table's arguments for limiting access to ARTs are adjusted to the aims and, moreover, used inconsistently.

Conclusion

In order to justify legislative intervention on ARTs in Russia, policy-makers represent the "problem" as this: wide access to ARTs threatens the "traditional family" and therefore the state. By policing access to parenting, the state protects "the family" icon and its own investment in it with help from the Orthodox Church.

Representing ARTs as a moral problem, as suggested by Mizulina's Committee, is a rather recent phenomenon in Russian policy-making. The *Concept of Demographic Policy until 2025* still describes ARTs as measures for stimulating the birthrate. This has changed in the discourses of the Round Table and its promotion of "traditional values." As demonstrated in my analysis, the latter discourses are full of inconsistencies. The discourses of the Round Table explicitly focus on "traditional family values." Limiting access to ARTs to married couples (of a man and a woman) contributes to the simplistic paradigm of the nuclear/sexual family. It generates social pressures and expectations of procreation and happiness that are sometimes unattainable. It abjectifies queer people in Russia and stigmatizes those who fall outside "the family" ideal by rendering some practices normative: i.e., those that relate to engaging in a heterosexual conjugal union (preferably orthodox) as the only way of parenting. Finally, "the nation" is paradoxically represented in this rhetoric as both the follower of an alleged "Western trend" to restrict access to ARTs and as an active opponent of "Western values." In this way, the arguments are clearly adjusted to the ends.

Even if the initiative to amend the existing legislation, represented by the Round Table and the *Recommendations*, does not enter into legal force in the near future, my analysis demonstrates the process of "problem" shaping for the sake of legislative intervention and reveals normativities of current family and ART policy in Russia.

Notes

1 Komitet Gosudarstvennoi Dumy po voprosam Semji, Zhenchin i Detei [Committee on Family, Women, and Children of the Russian Parliament] n.d.
2 Zhurzhenko 2004; Teplova 2007; Gurko 2008; Jarskaya-Smirnova 2010; Rivkin-Fish 2010; Shpakovskaya and Chernova 2010; Leykin 2011; Rozenholm and Savkina 2011; Denisov, Sakevich, and Jasilioniene 2012; Sperling 2015.
3 Rossiiskaya Associaciya Reprodukcii Cheloveka [Russian Association of Human Reproduction] n.d.
4 Even though registration is required to access some content of the webpage of the Association, the report can be found with a simple web search. I provide a web link to the document in the literature list (*Verbatim Report of the Round Table* 2014; Moskovkin 2014).
5 *Osnovy zakonodatelstva Rossiiskoi Federacii ob ohrane zdorovja grazhdan* [Fundamentals of Legislation on the Health Care of the citizens of the Russian Federation] 1993.
6 *Federalnyi Zakon №323 "Ob osnovah zdorovjya grazhdan v Rossiiskoi Federatsii"* [Federal Law №323 "On the basics of health protection of citizens in Russian Federation"] 2011.

7 Ibid.

8 This sphere is also regulated by:

- *Semeinyi Kodeks Rossiiskoi Federatsii* [The Family Code of the Russian Federation] 1995.
- *Federalnyi Zakon ob aktah grazhdanskogo sostoyanija №143* [The Federal Law on the Acts of Civil Status №143] 1997, Part 5, art.16.
- *Federalnyi Zakon №323 "Ob osnovah zdorovjya grazhdan v Rossiiskoi Federatsii"* [Federal Law №323 "On the basics of health protection of Russian Federation citizens"] 2011, art.55.
- *Prikaz Minzdrava Rossii №107 "O poryadke ispolzovaniya vspomogatelnyh reproduktivnyh tehnologyi, protivokazaniyah i ogranicheniyah k ih primeneniju"* [The Executive Order of the Ministry of Health №107 "The order of use of ARTs, contradictions and limitations"] 2012.
- *Prikaz Minzdrava Rossii №556 "Ob utverzhdenyi standarta meditsinskoi pomochi pri besplodii s ispolzovaniem vspomogatelnyh reproduktivnyh tehnologyi"* [The Executive Order of the Ministry of Health №556 "On the approval of the standard of health treatment in cases of infertility by the use of ARTs"] 2012.
- *Postanovlenie Pravitelstva Rossiiskoi Federatsii №932 "O programme gosudarstvennyh garantyi besplatnogo okazaniya grazhdanam meditsinskoi pomoschi na 2014–2016"* [Decree of the Russian Federation Government №932 "About the state guarantees for the free provision of medical care for the citizens 2014–2016"] 2013.

9 Rus. "одинокая женщина" which connotes being lonely.

10 These were: (1) introducing a special board consisting of social workers and the Orthodox Church assignees, which was meant to decide whether a married couple was eligible for surrogacy or not; (2) prohibition of any intermediary services in regard to surrogacy; (3) only a relative of a couple could become a surrogate – see Lebedev 2014 for an overview.

11 One made by an individual Round Table participant and the other by representatives of the Russian Association of Human Reproduction, who were also present at the meeting. I will refer to the first one as it provides a better insight into the debate.

12 *Kontsepsiya Gosudarstvennoi Semeinoi Politiki Rossiiskoi Federatsii na period do 2025 goda* [Concept of Family Policy of the Russian Federation until 2025] 2013. This document is a public project which implies public discussion and the possibility of introducing changes. I am referring to the edition that is available on the official webpage of the Committee on February 9, 2015.

13 *Kontseptsiya Demograficheskoi Politiki Rossiiskoi Federatsii do 2025, utverzhdennaya Prikazom Prezidenta Rossiiskoi Federatsii №1351* [Concept of Demographic Policy of the Russian Federation until 2025, approved by the Order of the President of the Russian Federation №1351] 2007.

14 *Federalnyi Zakon №135 "O zaschite detei ot informatsii, prichinyauschei vred ih zdorovju i razvitiju"* [Federal Law №135 "On Protection of Minors from Information Causing Harm to their Health and Development"] 2013.

15 This term was used in the wording of the law before the second Parliamentary Readings.

16 *Postanovlenie Pravitelstva Rossiiskoi Federatsii №932 "O programme gosudarstvennyh garantyi besplatnogo okazaniya grazhdanam meditsinskoi pomoschi na 2014–2016"* [Decree of the Government №932 "About the State Guarantees for the Free Provision of Medical Care for Citizens 2014–2016"] 2013.

17 *Postanovlenie Pravitelstva Rossiiskoi Federatsii №485 "O perechne socialnyh pokazanii dlya iskusstvennogo preryvaniya beremennosti."* [Decree of the Government of the Russian Federation №485 "About the List of Social Indications for Abortion"] 2003.

18 *Postanovlenie Pravitelstva Rossiiskoi Federatsii №98 "O socialnom pokazanii dlya iskusstvennogo preryvanija beremennosti"* [Decree of the Government of the Russian Federation №98 "About social indication for abortion"] 2012.
19 Fond Socialno-Kulturnyh Iniciativ [Socio-Cultural Initiatives Foundation] n.d.
20 Centr Natcionalnoi Slavy [National Glory Center] n.d.
21 Rus. ЗАГС.
22 *Postanovlenie Konstitutsionnogo suda Rossiiskoi Federatsii №496* [Supreme Constitutional Court order №496] 2006.
23 See Preamble and art.14 of *Konstitucija Rossiiskoi Federatsii* [Constitution of the Russian Federation] 1993.
24 Mizulina 2013, min. 31:50.
25 See the *Verbatim Report of the Parliamentary Readings* (2013) *Stenogramma rassmotreniya Federalnogo Zakona №135 "O zashchite detei ot informatsii, prichinyayushchei vred ih zdorov'yu i razvitiju"* [Verbatim Report of the Parliamentary Readings of the Federal Law №135 "On Protection of Minors from Information Causing Harm to Their Health and Development"].
26 See, for example, Mizulina 2013.
27 There are various religious and (geo)political interpretations of the concept, however.

References

Ahmed, Sarah. 2010. *The Promise of Happiness*. Durham: Duke University Press.

Bacchi, Carol. 2009. *Analyzing Policy: What's The Problem Represented to Be?* Pearson: Frenchs Forest.

Brednikova, Olga, and Nadya Nartova. 2007. "Narushaya molchanie: diskriminaciya zhenzchin v prostranstve novyh reproduktivnyh tehnologyi." [Breaking the Silence: Female Discrimination Within the Field of ARTs]. In *Sovremennaya Zhenshchina, Semja, Demographija* [Contemporary Woman, Family, Demography], edited by Olga Zdravomyslova, 156–181. Moscow: Zvenja.

Brednikova, Olga, Nadya Nartova, and Olga Tkach. 2009. "Assisted Reproduction in Russia. Legal Regulation and Public Debates." In *Making Bodies, Persons and Families. Normalizing Reproductive Technologies in Russia, Switzerland and Germany*, edited by Willemijn de Jong and Olga Tkach, 43–56. Berlin: LIT Verlag.

Butler, Judith. 2014. "Performing the Political." Paper presented at The First Super Symposium, Oslo, 2014. Accessed November 27, 2014. www.thefirstsuppersymposium.org/index.php/en/text-from-the-symposium.

Centr Natcionalnoi Slavy [National Glory Center]. n.d. Official Webpage. Accessed November 7, 2015. http://cnsr.ru/.

Chikin, Vladimir. 2008. "Semeino-Pravovoe Regulirovanie Primineniya VRT." [Family-Legal Regulation of ARTs Application]. *Juridichesky mir* [*Juridical world*] 11: 42–44.

Cutas, Daniela, and Sarah Chan. 2012. "Introduction. Perspectives on private and family life." In *Families: Beyond the Nuclear Ideal*, edited by Daniela Cutas and Sarah Chan, 1–12. London: Bloomsbury Academic.

Denisov, Boris, Viktoria Sakevich, and Aiva Jasilioniene. 2012. "Divergent Trends in Abortion and Birth Control Practices in Belarus, Russia and Ukraine." *PLoS ONE* 7 (11). Accessed October 8, 2015. http://journals.plos.org/plosone/article?id=10.1371/journal.pone.0049986.

Federalnyi Zakon №323 ot 11.21.2011 "Ob osnovah zdorovjya grazhdan v Rossiiskoi Federatsii" [Federal Law from 11.21.2011 №323 "On the Basics of Health Protection of Citizens in Russian Federation"]. 2011. Accessed October 24, 2014. http://base.consultant.ru/cons/cgi/online.cgi?req=doc;base=LAW;n=166059.

Federalnyi Zakon №135 "O zaschite detei ot informatsii, prichinyauschei vred ih zdorovju i razvitiju" [Federal Law from 06.29.2013 №135 "On Protection of Minors from Information Causing Harm to their Health and Development"]. 2013. Accessed November 26, 2014. http://base.garant.ru/70403756/.

Federalnyi Zakon ob aktah grazhdanskogo sostoyanija ot 11.15.1997 №143 [Federal Law on the Acts of Civil Status from 11.15.1997 №143]. 1997. Accessed October 24, 2014. http://base.consultant.ru/cons/cgi/online.cgi?req=doc;base=LAW;n=164546.

Fond Socialno-Kulturnyh Iniciativ [Socio-Cultural Initiatives Foundation]. n.d. Official webpage. Accessed November 7, 2015. www.fondsci.ru/.

Foucault, Michel. 2003. *Society Must Be Defended. Lectures at the Collège de France, 1975–1976*. New York: Picador.

Foucault, Michel. 2007. *Security, Territory, Population. Lectures at the Collège de France, 1977–1978*. New York: Picador.

Gurko, Tatiana. 2008. "Rossiya: Socialnaya Politika v otnoshenii molodyh roditelei" [Russia: Social Policy in Regard to Young Parents]. *Vlast* 6: 10–4. http://istoki-foundation.org/ru/programmers/holiness.

Jarskaya-Smirnova, Elena. 2010. "Cennostno-Simvolicheskoe Prostranstvo Semeinoi Politiki." [Axiological and Symbolic Space of Family Policy]. *Demoscope Weekly* 409–410. Accessed October 8, 2015. www.demoscope.ru/weekly/2010/0409/analit05.php.

Komitet Gosudarstvennoi Dumy po voprosam Semji, Zhenchin i Detei [Committee on Family, Women, and Children of the Russian Parliament]. n.d. Official Webpage. Accessed December 16, 2015. http://komitet2–6.km.duma.gov.ru/.

Konnov, Viktor, and Marina Gracheva. 2013. "Vsomogatelnie Reproduktivnie Tehnologii v Svete Garanty Prava na Uvagenie Chastnoi Zhizni. Analiz Rossyiskogo Zakonodatelstva i Praktiki Evropeiskogo Suda po Pravam Cheloveka." [Assisted Reproductive Technologies in the Light of Guarantees of Respect of Privacy. Analysis of Russian Legislation and Judicial Practice of European Court of Human Rights]. *Vestnik MGOU* 3. Accessed November 27, 2014. www.evestnik-mgou.ru/Articles/View/439.

Konstitucija Rossiiskoi Federatsii ot 12.12.1993 [The Constitution of the Russian Federation]. 1993. Accessed November 23, 2014. http://constitution.kremlin.ru/.

Kontsepsiya Gosudarstvennoi Semeinoi Politiki Rossiiskoi Federatsii na period do 2025 goda [Concept of Family Policy of the Russian Federation until 2025]. 2013. Accessed November 25, 2014. www.komitet2–6.km.duma.gov.ru/site.xp/050049124053056052.html and http://elenamizulina.ru/pdf/Book_1_preview.pdf. Accessed February 9, 2015.

Kontseptsiya Demograficheskoi Politiki Rossiiskoi Federatsii do 2025, utverzhdennaya Prikazom Prezidenta Rossiiskoi Federatsii ot 10.09.2007 №1351 [Concept of Demographic Policy of the Russian Federation until 2025, Approved by the Order of the President of the Russian Federation from 10.09.2007 №1351]. 2007. Accessed November 25, 2014. http://base.garant.ru/191961/.

Kruglyi stol v Gosudarstvennoi Dume. Vpechatlenia chlenov RARCh. "Pravovoe regulirovanie surrogatnogo materinstva: semeino-pravovoi aspekt" [Round Table in the State Duma. Impressions of the RAHR Members. "Legal Regulation of Surrogacy: A Family-legal Aspect"]. 2014. Accessed December 16, 2015. www.rahr.ru/d_index/report_ks.pdf.

Lebedev, Sergei. 2014. "Novosti iz parlamenta: surrogatnoe materinstvo po-mizulinski" [News from the Parliament: Surrogacy the Mizulina's Way]. Accessed September 24, 2015. www.probirka.org/surrogatnieprogrammy/7219-novosti-iz-gosdumy-surrogatnoe-materinstvo-po-mizulinski.html.

Leykin, Inna. 2011. "Population Prescriptions: (Sanitary) Culture and Biomedical Authority in Contemporary Russia." *Anthropology of East Europe Review* 29 (1): 60–81.

Mizulina, Elena. 2013. "Interview by Vladimir Pozner in 'Pozner.'" *Channel One Russia*, February 24. Accessed October 8, 2015. www.1tv.ru/sprojects_edition/si5756/fi21739.

Moskovkin, Lev. 2014. "Mizulina provela v k.830 krugly stol 'Pravovoe regulirovanie surrogatnogo materinstva'" [Mizulina Has Carried Out a Round Table "Legal Regulation of Surrogacy: A Family-legal Aspect in Auditorium"]. Accessed October 24, 2014. http://leo-mosk.livejournal.com/2095522.html.

Osnovy zakonodatelstva Rossiiskoi Federacii ob ohrane zdorovja grazhdan [Fundamentals of Legislation on the Health Care of the Citizens of the Russian Federation]. 1993. July 22. Accessed March 3, 2015. www.consultant.ru/document/cons_doc_LAW_122942/.

Pavlova, Julia. 2007. *Reproduktivnaya funkciya organizma kak forma realizacii konstitucionnogo prava cheloveka na zhizn* [Reproductive Function of the Body as a Form for Constitutional Human Right for Life]. Moscow: Moscowsky Gumanitarnyi Universitet [Moscow University for the Humanities].

Postanovlenie Konstitutsionnogo suda Rossiiskoi Federatsii ot 11.16.2006 №496 [Supreme Constitutional Court Order from 11.16.2006 №496]. 2006. Accessed March 3, 2015. www.law.edu.ru/article/article.asp?articleID=1277771.

Postanovlenie Pravitelstva Rossiiskoi Federatsii ot 02.06.2012 №98 "O socialnom pokazanii dlya iskusstvennogo preryvanija beremennosti" [Decree of the Government of the Russian Federation №98 from 02.06.2012 "About Social Indication for Abortion"]. 2012. Accessed October 12, 2015. http://base.garant.ru/70137312/.

Postanovlenie Pravitelstva Rossiiskoi Federatsii ot 08.11.2003 №485 "O perechne socialnyh pokazanii dlya iskusstvennogo preryvaniya beremennosti." [Decree of the Government of the Russian Federation №485 from 08.11.2003 "About the List of Social Indications for Abortion"]. 2003. Accessed March 23, 2015. www.consultant.ru/document/cons_doc_LAW_43773/.

Postanovlenie Pravitelstva Rossiiskoi Federatsii ot 10.18.2013 №932 "O programme gosudarstvennyh garantyi besplatnogo okazaniya grazhdanam meditsinskoi pomoschi na 2014–2016" [Decree of the Government from 10.18.2013 №932 "About the State Guarantees for the Free Provision of Medical Care for Citizens 2014–2016"]. 2013. Accessed February 23, 2015. www.rg.ru/2013/10/22/medpomosch-site-dok.html.

Prikaz Minzdrava Rossii from 08.30.2012 №107 "O poryadke ispolzovaniya vspomogatelnyh reproduktivnyh tehnologyi, protivokazaniyah I ogranicheniyah k ih primeneniju" [Executive Order of the Health Ministry from 08.30.2012 №107 "The Order of Use of ART, Contradictions and Limitations"]. 2012. Accessed October 19, 2014. http://base.consultant.ru/cons/cgi/online.cgi?req=doc;base=LAW;n=142595.

Prikaz Minzdrava Rossii ot 10.30.2012 №556 "Ob utverzhdenyi standarta meditsinskoi pomochi pri besplodii s ispolzovaniem vspomogatelnyh reproduktivnyh tehnologyi" [Executive Order of the Health Ministry from 10.30.2012 №556 "On the Approval of Standard of Health Treatment in Cases of Infertility by the Use of ART"]. 2012. accessed October 19, 2014. http://base.consultant.ru/cons/cgi/online.cgi?req=doc;base=LAW;n=145731.

Recommendations. 2014. *Proekt Rekommendatsii kruglogo stola "Pravovoe regulirovanie surrogatnogo materinstva: semeino-pravovoi aspekt"* [Project of Recommendations to the Parliament from the Round Table "Legal Regulation of Surrogacy: A Family-Legal Aspect"]. 2014. Accessed November 24, 2014. www.komitet2–6.km.duma.gov.ru/site.xp/051053055124056050057.html.

Reglament komiteta Gosudarstvennoi Dumy po voprosam Semji, Zhenchin i Detei [Regulations of the Committee on Family, Women, and Children of the Russian Parliament]. n.d. Accessed December 16, 2015. www.komitet2–6.km.duma.gov.ru/site.xp/052048055.html.

Restriction of Reproductive Rights in Russia, 2011–2012: Populist Politics at the Expenses of Women's Health and Welfare. 2012. Written statement by the Heinrich Böll Foundation (Moscow Office) for the 56th Session of the UN Commission on the Status of Women. Accessed February 26, 2015. http://genderpage.ru/?p=588.

Rivkin-Fish, Michele. 2010. "Pronatalism, Gender Politics, and the Renewal of Family Support in Russia: Toward a Feminist Anthropology of 'Maternity Capital.'" *Slavic Review* 69 (3): 701–724.

Romanovsky, Georgy. 2010. "Demographiya i vspomogatelnye reproduktivnye tehnologii: perspektivy pravovogo regulirovaniya." [Demography and ARTs: Prospects of Legislative Regulation]. *Vestnik NGU* 6 (2): 148–154.

Rossiiskaya Associaciya Reprodukcii Cheloveka [Russian Association of Human Reproduction]. n.d. Official Webpage. Accessed December 16, 2015. www.rahr.ru/.

Rossiiskoe Informacionnoe Agentstvo [Russian Informational Agency]. 2013. "EKO v Rossii: chastnye i gosudarstvennye centry borutsya za pacientov." [IVF in Russia: Private and State Centers Fight for Patients]. Accessed October 11, 2015. http://ria.ru/society/20130725/951958026.htm.

Rozenholm, Arja and Irina Savkina. 2011. "We Must All Give Birth: That's an Order! The Russian Mass Media Commenting on V. V. Putin's Address." In *Russian Mass Media and Changing Values*, edited by Arja Rozenholm, Kaarle Nordenstreng and Elena Trubina, 79–102. New York: Routledge.

Samoilova, Valentina. 2012. *Semeino-Pravovie Aspekty Realizacii Reproduktivnyh Prav pri Priminenii Vspomogatelnyh Reproduktivnyh Tehnologyi* [Family and Legal Aspects of Reproductive Rights with Application of ARTs]. Moscow: MESI.

Semeinyi Kodeks Rossiiskoi Federatsii ot 12.29.1995 №223 [Family Code of the Russian Federation from 12.29.1995 №223]. 1995. Accessed October 24, 2014. www.consultant.ru/popular/family/.

Sergeev, Yury and Julia Pavlova. 2006. "Problemy Pravovogo Regulirovaniya Primineniya VRT." [Problems of Legal Regulation of ARTs]. *Medicinskoe Pravo [Medical Law]* 3: 3–8.

Shpakovskaya, Larisa and Zhanna Chernova. 2010. "Molodye Vzroslye: Brak, Partnerstvo, and Roditelstvo. Diskursivnye Predpisaniya i Praktiki v Sovremennoi Rossii." [Young Adults: Marriage, Partnership and Parenthood. Discursive Practices in the Contemporary Russia]. *Laboratorium* 3: 19–43.

Sokolova, Natalia, and Anna Mulenko. 2013. "Novelly Rossiiskogo Zakonodatelstva o Priminenyi Vspomogatelnyh Reproduktivnyh Tehnologyi." [Innovations of the Russian Legislation on ARTs]. *Medicinskoe Prav [Medical Law]* 1: 26–30.

Sperling, Valerie. 2015. *Sex, Politics and Putin. Political Legitimacy in Russia.* New York: Oxford University Press.

Spilker, Kristin Hestflått. 2008. Assistert slektskap. Biopolitikk i reproduksjonsteknologienes tidsalder [Assisted Kinship. Biopolitics in the Age of Reproductive Technologies]. PhD diss., Norwegian University of Science and Technology.

Spravedlivaya Rossiya [A Just Russia party]. n.d. Official Webpage. Accessed December 16, 2015. www.spravedlivo.ru/.

Verbatim Report of the Parliamentary Readings. 2013. *Stenogramma rassmotreniya Federalnogo Zakona ot 06.11.2013 №135 "O zashchite detei ot informatsii, prichinyayushchei vred ih zdorov'yu i razvitiju"* [Verbatim Report of the Parliamentary Readings of the Federal Law №135 "On Protection of Minors from Information Causing Harm to Their Health and Development" from 06.11.2013]. Accessed November 27, 2014. www.cir.ru/docs/duma/302/2605062?QueryID=5225142.

Svitnev, Konstantin. 2010. "VRT I Pravo na Materinstvo." [ARTs and a Right for Motherhood]. *Medicinskoe Pravo* [*Medical Law*] 3 (31): 5–9.

Svitnev, Konstantin. 2012. "Obzor pravopriminitelnoi praktiki po delam, svyazannym s osparivaniem otkazov organov ZAGSa v registracii detei, rozhdennyh v rezultate primineniya programm surrogatnogo materinstva." [An Overview of Judicial Practice Regarding Cases of Litigation of Refusals of the Civil Registry Office to Register Children Born as a Result of Surrogacy Program]. *Semeinoe i Zhilischnoe Prav* [*Family and Housing Law*] 1: 12–15.

Teplova, Tatyana. 2007. "Welfare State Transformation, Childcare and Women's Work in Russia." *Social Politics* 14 (3): 284–322.

Thompson, Charis. 2005. *Making Parents: The Ontological Choreography of Reproductive Technologies*. Cambridge: MIT Press.

Vserossiiskaya Programma "Svyatost Materinstva" [All-Russia Sanctity of Motherhood Program]. n.d. Official Webpage. Accessed June 22, 2016. www.fap.ru/programs/svyatost-materinstva/.

Zhurzhenko, Tatiana. 2004. "Staraya ideologiya novoy semyi: demographicheskiy natsionalizm Rossii i Ukrainy" [Old Ideology of a New Family: Demographic Nationalism of Russia and Ukraine]. In *Semeinye uzy: Modeli dlya sborki* [Family Ties: Models for Assembling], edited by Sergei Ushakin. Vol. 2. 268–296. Moscow: NLO.

Part V

"New Normals" and their Discontents

18 Lesbian Kinship and ARTs in American Popular Culture

The L Word and *The Kids Are All Right*

Julianne Pidduck

This chapter examines *The L Word* (2004–2009) and *The Kids Are All Right* (2010), two recent American cultural productions depicting lesbian couples who use ARTs to conceive. Produced by the premium cable network Showtime, *The L Word* is a TV series about affluent and glamorous Los Angeles lesbian lives. While the series is probably best remembered for its explicit lesbian sexuality, this chapter explores a plotline from the first season in which mixed-race couple Bette and Tina seek a suitable sperm donor to conceive a child. Meanwhile, the feature film *The Kids Are All Right* recounts how two teenage siblings brought up by their lesbian mothers contact the sperm donor (their biological father) with unforeseen consequences. Both productions were spearheaded by established lesbian cultural producers who are also parents: Ilene Chaiken acted as executive producer, creator and writer of *The L Word*, while Lisa Cholodenko is credited as director and co-writer of *The Kids Are All Right*. Partly inspired by personal and collective experiences of lesbian parenting, these productions are also carefully crafted narratives that navigate the changing conditions of lesbian representation within American popular culture during the first decade of the 2000s.

The L Word and *The Kids Are All Right* were produced within a sociopolitical context in which the enduring American cultural fantasy of the heteronormative nuclear family coexists uneasily with emergent practices of reproduction and kinship: assisted conception, lesbian and gay "families of choice," and legal battles over the recognition of same-sex marriage and lesbian and gay parenting rights. I have argued elsewhere that, alongside everyday performative practices of kinship and political and legal struggles, the field of cultural production is pivotal to the reproduction and reimagining of kinship (Pidduck 2009). At once conventional and highly adaptive, the narratives and genres of popular culture stage the symbolic negotiation of core cultural tensions (Altman 1984). In this light, this chapter studies how *The L Word* and *The Kids Are All Right* represent lesbian appropriation of ARTs, and queer women's sexuality and kinship more broadly, in relation to changing norms of kinship, gender, and sexuality in the USA.

The L Word and *The Kids Are All Right* articulate how female same-sex desire connects with reproduction and kinship by dramatizing controversial practices and themes, including lesbian appropriation of ARTs, queer female sexuality and motherhood. While these themes are novel to the heteronormative domain of American popular culture, the lesbian baby boom is an established sociological phenomenon in the United States and many other affluent countries. Since the late 1970s, queer women have routinely used non-medicalized donor insemination (also known colloquially as the "turkey baster" method), but from the mid-1980s they have increasingly turned to ARTs for the management of information and medical risks associated with HIV and other sexually transmitted diseases (Sullivan 2004, 32–34). The infertility clinics referenced in these productions are typical of a privatized American health-service sector operating without any regulation of cost, access, scope or quality of treatment (Asch and Marmor 2008). Ethical, economic and political problems of access to ARTs are not broached directly, as both works take for granted the access of their well-off lesbian protagonists to a private ART industry operating on a user-pay basis that is indifferent to sexual orientation. The low-key but pivotal role of ARTs in these productions enables fictional explorations of changing practices of biological and other forms of relatedness.

These mainstream representations of lesbian procreation and kinship were released in a context where LGBTQ individuals and communities are profoundly ambivalent toward norms of heteronormative and biological kinship (Pidduck 2009). Kath Weston (1991) argues that the discourse of "families of choice" involves a deliberate refusal or decentering of biological relatedness in a context where lesbian, gay and queer subjects are frequently rejected by their blood families, and have been figured individually and collectively as "exiles from kinship." The refusal of mainstream society to recognize LGBTQ kinship has proven devastating for the legal recognition of queer parents, and for LGBTQ access to health-care benefits (notably during the AIDS pandemic). Both productions are situated in early 2000s California, a context marked by high-profile political and legal battles over the legal recognition of same-sex marriage and lesbian and gay parenting: Same-sex marriage was briefly legalized in 2008 in California, only to be banned by Proposition 8, a State constitutional amendment barring same-sex marriages.

As popular culture productions, *The L Word* and *The Kids Are All Right* resolutely avoid explicit political references. Even so, their novel and self-conscious treatment of contested themes of lesbian sexuality and kinship need to be framed in an ideological context in which the State and the Christian Right have aggressively shored up heteronormative political, legal and sociocultural definitions of family. These forces have systematically vilified same-sex marriage and parenting, drawing on "a persistent cultural narrative denying the naturalness of lesbian and gay sexuality … because it is perceived to be inherently nonprocreative" (Hayden 1995, 56). In this context, the juxtaposition of a seemingly "perverse" and nonprocreative lesbian sexuality with assisted reproductive technologies presents a particularly potent cocktail. Queer women's appropriation of assisted conception, represented for the first time in these works, challenges and rearticulates cultural norms of gender, sexuality and motherhood.

Assisted Reproduction in *The L Word*: Two "Primal Scenes"

The opening sequences of the pilot episode of *The L Word* introduce its ensemble cast of friends, neighbors and lovers who live in a comfortable residential West Hollywood neighborhood. First, we see a young white man (Tim) as he carefully tidies up his home in preparation for the arrival of his girlfriend Jenny. Next, Tim's neighbors are introduced through a high-angle shot of two young women, one white and blonde and the other with darker skin and black hair, as they awaken naked and intertwined in their bed. Cut to Tina (the blonde woman) as she calls her girlfriend Bette into the bathroom to see her fertility monitor. "You're ovulating, let's make a baby," Bette coos, kissing Tina passionately on the mouth. In the next scene, the couple meet their friends Alice, Shane and Dana at a coffee bar and Tina announces "Today's the day!" Typical of the series' ongoing juxtaposition between intimate and public spaces shared by queer women, this scene embeds Bette and Tina's project to conceive a child within a close-knit "family of choice."

This episode is carefully scripted to initiate mainstream viewers into an unprecedented and expansive queer female televisual world. *The L Word* and, in a different way, *The Kids Are All Right* are ground-breaking and problematic instances of lesbian visibility in American popular culture. Watched avidly by "insider" lesbian and queer American and transnational audiences, they were also produced to attract "outsider" mainstream American audiences (Moore 2007). While explicit scenes of lesbian sexuality and assisted reproduction offer erotic spectacles and novel plotlines respectively for heterosexual viewers, queer female viewers read these works as welcome, although not necessarily totally accurate accounts of lesbian lives, which are still rarely portrayed in popular culture. In this light, *The L Word* presents a queer female frame of reference on assisted conception, sexuality, gender and kinship, while offering a "pedagogical" account of lesbian lives to uninitiated viewers.

Returning to the ART plotline in the pilot episode, later that day Tina and Bette visit a white artist friend and ask him to ejaculate into a plastic cup, then continue on to the infertility clinic. A Black female doctor in a white lab coat welcomes Tina and Bette into a cubicle, then leaves to test the sperm. She remarks to Bette, with a wink: "It's more likely to take if you're aroused." Lying on a gurney covered with a white paper sheet with her legs apart, Tina prompts a reluctant Bette to perform cunnilingus. Put off by the clinical setting, Bette reluctantly acquiesces, only to be interrupted by the doctor's swift return with the announcement: "That stuff wouldn't get anyone pregnant. Those little fellas just don't have what it takes." If conception has been insistently naturalized as a product of heterosexual intercourse, and consecrated in the intimate scene of the marital bed, the artificiality of the clinic is explored with the series' signature self-reflexive humor.

While scientific and cultural accounts of assisted conception often depict white male doctors as symbolic progenitors and female patients as passive vessels (Bouquet 2001), this interracial scene is unusual for its staging of a sympathetic encounter between an African-American doctor and a mixed-race lesbian couple. Biracial actress Jennifer Beals (Bette) is widely credited with introducing considered articulations of race, gender, class and sexuality into a predominantly white series (Warn 2009). In a series fascinated by powerful female figures, it is the biracial character Bette who incarnates a successful career woman, while Tina is the stay-at-home girlfriend and mother. This scene introduces a complicity between the doctor and Bette, both confident and successful African-American professionals. Furthermore, the doctor's disparaging comment about sluggish sperm challenges the accounts of male sexual and reproductive dynamism that are prevalent in ART discourses.

Do-It-Yourself Lesbian Conception: Desperately Seeking Sperm

The assisted conception plotline continues as Bette and Tina seek a suitable donor with viable sperm. The couple actively seeks the sperm of a prominent artist in order to maximize their chances of a gifted child, a choice implying a consumerist approach to reproduction in a neoliberal setting. Two promising volunteers eventually decline: The first is disappointed when he learns that he is to ejaculate into a cup rather than participate in a threesome; the second, who is invited into Bette and Tina's bedroom and engages enthusiastically in foreplay with the two women, is outraged to learn that they want his sperm. Rather than the gay male donors frequently privileged by many real lesbian couples (as in the comedy *Happy Endings* (2005)), Tina and Bette privilege heterosexual male donors; this plotline wryly acknowledges heterosexual male voyeurism and pornographic fantasies of lesbian sexuality. It is important to note that Chaiken and Showtime conceived *The L Word*'s "quality drama" and explicit sexuality between women not only to address lesbian and gay audiences, but also to offer "added value" to premium audiences, including heterosexual men (Ilyasova 2009).

Later in season 1, Bette proposes an African-American donor, Marcus Allen Woods, another successful artist. Tina initially objects on the grounds that she isn't "qualified" to mother an African-American child. An emotional discussion follows, in which Bette feels rejected by Tina's ambivalence toward conceiving a biracial child; Tina finally agrees to conceive a biracial child who, while not biologically related to Bette, "would be more like our child." She then proposes a different "scene" of insemination that would more fully include Bette, the non-biological parent: "You and me, sexy in love, with no doctors, no fluorescent lights, no paper gowns." Moved, Bette responds: "I would love to make a baby with you. Tonight in our home, in our bed, just you and me." This exchange establishes a sharp contrast between the initial clinical insemination and the "do-it-yourself" lesbian conception that follows.

This second "primal scene" eschews the artificiality of the clinic for a more "natural" conception through sexual intercourse in the intimacy of the monogamous couple's bed. Stylistically and symbolically worlds away from the clinic with its artificial and commercial connotations, the scene is shot in soft focus with candlelight and romantic music with the lovers drinking red wine. Tina toasts "Marcus Allen Woods' unbelievably high sperm count." (This comment refers, tongue-in-cheek, to the myth of Black male sexual potency, where Woods' sperm dramatically outperforms the first, white, donor's sperm.) Framed in a tight 2-shot with the vial between them, Bette and Tina scrutinize the sperm that was collected, cleaned and frozen at the infertility clinic.

BETTE: "Don't be grossed out, we have to honor it." In a wide-angle shot from the point of view of the vial of sperm, they each bow, in amused deference, to the sperm.
BETTE: "We honor you."
TINA: "We honor you. All 75 billion of you."
BETTE: "Do we have everything we need?"
TINA: "Syringe, diaphragm."
BETTE: "Magical juice." They hold up each item in turn.

The lovers kiss, moving toward the bed as romantic music fades up. After a short while, they each say in turn "Let's do it." Cut to a close-up of Bette's hand drawing the sperm into the syringe and deliberately releasing it. The scene concludes with a close-up on Tina's eye. This unusual sequence combines a pedagogical address (how two women can conceive a child in their own home), an erotic scene of lesbian sexuality and a "naturalized" dramatization of lesbian conception.

Mediating Conception and Kinship

In his influential study, David M. Schneider argues that "the cultural universe in American kinship incorporates elements from two major cultural orders, the *order of nature* [blood or more broadly biogenetic materials] and the *order of law* [marriage, culture]" (Schneider 1980, 27). For Schneider, blood relations and cultural kinship sanctified by marriage point to two oppositional and complementary types of "relation": on the one hand, *natural* relations based in substance or shared biogenetic material, and on the other *symbolic* relations founded in law, culture, or codes of conduct. In this structuralist analysis, the two codes are potently articulated in heterosexual intercourse.

> All of the significant symbols of American kinship are contained within the figure of (hetero)sexual intercourse, itself a symbol, of course. The figure is formulated in American culture as a biological entity and a natural act.... As a symbol of unity, or oneness, love is union of the flesh, of opposites, male and female, man and woman. The unity of opposites is not only affirmed in the embrace, but also in the outcome of that union, the unity of blood, the child.
>
> (Schneider 1980, 39–40)

Lesbian conception is not easily intelligible within a dominant American cultural discourse that privileges the "immutability" of blood kinship anchored in heterosexual intercourse and marriage.

Bette and Tina's second (and ultimately successful) conception scene works both with and against cultural codes of gender, nature, sexuality and race. In some ways, the scene equates lesbian conception with the powerful symbolism of procreation through (hetero)sexual intercourse as pivotal to reproduction and, more broadly, to American kinship. The second "primal scene" unfolds in the intimate setting of the bedroom of a monogamous couple, at a remove from the "artificial" scene of the clinic – and the male biological parent (Woods donates his sperm while passing through town, and has no interest in parenting). In her account of lesbian assisted conception, Corinne P. Hayden observes "an intriguing attempt to locate the metaphor of biological, *generative* power in the co-parent … [enabling] lesbians and gay men to claim an active role, both figuratively and literally, in the creation of the child" (Hayden 1995, 51). In *The L Word*, Bette's participation in the conception of the couple's child is carefully scripted through her choice of an African-American sperm donor, and through the scripting of Bette as an active sexual partner and the agent of insemination at the moment of conception. In contrast with "the cultural narrative of paternity as authorship [which] positions the male contribution as central and irreplaceable to the identity of the production of conception" (Hayden 1995, 51), *The L Word* offers a novel and provocative articulation of lesbian sexuality and assisted reproduction, and a savvy reworking of codes of race and gender.

To conclude this analysis, let me discuss briefly how Bette and Tina's procreative journey is embedded within an expansive lesbian televisual world. The unprecedented temporal and dramatic scope of *The L Word* facilitates a multiple and self-reflexive exploration of queer women's sexuality and kinship. Produced three decades into the lesbian baby boom, *The L Word* was first broadcast at the height of the lobby for same-sex marriage and parental rights in California; this dominant liberationist lobby for State recognition of lesbian and gay marriage and parental status was widely critiqued by queer activists and intellectuals as a form of "homonormativity" (Duggan 2002). Both representing and addressing LGBTQ viewers and communities preoccupied by debates around queer family, kinship and relationality, *The L Word* dramatizes many other queer bonds, including friendship, ex-lovers, fuck buddies, non-monogamous or casual sex, and so on. Not an isolated couple, Tina and Bette are firmly anchored in a close-knit "family of choice," made up of half a dozen friends and ex-lovers, within a broader field of nonprocreative queer female friendships and sexual encounters.

As mentioned above, Bette and Tina's initial pact to conceive is immediately shared with friends at a coffee shop. And again, their "inner circle" arrives unannounced shortly after Tina and Bette's second conception scene. With Tina lying on the floor with her legs up against the wall to facilitate conception, the friends discuss Dana's latest dating dilemma. Alice casually picks up the syringe, asking "What's this?" Bette responds "Marcus Allen Woods," just as Alice accidentally squirts the sperm across the room onto Dana, who squirms. Shane comments:

"Oh wait, you mean we could be here at the moment of conception?" Here, conception is not an intimate couple moment, but rather an experience to be shared with a tight-knit group of friends. Later in the series, with Tina well on in her pregnancy and the couple heavily focused on the imminent birth of their child, their friends stage an "intervention," reminding Bette and Tina to remain responsive to their friends – a wry reminder for the initiated of the dangers of homonormativity.

Ultimately, it is not the monogamous couple with a child, but rather *The L Word*'s "family of choice" that offers the series' most compelling figure of queer female kinship. In a series centrally organized around the exploration of queer female sexuality, monogamous couples, including Bette and Tina, prove unstable. Bette and Tina's parenting of their child Anjelica continues as one of several core plotlines: The couple separates, bisexual character Tina gets involved with a man, and a nasty custody battle ensues culminating in Bette's kidnapping of Anjelica. Deeply threatened by Tina's heterosexual relationship, Bette panics because she has no legal status as Anjelica's co-parent. Here, the series indirectly broaches the precarious legal status of lesbian and gay parents in the United States. While access to ARTs is established for those who can afford them, second-parent or step-parent adoption only became possible in California in 2013, alongside the legalization of same-sex marriage.

The Kids Are All Right: The Lesbian "Every-Family" and the Sperm Donor

As a premium series produced within the relatively permissive industrial context of American pay television, *The L Word* offered a dense and multiple exploration of queer female sexuality and kinship. In contrast, *The Kids Are All Right*, released in 2010, marks the first American popular lesbian family film made by the highly conservative Hollywood film industry. Financing was by no means assured for this potentially controversial script about how lesbian parents deal with the sudden appearance of the anonymous donor whose sperm they used to conceive their two children. Cholodenko describes in an interview how she pitched the film, smuggling in the "difference" of a lesbian family on the strength of an "every-family" storyline intelligible within the conservative framework of American popular culture:

> We were very conscious from the outset [that] this is an every-family. Parents that are together with certain values and hopes and dreams for their kids, certain issues in their own marriage. They're from a certain social economic class – I felt that would be an easier access point for people who would go see it. It was clearly intentional.
>
> (Cholodenko 2010, n.p.)

This conventional scripting of a white, middle-class lesbian family enables a ground-breaking naturalistic and nuanced dramatization of a life partnership between mature women, Nic and Jules, who are also parents. On the other hand, the normative articulation of gender and sexuality leaves the film open to criticism of its conservative defense of the nuclear family.

Film genre can be understood as a system of industrial classification enabling a certain alignment between film production and audience expectations; at the same time, film genre is often seen as a social "ritual" (Altman 1984, 8–10), where cultural productions symbolically work through problems of common concern. Part of the resilience of popular genres lies in their familiarity, alongside a capacity for renewal through the incorporation of new elements (the cowboy romance of *Brokeback Mountain* or indeed the lesbian family drama such as Cholodenko's film or the television series *The Fosters* (2013–)). Novel to *The Kids Are All Right* are the "every-family" headed by two women, and the potent narrative twist of the sperm donor. Like *The L Word*, Cholodenko's film probes tensions in the traditional discourses of family and kinship exemplified by the now-established practices of assisted reproduction, high divorce rates, and debates about same-sex marriage and parenting.

Cholodenko presents a frank portrait of a bickering couple fiercely dedicated to their teenagers, while struggling with the nagging tensions of a long-term relationship, including a failing sex life. The decision of teenager Joni to contact her biological father upsets the delicate equilibrium of this conventional family unit. The sudden arrival of the unknown sperm donor presents a threat to the legitimacy of the lesbian parents in a context where same-sex couples and lesbian and gay parents are not legally recognized, and where they are often seen as inadequate imitations of a heteronormative ideal (Weston 1991).

In this light, consider a pivotal scene in which, after an initial meeting with Joni and Laser, Paul is invited to the family home for dinner. Greeted by Nic at the door, Paul compliments the couple on their home and offers them a good bottle of red wine. Nic goes into the kitchen to pour the wine, accompanied by Jules who admonishes her: "Go easy on the wine, hon. It's daytime." Nic replies sharply: "Same goes for the micro-managing. OK?" This exchange exemplifies the tensions between the two women as they try to present a united front to Paul. In the next scene, the two mothers, two children and biological father are pictured dining together in the back yard. Widely reproduced in the film's publicity, this title image extends the visual iconography of the American nuclear family breaking bread together in the open air; this image evokes a "queer" kinship that could potentially challenge the norm of the heterosexual nuclear family.

In the conversation that follows, Nic plies Paul with a series of questions about his employment, social life, age, and so on. When Paul says that he runs a restaurant, Nic pointedly mentions that while looking for a sperm donor the couple had read in his file that he was studying international relations. Paul replies that he dropped out of college, which he found to be "a massive waste of time," in order to engage in more practical pursuits. As in *The L Word*, this exchange reveals the couple's middle-class values and aspirations in "shopping" for sperm within a privatized model of assisted reproduction. Nic in particular upholds the importance of respectability, a college education and social standing as she pushes Joni and Laser toward academic achievement.

Lesbian Motherhood, Lesbian Sexuality

As with the depiction of Bette and Tina's relationship in the first season of *The L Word*, this scene consolidates a portrait of a strongly gendered relationship: Nic, an assertive and at times controlling soft butch character with a demanding career as a gynecologist, is head of the family, while Jules is awkward and unsure of herself as a stay-at-home mom who has failed in a series of small business ventures. This scene also charts an escalating power struggle between Nic's abrasive and controlling personality and Paul's self-deprecating yet smug assurance as the owner of a successful organic restaurant. The improbable narrative twist of an affair between Jules and Paul pushes these tensions to a crisis point. Unable to measure up to Nic's expectations, Jules finds comfort in the arms of the easy-going and supportive Paul. Jules' sexual satisfaction with her children's biological father is dramatized through several awkward, noisy and enthusiastic sex scenes that contrast starkly with the film's pointed account of Jules and Nic's lackluster sex life – notably a comedic scene in which the women watch gay male porn in order become aroused, without success.

This unlikely scenario sets in play a potent mix of signifiers. Central to the film's marketable uniqueness, this narrative twist ensures a certain appeal for mainstream audiences – as well as a certain unease among queer female viewers. Paul's arrival on the scene sets this ground-breaking portrait of a lesbian relationship and parenting in dialogue with heteronormative accounts of gender, sexuality and kinship. The lesbian family is reframed as potentially "lacking" in at least two ways: the teenagers' "missing" biological father associated with the cultural norm of the heterosexual family, and the "lacking" phallus. Ellen Lewin argues that the cultural figure of the lesbian mother is highly problematic in American culture given that "lesbians, after all, were assumed to be creatures defined by their sexual appetites" and consequently "at odds with the … selfless devotion expected of mothers" (Lewin 1995, 193). With its wry depiction of what is known colloquially among queer women as "lesbian bed death," Cholodenko's film privileges a representation of devoted lesbian mothers at the expense of a fulfilling lesbian sexuality.

This negotiation of certain clichés around lesbian sexuality and families in *The Kids Are All Right* led to a mixed reception among queer and lesbian critics and audiences. For instance, Jack Halberstam (2010), argues that

> the naturalization of [Paul's] sexual power and the naturalization of the lack of charisma of the moms again stabilizes a grid of desire that always tips in favor of male heterosexuality and leaves lesbians stranded. With the scales tipped this way, it becomes inevitable that Jules will sleep with Paul, that she will become dick-obsessed, that Nic will be cast as the sad, slightly butch partner who loses out to the dynamic, phallic dad.

In contrast with Cholondenko's film, *The L Word* deliberately stages the primal scene of lesbian conception that emphasizes pleasure and the generative sexual role of the non-biological parent; here, the biological father figure in assisted reproduction is sidelined to re-center the two lesbian parents. In *The Kids Are All Right*, the return of the male progenitor unleashes a head-on collision between the emergent and contested lesbian family and what Schneider calls the "immutability of blood kinship."

Beginning a sexual relationship with Jules and assuming a fatherly role with Joni and Laser, Paul begins to occupy the symbolic place of the patriarch of a reconstituted heterosexual nuclear family. After Nic discovers Jules' infidelity and the devastated family cuts all ties with Paul, he returns one last time to see Joni before she leaves for college. Nic stands up to Paul in a climactic confrontation.

NIC: "Let me tell you something, *man*, this is not your family. This is my family."

PAUL: "I know that, Nic."

NIC: "No, you don't know. You don't know, and you know why? Because you're a fucking interloper. If you want a family so much, you go out and make your own!"

Slamming the door in Paul's face, Nic bravely defends the integrity of the lesbian nuclear family and her place at its head. Within the generic logic of the family comedy drama, the casting out of the "interloper" leads to a new narrative equilibrium with the symbolic defense of the integrity of the (lesbian) every-family.

In a social context where same-sex marriage and queer families struggle for legitimacy, Cholodenko's film foregrounds the vulnerability of the lesbian family, while ultimately defending it. Toward the end of the film, Jules makes a heartfelt speech to the effect that "marriage is fucking hard," leading to a tentative truce with Nic: In the car after dropping Joni off at college, the film closes on a shot from Laser's point of view in which Nic takes Jules' hand. In the end, the hard labor of "marriage" and parenting trump the sperm donor's claim to blood kinship. If the film's title seems to flag up the well-being of children raised by lesbians, its dénouement works overtime to ensure that (lesbian) "marriage" is all right. Although, in the film's present, same-sex marriage is not recognized by the state of California, the fictional couple "performs" conventional marriage and parenting in a manner that is intelligible to a mainstream American audience.

Conclusion

As established cultural producers, Chaiken and Cholodenko draw on personal and collective experience of a well-established but relatively invisible lesbian baby boom to represent queer women's experiences of reproduction, parenting and kinship. This chapter has explored how *The L Word* and *The Kids Are All Right* navigate the industrial contexts of premium cable television and genre film, as well as a doubled address to queer "insider" and "mainstream" or "premium" audiences (Moore 2007) that both enabled and delimited these productions. I have identified core cultural tensions arising in and around these representations of lesbian conception, parenting and kinship, notably Lewin's argument that lesbian sexuality with its connotations of perversity is incommensurable with American cultural expectations of motherhood. With its explicit depictions of desire and sexual encounters between women, *The L Word* stages a passionate lesbian sex scene that foregrounds the agency of both partners at the moment of conception. Emphasizing how the series plays deliberately to heterosexual male viewers, I suggest that *The L Word*'s dramatic scope and explicit sexuality were bartered against a certain renewed objectification of lesbian sexuality. *The Kids Are All Right*, in contrast, depicts devoted lesbian mothers plagued by "lesbian bed death." With her lesbian "every-family," Cholodenko chose to work within the more conservative Hollywood film industry, which allowed her to reach broad audiences; it is important to underscore that, within this context, explicit (and especially lesbian or gay) sex leads to restricted ratings.

Given that the representation of queer women's sexuality, conception and kinship is a delicate business in a puritanical and heteronormative American context, these productions must carefully consider how their narratives articulate the place of men as fathers and sperm donors and in the projected audience. While male characters are rare in *The L Word*'s lesbian televisual world and the question of paternity is sidelined in the ART plotline, the series sought out a heterosexual male audience, while seeking to "manage" it diegetically through humor and self-reflexive commentary. In the case of *The Kids Are All Right*, interviews with Cholodenko underscore how the financing of the film was contingent on the inclusion of a strong male lead character that male viewers could relate to. As in other popular productions addressing ARTs (feature films *21 Grams* (2003), *Happy Endings* (2005), and the ABC series *The Fosters* (2013–)), *The Kids Are All Right* insists on the point of view of the sperm donor or biological father. While artificial insemination as the "new normal" enables autonomous conception for women, many of these productions demonstrate a preoccupation or anxiety concerning the appropriation of male biogenetic material and men's roles as parents.

References

21 Grams. Film. United States: Alejandro González Iñárritu, 2003.

Altman, Rick. 1984. "A Semantic/Syntactic Approach to Film Genre." *Cinema Journal* 23 (3): 6–18.

Asch, Adrienne, and Rebecca Marmor. 2008. "Assisted Reproduction." In *From Birth to Death and Bench to Clinic: The Hastings Center Bioethics Briefing Book*, edited by Mary Crowley, 5–10. Garrison, NY: The Hastings Center. Accessed May 6, 2014. www.thehastingscenter.org/Publications/BriefingBook/Detail.aspx?id=2210.

Bouquet, Mary. 2001. "Making Kinship, with an Old Reproductive Technology." In *Relative Values: Reconfiguring Kinship Studies*, edited by Sarah Franklin and Susan McKinnon, 85–115. Princeton: Duke University Press.

Cholodenko, Lisa. 2010. Lisa Cholodenko Interview: "The Kids Are All Right" Director Makes a Lesbian Domestic Comedy. Interview by Ella Taylor. *San Francisco Weekly*. Accessed February 4, 2012. www.sfweekly.com/sanfrancisco/lisa-cholodenko-interview-the-kids-are-all-right-director-makes-a-lesbian-domestic-comedy/Content?oid=2177833.

Duggan, Lisa. 2002. "The New Homonormativity: The Sexual Politics of Neoliberalism." In *Materializing Democracy*, edited by Russ Castronova and Dana D. Nelson, 175–194. Princeton: Duke University Press.

Halberstam, Jack. 2010. "The Kids Aren't Alright." *Bullybloggers*, July 15, 2010. http://bullybloggers.wordpress.com/2010/07/15/the-kids-arent-alright.

Happy Endings. Film. United States: Don Roos, 2005.

Hayden, Corinne. 1995. "Gender, Genetics, and Generation: Reformulating Biology in Lesbian Kinship." *Cultural Anthropology* 10 (1): 41–63.

Ilyasova, Alex K. 2009. "Show Time: Sundance Meets Corporate America." In *The Business of Entertainment: Television*, volume 3, edited by Robert C. Sickets, 101–123. Westport CT: Praeger.

Lewin, Ellen. 1995. "On the Outside Looking In: The Politics of Lesbian Motherhood." In *Conceiving the New World Order: The Global Politics of Reproduction*, edited by Faye D. Ginsburg and Rayna Rapp, 103–121. Berkeley: University of California Press.

Moore, Candace. 2007. "Having It All Ways: The Tourist, the Traveler, and the Local in *The L Word*." *Cinema Journal* 46 (4): 3–23.

Pidduck, Julianne. 2009. "Queer Kinship and Ambivalence: Video Autoethnographies by Jean Carlomusto and Richard Fung." *GLQ: A Journal of Lesbian and Gay Studies* 15 (3): 441–468.

Schneider, David M. 1980. *American Kinship: A Cultural Account*. 2nd Edition. Chicago: Chicago University Press.

Sullivan, Maureen. 2004. *The Family of Woman: Lesbian Mothers, their Children, and the Undoing of Gender*. Berkeley: University of California Press.

The Fosters. Television series. First broadcast in June, 2013 by ABC. (2013–).

The Kids Are All Right. Film. United States: Lisa Cholodenko, 2010.

The L Word. Television series. First season. First broadcast January–April, 2004 by Showtime.

Warn, Sarah. 2009. "Radical Acts: Biracial Visibility and The L Word." In *Reading The L Word*, edited by Kim Ackass and Janet McCabe, 189–197. London: I. B. Tauris.

Weston, Kath. 1991. *Families We Choose: Lesbians, Gays, Kinship*. New York: Columbia University Press.

19 Naturalization and Un-Naturalization

ARTs, Childlessness and Choice

Malin Noem Ravn

In this chapter I illuminate questions of childlessness, ARTs and choice in a Norwegian context. My argument revolves around the naturalization of IVF in Norway, and how this leads to the un-naturalization of childlessness.

Lending her voice to the chapter is Lise, a woman I interviewed while she was pregnant by IVF.[1] I use her story to explore the wider reproductive context of decisions concerning IVF made by those who use ARTs in post-millennium Norway. In contemporary Norway, Lise is considered normal and conspicuously unprovocative – she is in a heterosexual relationship, and both she and her husband Lars are of reproductive age. After undergoing three cycles of treatment, they successfully conceived with IVF, using Lise's egg and Lars' sperm. Finally, Lise gave birth to a healthy child. In the context of the body of studies on reproductive technologies, and in this specific cultural context, Lise's story is not controversial. Precisely for this reason, I find it relevant for illustrating what is now conventional in our cultural environment. In the twenty-first century, Lise's story is an example of what has become one of several "natural" stories of conception.

Following my presentation of Lise's personal narrative, I explore her specific process of delineation between normal and abnormal, understandable and unintelligible, acceptable and unacceptable, through which she struggled to construct herself and her choices as "normal" and "natural." At the same time, she was inadvertently suggesting that other actions and choices were "not normal" and "unnatural."

Feminism and Reproductive Choices

Western feminist scholarship in the field of reproduction and reproductive technologies has been preoccupied with questions of reproductive choice. These questions have evolved in parallel with the development of new reproductive choices – that is, the technologies, tests and screenings available. From arguing that access to reproductive choice is predominantly positive and that feminists should fight for women's right to control their reproductive bodies, discussions about choice have become more nuanced and the concept of choice, itself, has been problematized. For instance, women who have been forced to make difficult reproductive choices have been labeled "moral pioneers" (Rapp 1988), and the importance of the right *not* to choose has been asserted (Hubbard in Franklin and McNeil 1988). Furthermore, it has been argued that reproductive choices are elements of consumerism, partaking in the liberal construction of reproductive bodies and substances as though they were commodities in a global market. Feminists have also discussed how the social practice of ARTs both makes choices possible and effectively limits them through, for example, the availability of technologies and legal restrictions on their use. This, in effect, normalizes certain kinds of behavior (Sawicki 1999; Throsby 2004; Thompson 2005) and leads one to question the ontological status of reproductive choices as *choices*.

In this chapter, I explore the meaning of reproductive choice in a specific Norwegian cultural, regulatory, medical and personal context. I also indicate some effects of the choices made in this context. I am inspired by Jana Sawicki's (1999) conceptualization of ARTs as disciplinary technologies that produce new objects and subjects of knowledge, but also new sites of resistance. Sawicki argues that ARTs produce new norms of motherhood, by attaching women to their identities as mothers and offering specific kinds of solutions to problems (Sawicki 1999, 194). I explore the intersections between IVF technology, state regulation and the cultural environment that constitute a particular form of disciplinary context within which individuals and couples navigate. The individuals and couples who are situated in a specific medico-cultural disciplinary context do not merely comply with their situation. Rather, they actively construct specific situations, as infertile couples' engagement with ARTs is fundamental to the production of these technologies and their meaning (Throsby 2004).

The disciplinary reproductive context generates certain normalizations and naturalizations: some choices and actions become self-evident. For example, IVF's "difference" from "natural" conception is downplayed, legal access to IVF delineates the couples who are "legitimate" reproducers and those who are not, and the IVF process is domesticated and interpreted as "new examples of old things" (Thompson 2005, 141). Subsequently, IVF becomes part of the appropriate repertoire of conception (Lie *et al.* 2011), blurring the line between nature and culture (Lie 2002). In this chapter, I discuss the choices available to Lise, in the particular disciplinary context of contemporary Norway, and investigate the consequences of her active engagement: what positions and meanings did her choices and reflections produce?

New Situations, New Choices

Lise was 30 weeks pregnant the first time she spoke with me about being pregnant and conceiving with the aid of IVF. Although her story of infertility, IVF and pregnancy is unique and utterly personal, it also follows a generally recognizable storyline: Lise met Lars, her husband, when she was in her late 20s. After they became a couple the diffuse notions Lise had of future family life slowly solidified into concrete wishes and hopes that, together, they could form their own nuclear family. The realization that they were infertile slowly dawned on them, as a result of months of futile attempts to conceive. It did not really come as a shock to Lise, but, since it was a lengthy and gradual process, she could not pinpoint exactly when they started to suspect that a child would not come without active intervention. "Active intervention," when it comes to conception, advances through many stages. Lise and Lars first did internet research to find tips on getting pregnant, then later engaged in planned sexual intercourse according to a calendar of ovulation. When this failed, they turned to their doctor. After a medical examination, they were transferred to the local fertility clinic. Lise and Lars continued to discuss their options, both with the medical experts and with each other. They also discussed their resources, preferences and limits. Lise said:

> When you find yourself in such a situation, you have to discuss *everything*. Nothing of what you have taken for granted counts, the situation just isn't what you thought it was, so we had to discuss every possible and impossible move thoroughly: "Is it an option to adopt?", "Is Lars too old to apply for adoption?", "Will we go for ICSI if we need to?", "Will we go abroad for egg donation?", "How many cycles of treatment are we willing to take?" In short, we discussed a lot!

Many of these questions were hypothetical, and Lise emphasized that the position she and Lars were creating was temporary and contextual – what was a "no" to sperm donation at one point (before it was actualized as an option) could have been turned into a "yes" at a later date. Still, Lise felt it was important for them to start their discussions.

> We agreed, for instance, that we should start the adoption process alongside the IVF process. Because we knew that it could take some time, and we had decided and agreed that to have a child was the most important thing, not whether it was biologically related or not.

Lise emphasized entry into the adoption process as a discussion and a specific choice, something they wanted to do "alongside the IVF process," while the IVF process, in itself, was not marked as an explicit choice. I prompted her by asking whether she had had any doubts about starting the IVF process. When I asked whether she had ever considered not going ahead with IVF, Lise slowly replied:

> No, not really. Like I said, I only have one life, and ... no, it didn't feel right not to try. I mean, we were well aware that it might not work ... we had reconciled with that fact, and that we might end up childless. But we never considered *not* trying in the first place.... We actually know a couple who decided not to try IVF.... It was some sort of religious reason and I think ... I seriously do not understand it. If it were us, I think we would have spent the rest of our lives wondering ... whether it maybe *could* have worked.

In what was otherwise an unexpected and "unnatural" situation, for Lise and Lars there was at least one "natural" course of action: IVF. Two interrelated themes emerge from Lise's narrative. The first is the obviousness with which she describes her vision of a future with children (Ravn 2005). The second is the obviousness with which she and Lars, in her recounting of the events, decide to begin IVF, which I discuss in the following section.

Naturalization of IVF

Assumptions about future parenthood are immediately altered when one finds oneself unable to conceive. "Infertility," in a medical sense, can be understood as the physical inability to conceive, while "involuntary childlessness" can be defined as "the active but frustrated desire for a ... child" (Throsby 2004, 14), a desire that can be resolved in several ways. Although Lise and Lars were forced to come to terms with a *possible* childless future, they felt it was obvious that they should try to remedy the situation rather than accept childlessness. Inactivity was not perceived as a possible choice. Instead, their choice was between adoption and reproductive technology.

ARTs and adoption belong to the same procreative universe of "unnatural" but naturalized options (Melhuus and Howell 2009) and, for some time, both adoption and IVF existed as parallel possibilities for Lise and Lars. The adoption process is lengthy, complicated and costly, partly because it is carried out in accordance with an increasing number of procedures, regulations and national and international laws (Howell 2006). Prospective parents are investigated and evaluated: they are interviewed by child welfare authorities and required to provide medical certificates, financial certificates and certificates of good conduct from the police. The process is described as emotionally strenuous and exhausting, and usually takes three years or more. The process of applying for fertility treatment, on the other hand, is less regulated and mainly involves a medical examination which, in contrast to the evaluation process connected with adoption, focuses little attention on the couple's social or emotional capacity.

Lise described the adoption process and the medical examination and fertility treatment as "strenuous in completely different ways." The physical process of fertility treatment was perceived as painful at times, physically invasive and time consuming, but when she recounted her experiences to me, Lise did not place much emphasis on these factors. Lise and Lars were accepted for public treatment, and the preferred way forward seemed obvious: they had access to medical help, they could afford it and they would use it. For several reasons, such as anticipation of the experience of pregnancy, the biological bond between parents and child, the "control" over and knowledge of the prospective child's early life and the economics involved, they chose IVF over adoption.

Thus, in Lise's narrative, both IVF and adoption were clearly *legitimate* ways to alleviate childlessness. At the same time, however, she "had to try" IVF. This formulation is recognizable from many studies of infertility and ARTs. Reproductive desire is often naturalized as an inherent human or parental drive, and this formulation reveals that the pursuit of reproductive desire is at the core of the experience of IVF (Franklin 1997, 103). The obviousness of "having to try" IVF indicates that it is not only a legitimate, but also an expected and normalized behavior for involuntarily childless couples. Furthermore, recipients of the treatment interpret their engagement with IVF in light of their naturalized reproductive desire, so "the key issue is not *whether* or not you engage with technology for reproduction, but *why*" (Throsby 2004, 63 emphasis in original). The choice to undergo ART treatment, then, is naturalized "through the perceived naturalness of the *intention* with which they were engaging with that technology" (ibid., emphasis in original). The wish to have children is understood as a natural urge. Hence, acting upon this urge is also considered natural. Reproductive treatment can result in the bodily experience of pregnancy and a biologically related child; therefore, the treatment is interpreted as being closer to "nature" than adoption.

In the medical definition of infertility, diagnosis depends on a normal, heterosexual sex life over a period of a year, resulting in no conception. But the *cultural* definition of infertility is different. It has previously been argued that ARTs have become a "natural" (in the sense of normal or expected) way to have children (Lie *et al.* 2011). In this sense, one is not, culturally speaking, regarded as infertile unless one has "tried everything," including attempting conception by using available reproductive technologies.

Lise expressed this cultural definition in her narrative, both in the sense that she had a pragmatic view of the technological help she received, and that she regarded her pregnancy as "normal" after the first few months. But she also demonstrated it in the way in which she spoke about the other couple; she did not understand why they chose *not* to attempt IVF.

Lise indicated that she would not have *known* whether she was infertile had she not tried IVF. Through this logic, IVF treatment becomes almost as normal and natural as the wish for children itself. In effect, IVF is not really a choice. In Lise's narrative, the unexpected behavior is to *not* attempt IVF.

A "Normal" Pregnancy with the Aid of a "Helping Hand"

So far, I have shown how IVF became naturalized for Lise. Some of the arguments that she used in her decision to try IVF before adoption are specifically grounded in notions of the body and the "natural," such as anticipation of the experience of pregnancy and the emphasis on a biological bond between parents and child. In this section, I explore how Lise's choice of IVF constructs the meaning of these biological values. I will show how she uses these values, together with her construction of technology and medical experts as a "helping hand," to view her pregnancy as primarily a "normal" pregnancy, herself as a "normal" pregnant woman, and her child as a "normal child."[2]

ARTs are often framed as a helping hand – offering assisted rather than artificial conception (Lie 2002) – by regulatory authorities, the medical establishment and recipients. This formulation defines IVF as assisting nature when it does not function in the way it normally should (ibid.). Furthermore, it implies that the categories, entities and positions produced by IVF are natural (Throsby 2004, 54). One of the reasons Lise gave for choosing IVF over adoption was the possibility of having "her own" children, a phrasing which, in this context, connotes biologically related children. Biology is important for understanding genetic relatedness and personal identity (Spilker 2008; Melhuus 2009; Ravn 2009) and I understand the idealization of biological ties to be a contributory aspect of the naturalization of IVF. In the following, I explore how Lise emphasized the results of IVF as "natural" and "biological."

IVF is constructed as a neutral or merely facilitating technology that is not understood to transform any of the cultural or biological dimensions of the relationship between child and parents. Lise presents this as important. When I prompted her on the question of whether her child was "special," she commented rather indignantly on the out-of-date terminology that marks children born by the aid of IVF as "a special kind of children":

> You know, I think about the word they used before: "test-tube babies" – that really gives the wrong associations! They're not babies nurtured and born from a test tube; we only needed help to *conceive* them. Everything else happened here, in my body, not in a test tube.

This leads to another, but related, reason why Lise preferred IVF over adoption: she wanted to feel "how it is to be more than me, both physically and socially." The urge to experience a pregnancy is presented as a driving force (or a loss) in several studies on involuntary childlessness and ARTs (Franklin 1997; Tjørnhøj-Thomsen 1998; Throsby 2004). I interpret Lise's statement in the context of a cultural interpretation of the physical state of pregnancy as a meaningful experience in itself, exceeding the interpretation of pregnancy as the process of having a child (Ravn 2004). The meanings that pregnancy and the pregnant body produce are multiple, but of particular interest here are the ways in which the pregnant body is presented as extraordinarily natural and how the experience of pregnancy is portrayed as a way to learn something about oneself, both as a person, generally, and as a woman, specifically. Lise said:

> There are of course many women who don't have biological children; I don't know how they think about it. I mean, I could have become one myself, but I … it's hard to say now. I guess motherhood is the same regardless of the way you get the children, but … to go through a nine-month pregnancy is clearly something extraordinary. To grow and feel life within your own body, that's … only those who have done it understand it properly.… But I don't mean that I wouldn't have been a "real woman" if I hadn't given birth. I just think I would have been a slightly *different* woman. That's all.… Or, I don't know.

Lise struggled with the importance she gave to the experience of pregnancy. She stated explicitly that becoming a mother was *the* most important aspect, regardless of the manner in which it happened. I believe this is a stand taken on principle toward how she thought motherhood *should* be understood. At the same time, she valued the experience of pregnancy. In giving weight to this experience, she supported her own choice of employing IVF. The "natural" pregnant body became something she achieved through her choices, work and sacrifices. Emphasizing the naturalness of pregnancy was a way to show that her choice had produced a natural pregnancy and a natural child. She had "invited" nature into her body *through* IVF – so that IVF became her link with the natural.

In her narration, Lise was not willing to give IVF much transformative power. At one point, she explicitly stated that it helped her only by functioning as a spare fallopian tube. In her narrative, this became an insignificant event – not in its *effect*, since she arguably succeeded in becoming pregnant with this help, but in what was meaningful for her in the process of understanding her pregnancy, her situation and herself. She stated that her pregnancy was "normal":

> In the first few months, I was really eager to talk to people who had conceived through IVF – especially before we were lucky ourselves. But after that … I don't find it of particular importance or interest any more – I have just as much pleasure talking to a "naturally" pregnant woman about pregnancy – the IVF doesn't really count any more. It feels just like a normal pregnancy. But of course … if I meet someone who is where I have been, who is trying, and under treatment – and who is wondering about the process and such things, I surely will help in any way I can, telling about my experiences and all. But for my own sake? No, right now I care most about birth – I devour birth stories [laughs]. Conception stories are so passé! [laughs]

Pregnancy has a dual character: it is a condition, but it is also most definitely a process. The process aspect of pregnancy can be seen in the fact that narratives of pregnancy regularly place emphasis on that which is to come, not on that which has passed. Both pregnancies in general (Ravn 2004) and IVF pregnancies in particular are often framed as "obstacle courses," in that each stage is broken down into further stages where there are more hurdles to overcome and more things that can go wrong (Franklin 1997, 104). But the present and future obstacles, not those that have already been overcome, seem most relevant for both the story and the experience of pregnancy. A pregnant woman primarily looks ahead. In that way, since IVF is a procedure of conception, and since the medical establishment emphasizes technology-assisted pregnancies as "normal" after the first few months, Lise's preoccupation with birth rather than conception shows an adherence to the "normal" narratives of pregnancy, which inherently under-communicate the "assisted" aspect.

So far, I have discussed how Lise's choices and her reflections upon those choices served to naturalize IVF and produce "natural" categories. In the remainder of the chapter I look at how she created boundaries between her own choices and the options she rejected: how, through establishing her own position, she also generated other positions that contrasted with hers and thus produced alternative meanings and categories, such as the "un-naturalization" of infertility.

Constructing Limits

Lise and Lars reflected a great deal on how far they were willing to go, in terms of both types and number of treatments. Lise emphasized that they established a position that was theirs, personally: "in our specific situation," as she repeatedly formulated it. She insisted that she did not want to make any general moral judgments in this context. Lise's statements imply a sensitivity and understanding that the situation of childlessness is very difficult, and she did not want to condemn those who chose differently from her. Even so, through the discussion of her choices and limitations she generated certain other positions that were presented as being understandable or legitimate to a greater or lesser extent.

During one part of the interview, we discussed sperm and egg donation.[3] Lise stated, with reference to the problem of the "third party" (the donor), that both procedures would have been going too far: "For me they're principally the same, but then again, for me personally they're both beyond the limit. But not generally. I want to emphasize that. For some people it's probably the right thing to do." She also discussed what she presented as variations of IVF, some of which she saw as going "further" than regular IVF:

> [T]here are so many options nowadays that you have to think through to be able to take your stance. But I had no reservations whatsoever about regular IVF. It's all very pragmatic. Like, I think of it as if they helped us by being a fallopian tube. That's it, really. But of course, there are many variations of IVF as well. You have ICSI [microinjection] which means that they help you *a bit* more, and … yes, there are many variations. I believe that, for our part, microinjection would have been fine.… Probably we would have gone that far, it we had had to. But I think our limit would have been there, after ICSI. *Our* limit that is. In *our* situation.

Lise contextualized her position in relation to these possible treatments as hypothetical, meaning that it was not really tested before she became pregnant and the choice became a reality. She said: "These are very difficult questions, and you *never* know what you would have done if you were desperate enough." Lise's statements communicate two messages: on the one hand, through the use of phrases such as "beyond the limit," "go that far" and "desperate enough," she implicitly questions the morality and sustainability of venturing down the path of technological assistance. These phrases also communicate her limits and demarcate her position within the limits – *not* too far and *not* desperate. On the other hand, she does not rule out the possibility that she could have been in the same situation herself, thus separating the position of desperation from her own experience, yet understanding it as something with which she might have been able to identify.

Lise also identified limits and, thus, different positions in relation to those limits when she discussed a number of treatments. In those discussions, the influence of the disciplinary context became tangible. Lise said that she and Lars "got lucky at our last try." In the context of public treatment in Norway (i.e., treatment provided free by the public health-care system), this usually means the third cycle of IVF. I asked her whether they had considered stopping before that, after the first or second cycle, but she said no. "That was not an option for us. We knew we had three 'goes' at it, and we wanted to use them." Furthermore, Lise said that she and Lars would have stopped after the third cycle. "Three cycles was our limit. Then it would have been enough. Then we would rather have continued the adoption process." For Lise and Lars, it would have been financially possible to continue with more IVF cycles, either abroad or privately, so her argument was not based on economics. Rather, she perceived the state's offer and limits as being somehow "normal" and "reasonable." This was further demonstrated by a story she told about a couple who stopped treatment after one cycle:

> I don't know in detail why they didn't continue. But I do know that they found the thought of further treatment too much, and they regarded a life without children as an alternative good life. But I of course respect their choice. And I sort of understand it. People put in such a difficult situation shouldn't be questioned about their choices. It is tough enough as it is. But for *us* that wasn't an option. We had to at least try [the cycles we were offered]. Otherwise we would always have wondered, wouldn't we?

Lise's comments on this case resonate with her comments on the couple who chose not to go through with IVF treatment at all. Again, Lise indicated that the active choice in this context was to *not* go into treatment, as in the former case, and to *stop* treatment before it was "normal" to do so, as in the present case. In her argument, she gave much credit to the medical establishment and the state, in that they "probably know what they're doing." She believed there was a reason for the three cycles, and that it amounted to a "*reasonable* number of cycles." To add one more turn to the interpretation, I argue that, in Lise's view, guided by her particular political-medical context, not venturing into treatment or stopping treatment before the end of the state-sponsored cycles amounts to an active choice to remain childless.

Lise created another position when it came to number of treatments: she believed that exceeding the "normal" limit of three cycles was potentially dangerous. She told the story of someone she knew, for whom "the IVF project," as she called it, "got out of control."

> They're going [abroad] for their tenth cycle now, and it has become part of their lifestyle, really. They don't do anything else, no holidays, no parties, nothing. Because they always have to think of the cycles, and to eat healthily, and … not drink and … it's become their, or maybe only her, only focus. I don't think it's healthy for them. Not for them individually. Not for the relationship. But then again…

Again, three cycles was considered the "normal" number, through which Lise created meaning. She did not explicitly state that she believed the couple she mentioned would never be successful, but rather that their project wasn't worth it – it cost them too much. She presented their position as desperate, and, even though Lise identified with a certain *degree* of desperation, the story above was presented as a case in which the child wish was no longer natural, but rather unintelligible and unhealthy.

Lise used her own understanding and evaluation of the child wish as an interpretative device to assess other people's choices, choices she perceived to be understandable to a greater or lesser extent in relation to her own. The explicit story Lise told was one in which the situation of childlessness was so emotionally and socially difficult, filled with so many questions, that she did not want to judge the subjects for choosing differently from her. But, at the same time, she implicitly created positions of "not trying hard enough" and "trying too hard" to alleviate childlessness, with her own position lying at the balance point in between. In the last section, I round off the discussion with a brief analysis of how Lise's story creates a particular understanding of childlessness.

Naturalizations and Un-Naturalizations

Throughout the recounting of Lise's story, I have made visible a position that was produced by the disciplinarian context and by her choices. Lise presented her own choices as "normal" and "natural." She drew lines between what were, for her, acceptable and less acceptable technologies, justifiable and less justifiable choices. She established a position both in relation to and in contrast with those who made different choices – both those who did not go as far as she had and those who went further. Her choices positioned her as active yet not desperate, understanding but not condemning; they were presented as "natural" ways to cope with childlessness. But do naturalizations of actions and choices of this kind inadvertently also produce un-naturalizations?

The normalization and naturalization of IVF in this story create a particular understanding of childlessness and generate different degrees of legitimate, socially accepted childlessness. To act on infertility in a bodily way, as Lise did, is presented as the most obvious way to act within a context characterized by biologism and medicalization, where the desire for children is understood as a biological urge and where technology and expertise are available. Motherhood, family life, the desire for children, and IVF are all perceived as natural, so what becomes "unnatural" is, rather, the state of childlessness. Childlessness becomes both socially and medically unnatural – more unnatural than the steps taken to alleviate or cure it. Infertility becomes un-naturalized in the sense that, although it is perceived as a medical, and hence abnormal but nature-given condition, the fact that one *by choice* does not "do" what is possible to alleviate it makes infertility appear to be a chosen and human-generated condition, un-naturalized because one has not followed one's natural drives to the culturally appropriate lengths.

Through her story, Lise tried to make sense of her situation and choices. All of her choices and reflections on limits could, of course, be questioned: why did she construct the limits where she did? But, through her argument, she constructed them as reasonable, logical – and "natural." Hers is not necessarily a hegemonic position but, through her narration, it is clearly understandable and logical within her cultural context. At the same time, her choices and the stories she tells about them in this specific context produce other, unintentional effects, such as the un-naturalization of childlessness. This, I believe, is indicative not only of Lise's story, but also of the many stories contributing to cultural constructions of reproduction and ARTs within different cultural contexts.

Notes

1 The project's main aim was to study lay people's understanding of the intersection of gender, genes and reproduction in a Norwegian context. The researchers involved in the project were project leader Prof. Merete Lie, Kristin H. Spilker and myself. The project was funded by the Norwegian Research Council. Altogether we conducted 15 interviews with Norwegian heterosexual couples for the project. The interviews were conducted in Norwegian, and the quotes have been translated into English by the author.

2 "Normal" must here be understood as "not specifically marked by IVF technology," as of course pregnancies, pregnant bodies, and children can deviate from any definition of "normal" in a multitude of ways.

3 Sperm donation is legal and egg donation is illegal in Norway, as discussed in other chapters of this book.

References

Franklin, Sarah. 1997. *Embodied Progress: A Cultural Account of Assisted Conception.* London: Routledge.

Franklin, Sarah, and Maureen McNeil. 1988. "Review: Reproductive Futures: Recent Literature and Current Feminist Debates on Reproductive Technologies." *Feminist Studies* 14 (3): 545–560.

Howell, Signe. 2006. *The Kinning of Foreigners: Transnational Adoption in a Global Perspective.* New York: Berghahn Books.

Lie, Merete. 2002. "Science as Father? Sex and Gender in the Age of Reproductive Technologies." *The European Journal of Women's Studies* 9 (4): 381–399.

Lie, Merete, Malin Noem Ravn, and Kristin Spilker. 2011. "Reproductive Imaginations: Stories of Egg and Sperm." *NORA – Nordic Journal of Feminist and Gender Research* 19 (4): 231–248.

Melhuus, Marit. 2009. "Conflicting Notions of Continuity and Belonging: Assisted Reproduction, Law, and Practices in Norway." *Social Analysis: Journal of Cultural and Social Practice* 53 (3): 148–162.

Melhuus, Marit, and Signe Howell. 2009. "Adoption and Assisted Conception: One Universe of Unnatural Procreation. An Examination of Norwegian Legislation." In *European Kinship in the Age of Biotechnology*, edited by Jeanette Edwards and Carles Salazar, 144–161. New York and Oxford: Berghahn Books.

Rapp, Rayna. 1988. "Moral Pioneers: Women, Men and Fetuses on a Frontier of Reproductive Technologies." *Women & Health* 13 (1–2): 101–117.

Ravn, Malin N. 2004. "En kropp: To liv: Svangerskapet, fosteret og den gravide kroppen – en antropologisk analyse." [One Body: Two Lives. Pregnancy, the Fetus and the Pregnant Body – An Anthropological Analysis]. PhD diss., Norges teknisk-naturvitenskapelige universitet.

Ravn, Malin N. 2005. "A Matter of Free Choice? Some Structural and Cultural Influences on the Decision to Have or Not to Have Children in Norway." In *Barren States: The Population "Implosion" in Europe*, edited by Carrie B. Douglass, 29–47. Oxford, New York: Berg Publishers.

Ravn, Malin N. 2009. "Substances of the Body: Blood, Genes and Personhood." In *Contested Categories: Life Sciences in Society*, edited by Susanne Bauer and Ayo Wahlberg, 31–48. Farnham: Ashgate.

Sawicki, Jana. 1999. "Disciplining Mothers: Feminism and the New Reproductive Technologies." In *Feminist Theory and the Body: A Reader*, edited by Janet Price and Margrit Shildrick, 190–202. Edinburgh: Edinburgh University Press.

Spilker, Kristin H. 2008. "Assistert slektskap: biopolitikk i reproduksjonsteknologienes tidsalder." [Assisted Kinship: Biopolitics in the Time of Reproductive Technologies]. PhD diss., Norges teknisk-naturvitenskapelige universitet.

Thompson, Charis. 2005. *Making Parents: The Ontological Choreography of Reproductive Technologies*. Cambridge: MIT Press.

Throsby, Karen. 2004. *When IVF Fails: Feminism, Infertility and the Negotiation of Normality*. Basingstoke: Palgrave Macmillan.

Tjørnhøj-Thomsen, Tine. 1998. "Tilblivelseshistorier: barnløshed, slægtskab og forplantningsteknologi i Danmark." PhD diss., Københavns Universitet.

20 Sperm Stories[1]

Sociotechnical Imaginaries of Sperm Donation and Sperm Banking in Denmark

Stine Willum Adrian

Introduction

> We only have donors who carry both wonderful characteristics and risks of genetic illnesses. We have no "clean" donors.
>
> (CEO of the Viking Bank, November 2015)

With two of Europe's largest sperm banks exporting sperm worldwide, and liberal regulations regarding sperm donation, Denmark has emerged as a popular destination for fertility travelers in need of donor sperm. Internationally, media stories have taken up the news, and headlines of Viking babies are regularly circulated (Johnston 2015; Aldridge 2015). When I conducted an interview with the CEO of the Viking Bank, the argument that "donors are not clean" surprised me because the statement differed from the stories I had encountered when I interviewed him ten years earlier (Adrian 2006, 2010). His perspective on sperm, genes, and technologies seemed to have shifted during the ten years that had passed and this directed my interest to analyze what was at stake as new technologies and imaginaries are emerging regarding sperm donation. In this chapter I ask: What are the sociotechnical imaginaries narrated in relation to Danish donor sperm, and what effects do these have as they become entangled in policies and practices?

My interest in sociotechnical imaginaries is inspired by Sheila Jasanoff's conceptualization of the term. She argues that, although sociotechnical imaginaries are collective, they may have different origins, and include technological agencies, social practices, and cultural imaginaries (2015, 1–33). I particularly draw on the term to understand how different conceptualizations of sperm donation in the empirical material I analyze emerge along a continuum from technophobic to technophilic, and how these sociotechnical imaginations have effects on policies and practices.

Inspired by Franklin, Lury, and Stacey (2000), I perceive the sociotechnical imaginaries of sperm donation as entangled in different iconographic narrations and visualizations of the sperm. In terms of methodology, I approach these through visual analysis (Sturken and Cartwright 2001) and narrative analysis (Polkinghorne 1995). This methodological choice reflects the influence on this chapter of previous research within the fields of feminist technoscience studies and feminist medical anthropology analyzing the use of ARTs, for example Strathern (1992), Franklin (1997), Tjørnhøj-Thomsen (1999), Becker (2000), Inhorn (2003), and Thompson (2005).

Empirically, the chapter draws on two periods of ethnographic fieldwork ten years apart. The first period, from 2002–2004, focused on new stories of creation at fertility clinics and sperm banks in Denmark and Sweden (Adrian 2006). The second focuses on the globalization of Danish sperm (Adrian 2015). During both sets of fieldwork I conducted observations of and interviews with staff at fertility clinics and sperm banks, and women who, with or without partners, were seeking treatment with donor sperm. In addition, webpages, advertising material, websites, and newspaper articles are included in the analysis.

For analytical reasons and in order to anonymize my material, I have renamed the clinics and sperm bank where I conducted the fieldwork and interviews that I draw on in this analysis. I have chosen to call the Danish sperm bank "the Viking Bank," because it has used Viking mythology in its branding of sperm abroad.[2] I have called a Danish insemination clinic led by a midwife "The Alternative" because its focus is to create an alternative atmosphere, including offering alternative stories of family, kinship, and sexuality.

To provide a context for my analysis, I start with an introduction to the main features of Danish ART policies, focusing in particular on the ways in which they have changed regarding donor insemination between 1997 and 2015. In the main part of the chapter I first discuss how, in the sales strategy of the sperm bank, sperm is iconographically narrativized and visualized through hypermasculinized donors, represented as virile Vikings, and how the images of Viking sperm are entangled with stories of "better" genes. Second, I analyze how sperm from "donors," who are consciously not articulated as "fathers" at The Alternative, enables new sociotechnical imaginaries entangled with new understandings of kinship. Third, I discuss how the iconographic imaginary of donor sperm as "contaminated" or "not clean" both draws upon and challenges previous sociotechnical imaginaries. Finally, I sum up the analysis by discussing the different contradictory sociotechnical imaginaries that are at stake in the policies and practices of Danish sperm banking and sperm donation.

Changing Policies and Practices Relating to Donor Insemination in Denmark

The Danish legislation relating to ARTs was implemented in 1997. Since then, regulations and practices have changed significantly, and become increasingly complex (Mohr 2014; Adrian 2015). In a Danish context, the development of private sperm banks as part of a larger fertility industry is intriguing, as free public health care is a cornerstone of the welfare state. However, sperm banking and sperm donation have been at the forefront of privatization, and today two sperm banks selling donor sperm globally are situated in Denmark (Adrian 2015).

During my first fieldwork in 2002, the original legislation on ARTs, enacted in 1997, did not allow medical doctors to provide fertility treatment to lesbians or single women; this legislation was passed after acrimonious debates in the Danish Parliament (Lützen 2000; Bryld 2001; Stormhøj 2002; Albæk 2003). However, this was challenged in 1999 when the first insemination clinic was established by a midwife offering treatment to single women and lesbian couples. This was possible in practice because the legislation only prevented medical doctors from doing so.

In 2007, the EU Tissue and Cell Directive was implemented in Denmark (Sundhedsstyrelsen 2015). In the same year, medical doctors were permitted to give lesbians and single women fertility treatment, even at public hospitals (Petersen 2009). From 2006–2012, the midwife clinics began offering a broader choice regarding the selection of sperm from Danish donors. This was possible because Danish sperm banks were permitted at this point to offer sperm donation with non-anonymous donors and donors with extended profiles. Clinics owned by medical doctors, which were regulated by the law on assisted reproduction, were, in contrast to the unregulated midwife clinics, not allowed to market donor sperm with extended donor profiles back then. But recently, in 2012, this practice became legal for medical doctors, too.[3]

Donor Imaginaries of Better Sperm and Viking Masculinity

The first sperm story originates from my first day of fieldwork at the Viking Bank.

> A secretary followed me to the meeting room where I could hang my jacket. In the room was a whiteboard with a rather large drawing of an erect penis ejaculating into a test tube. The employee showing me around seemed both embarrassed and amused by the drawing. Since I had not expected any sexualized pictures of the donors, I was very surprised to see the penis, and started to giggle with her.
>
> (Fieldnote 2002)

The drawing of the penis was a sketch of a neon billboard that they were considering making in order to draw attention at a fertility conference. The penis lamp was initially intended to be made in neon, and go from non-erect to erect, with flickering neon lights representing the ejaculated sperm flowing into the test tube. Finally, the neon light was meant to fall to the floor to symbolize the sperm bank spreading sperm around the world. While I was carrying out observations at the annual meeting of The European Society of Human Reproduction and Embryology (ESHRE) in the summer of 2003, I saw that the lamp had been transformed into a more modest anatomical drawing of a cross-section of the erect penis. Small, blinking lights demonstrated how the sperm was constantly being ejaculated into a test tube.

Reading the picture as a continuous "money shot," a hard-core pornographic story indulging in visualization of the erect penis and sperm, one could argue, as Linda Williamson does in her analyses of pornographic movies, that:

> Perhaps in the money shot's repeatedly inflated, "spending" penis we can see condensed all the principles of late capitalism's pleasure-oriented consumer society: pleasure figured as an orgasm of spending; the fetish not simply as commodity but as the surplus value of orgasm.
>
> (Williamson 1989, 108)

By reading the lamp as pornography, we can see the sperm not only as money, or a commodity, but also as a sign of masculinity, virility, or as a sexual bi-product generating surplus value. The sociotechnical imaginary at play underscores the making of healthy children and connects the icon of sperm from hyper-virile donors with hyper-fertility. However, the other side of the coin is also implied in this imaginary: the myth of the infertile man, stigmatized as the impotent counter-image to the icon of the hyper-virile and hyper-fertile donor.

Interestingly, the iconographic focus on sperm from "virile" and "fertile" donors was connected to the increasing globalization of the product. In 2002, the Viking Bank was already an international sperm bank selling to more than 35 countries (a number that has increased to more than 80 today). Already back then, the international framing of the business had led to differentiated storytelling practices, targeted at markets that were defined by differing legislation and consumer demands.

In 2001, globalization and the diversity of markets influenced the development of two new webpages used for marketing: one for Denmark and a global market intended for sale to clinics, and one directed toward the USA, where sperm was sold and marketed directly to the parents-to-be, in which the donor profiles included information on the donors' academic merits, hobbies, and personal reflections on being a donor. The Viking Bank's website targeting the American market was seen in the Danish media as rather controversial and was criticized for being eugenic as the donor selection was not only based on phenotypes (Christensen 2001; Lade 2001).

When, in 2004, the Viking Bank redeveloped its webpage for the American market it even marketed the sperm by drawing on Scandinavian sagas and cultural imaginaries of Vikings (Adrian 2006, 2010; Kroløkke 2009). This meant that the American webpage was reinforcing the way in which the CEO of the sperm bank had described the imaginary relationship between the global migration of Vikings and the sperm bank's increased market sale in an interview with me in 2002:

> It's a repetition of what we did 1000 years ago [laughter]. We also spread our genes then.... We simply raped and robbed and so on, and spread our genes. And now we're doing this again in the same way, under less primitive conditions. And this time we're welcome.
>
> (Interview CEO 2002)

In the CEO's reference to the Viking adventure story, Viking sperm is presented as just as "naturally" vigorous today as it was, according to the legend, when the

Vikings were "spreading their genes" 1000 years ago. As in the pornographic story, the hyper-masculinity and virility of the Viking hero with whom the donor is associated reflects badly on his counterpart, the infertile man. Thus, the sperm bank presents an imaginary of donor sperm as better than "ordinary" sperm.

Sperm as "Donor" – Not "Father": Thinking Technologies of Kinship Differently

Subversive alternative stories of sperm donation have also been circulating, not least as a result of the legislation that only permitted medical doctors to treat heterosexual couples from 1997 to 2007. The Alternative was one of the insemination clinics established as a political protest against this discriminatory legislation. On top of this, The Alternative's mode of care is woman-centered and focused on demedicalization, emphasized by the homey décor of the clinic (Adrian 2006, 2014).

What made the sperm stories told at The Alternative different from those of other fertility clinics and the sperm bank's narratives, was among other things the way in which the origin of the sperm was narrated as coming from a "donor," not from a "father" (Adrian 2006, 281–288). This became clear to me when, in 2003, I interviewed Tilde who worked at The Alternative. She pointed out that I should not use the term "father" as synonymous with "donor," a habit I had developed during my fieldwork at other clinics and sperm banks. This point was central to the way in which sperm donation was discursively constructed, carried out, and made kin at The Alternative.

Tilde emphasized that, before the insemination, she would interview the future parent/parents. In so doing, she would focus not only on medical questions, but also on how they as parents would explain to the child how it was conceived. Tilde told me that she was especially careful with single women. She wanted to make sure that they were not secretly holding on to the dream of a nuclear family. She was afraid that if the parents were unable to explain their choice convincingly, it would be difficult for the child to grow up in a different type of family, and face societal prejudice. Occasionally, Tilde and her colleagues would decide not to treat a woman if they were uncertain whether the child would be supported during its upbringing. However, the selection was not based on exclusion of specific groups.

The stories about the making of alternative families at the clinic became important in terms of challenging the legislation, which from 1997 to 2007 excluded lesbians and single women from fertility treatment monitored by medical doctors. Although lesbian couples and single women were granted the right to treatment when the law was changed in 2007, from 2007 to 2012 The Alternative and other clinics run by midwives were still not regulated by law. So, just as The Alternative and other midwives' clinics had been instrumental in creating an alternative story of lesbian and single women as parents, they also took the opportunity to begin buying non-anonymous donor sperm from Danish sperm banks, including from sperm donors with extended profiles, in this way enabling greater consumer choice prior to 2012, when this practice also became legal for medical doctors.

Considering that The Alternative is drawing on a sociotechnical imaginary of demedicalization, it is interesting that it introduced treatment with sperm from non-anonymous donors and donors with extended profiles. In other words, the alternative narratives have been written in a strategic subversive alliance with the private sperm banks, challenging the premises of the existing legislation by not only enabling single women and lesbians to become parents, but also allowing them to choose sperm from both anonymous and non-anonymous donors, with or without extended profiles. In this regard, the sociotechnical imaginaries were more focused on how sperm donation is another means of making kin. Implicitly, they include technological critiques as sperm donation is imagined and performed differently than in a clinical setting, and the care is explicitly defined and practiced as woman-centered.

Sperm as "Contaminated" and Not "Clean"

Masculinity, virility and fertility were not the only criteria used to organize sperm in the Danish sperm bank. When I interviewed the CEO in 2002, he argued:

> There are a lot of things that need to be organized in terms of security. One may argue that there is nothing special in running a sperm bank. In other words, sperm is something a lot of people have. All men walking around have some. So what is it we have that others don't? It is security. We can be completely sure that the sperm we have here is not mixed up or contaminated … it's an entire set of genes that we have. If they get exchanged, it becomes completely different genes … so it is a lot of security control.
>
> (Interview CEO 2002)

The organization of the sperm bank, from the selection of donors to the handling and categorization of the sperm, is focused on producing "secure" sperm that is not contaminated, is defined by its "genes" and is organized in ways that minimize mix-ups in the laboratory.

Although sperm donation implies that the social father is not genetically linked to his child, the guidelines from the health authorities at the time underscored that donor selection had to mimic the phenotype of the soon-to-be social father. In other words, "race" and other physical characteristics that enable resemblance between father and child was seen as important for the making of kin.

Accordingly, the categorization of the donated sperm is described and organized in relation to the donors' physical characteristics such as eye color, height, and weight.

In the process of handling sperm, employees had to deal with the risk of contaminated sperm. In the storage process, the donor sperm is thus transformed into a potential "*health hazard*." This became clear in my observations at the laboratory. When the donor hands over the sperm to the lab technician, he does so on a cardboard tray. This tray is used as what employees call a "transport cart." This is done to enable the lab staff to move the sperm without wearing gloves, thus maintaining a relaxed atmosphere around the donor. However, on the other side of the counter, the lab technician's hands are gloved and the sperm is no longer a "normal" bodily fluid. Instead, it is handled as though a virus (such as HIV or infectious hepatitis) has contaminated it.

The gloves are just one of the devices that play a part in the practices of risk management. Such practices were also involved when the staff produced "secure" sperm using "high-security straws" for cryo-preserving and storing the sperm,[4] involving such diverse matters as handling pipettes carefully and disciplining the donor's sex life in order to decrease his chances of contracting sexually transmitted diseases.

Behind the concern shown by the CEO and the doctor when telling me about security measures was not only the wish that, through my research, I should publicly convey the story of the "secure sperm" that was commercially important for the Vikings Bank's image. The need to prevent the major disaster that would take place if somehow "contaminated" sperm from the sperm bank was used by mistake was also clear. This need was given greater urgency by the actual occurrence of a similar disaster in blood banks worldwide.[5] The story of possible disaster and potential contamination can hence be seen both as a possible threat and as a narrative that gives the sperm value and structures the purification ritual, from the moment it enters the bank until it has become a product worth being sold. Over time, this story has been reinforced by the implementation of the EU Cell and Tissue Directive that was implemented in Denmark in 2007. The regulatory changes have led to new practices in the lab as sperm, culture medium, and all the equipment used needs to be traceable. This implies increased documentation, better quality control systems, and audits demanded by the health authorities (Sundhedstyrelsen 2015). The premises implied in these practices and regulatory texts are sociotechnical imaginaries that focus on how technologies enable insecurity and disasters. However, one might also argue that what is implied in these narratives is a technological determinism that seems to promise more "secure" sperm (based on a genetic essentialism and purification).

During my fieldwork in 2002, the stories I was told presented the Viking Bank's sperm as more secure and thus also genetically better than other donor sperm. Thus, when I returned to the sperm bank in 2011 and interviewed the CEO in 2013, it surprised me that he argued that "no clean donors" exist.[6]

The interview in 2013 was conducted after a major media scandal. This scandal did not directly influence the legislation on treatment by ARTs that had already been passed in Parliament, but it did have an impact on the development of guidelines and the Danish interpretation of the legislation in the EU Tissue and Cell Directive.

The core of the news was a story about a sperm donor who turned out to be a carrier of neurofibromatosis type 1 (NF1). This is a variable genetic disorder which has many different symptoms that can vary from exhibiting café-au-lait spots on the body to the development of tumors (NFDanmark 2015).

By 2009, the donor had passed on NF1 to at least nine of the 43 children conceived using his sperm (Vaaben 2012). When the story broke in the Danish media, the case was already well known internationally, as the involved sperm bank had made the case public (Callum *et al.* 2012).

This story raised issues such as how many offspring a donor ought to have, who is responsible for reporting pregnancies to the health authorities, and what screening procedures can be expected. The combination of the high number of reported half-siblings, a high degree of non-disclosure to donor-conceived offspring, and anxiety about incest, consanguinity, and the spread of genetic diseases created fodder for media stories full of affect (Lytken 2012a, 2012b; Dahlgaard 2013a). In the first guidelines issued after the legislative changes in 2012, the maximum number of offspring allowed for each donor in Denmark was halved to 12 (which in practice is understood as a permit to donate to 12 families, but does not include children born outside Danish borders) (Sundhedsstyrelsen 2012). More importantly, sperm banks were identified as responsible for ensuring that this number of children was not exceeded. This became a controversial issue with one sperm bank, in particular, which found it technically impossible to fulfill the requirements of the legislation. The bank temporarily stopped delivering sperm in Denmark, and in the media warned that this legal change could develop into a "sperm drought" (Dahlgaard 2013b). Later, the controversy was overcome, and sperm banks continue to sell sperm internationally as well as nationally as the guidelines were changed (Ministeriet for Sundhed og Forebyggelse 2015).

However, the story of NF1 has also played an important role in how donors' genes are perceived by the public. Through the internet, the parents – predominately the mothers – of the children who had been diagnosed with NF1 got in contact with one another, and together they played an active role in voicing their concerns regarding how the sperm bank had managed the first reports on children born with NF1. On top of this, these parents have indicated their surprise that children born by sperm donation can have genetically inheritable diseases, inherited from the donor's side. This perspective is being used as a central argument in a court case that they have been pursuing against the sperm bank (Christensen 2014). The critique voiced against the sperm banks is embedded in the sociotechnical imaginaries implied in the stories of Viking sperm. Thus, the advertising on a global market that they had better sperm, indicated by stories of "Viking sperm," had left the parents unprepared for the possibility of this sperm carrying genetic diseases.

This critique evolved at the same time as technological advances in genetic testing and screening had made their use cheaper. Against this background, the CEOs of the sperm banks were considering if and how much they should make use of these technological developments, and what the consequences of these opportunities might be for sperm banking. If all donors come with a risk profile, will it be possible to recruit donors at all, as nobody is "clean"?

The story narrated by the CEO, that "donors are not clean," could in other words be seen as a shift in how the Viking Bank perceive genes. As a consequence of this new perception of genes, the Viking Bank has changed its practices regarding the reporting of illnesses or congenital defects inherited from the donor. While, previously, donor sperm was blocked from further use if it was discovered that the offspring had inherited diseases or malformations, the Viking Bank has now developed a new system in their donor selection search engine on their website.[7] It informs the consumer if there has been a report about the donor. The consumer can act on this information by choosing either to click to pursue it or not. The idea is to enable consumers to decide for themselves whether or not they want to know about the possible risks.

Conclusion

In this chapter I have analyzed sociotechnical imaginaries related to Danish donor sperm. I have explored how these sociotechnical imaginaries are entangled with policies and practices and how they are changing over time.

As I read the sperm stories, different and sometimes contradictory sociotechnical imaginaries are evoked. Several of them draw heavily on technophilic and technophobic imaginations that are inherently deterministic.

The iconographies of the super-virile, masculine donors developed through the illustration of the erect, ejaculating penis and the Viking donors, have been a successful sales strategy for the Viking Bank over the years. By drawing on imaginaries of masculinity, kinship, whiteness, heterosexuality, and secure sperm, the Viking Bank has ascribed an added value to the sperm in terms of producing babies connoting genetic enhancement. At the same time, this technoscientific imaginary draws implicitly, and probably without reflection, on the stigma of male infertility.

The general media criticism of sperm banking, to which the NF1 case gave rise, interestingly draws on the same sociotechnical imaginaries as the Viking stories. The critical discourses implied a belief that donor sperm ought to be better and more secure than "ordinary" sperm. However, in practice only a few genetic tests are carried out on sperm donors today – a practice which is being challenged at a time when the technologies of sequencing the genome are becoming economically viable. In order to meet this challenge, the Viking Bank has been going through a process of changing its perspective on genes and has tried to develop a method of donor selection in which the consumer chooses to learn or not learn about the known risks of inheritable diseases that this donor may carry. In this way, technological and scientific development has been a part of challenging the imagination of genes that was inherent in the previous Viking stories.

The technophobic or technophilic imaginaries that draw on genetic essentialism and technological determinism do not stand alone, however. Technologies can be imagined, practiced, and used in other ways. This is illustrated in The Alternative's stories of sperm. Their point of departure is to create woman-centered care, enabling more women to have children by supporting alternative narratives of kinship and family in a society where heteronormativity prevails.

The sociotechnical imaginaries that The Alternative draws upon are in this regard a critique of both the mode of care related to medicalization, and the exclusion and stigmatization of single women and lesbians that was a consequence of the law between 1997 and 2007. In this way, The Alternative's imaginaries of donor sperm as a product of technoscience were not focused on seeing the technology as a means of increasingly controlling reproduction, but instead as a way for women to have children without hetero-sex. In this respect, the practice of introducing donors with extended profiles can also be seen as a way to provide care for the future families, as extended profiles and open donors enable more information to develop when women tell the stories of their origin to their future children.

Exploring the different sociotechnical imaginaries in the sperm stories and their entanglement with policies and practices is interesting because it not only creates valuable understandings of how sociotechnical imaginaries are at stake as technologies are developed, used, and implemented, they are also illustrative of how sociotechnical imaginaries are not innocent. They are part of inclusions and exclusions, marginalizations and stigmatizations. In the case of sperm donation, these processes involve emergent technologies, donors, donor-conceived offspring, infertile men, the mothers (to be), and the sperm banks and fertility clinics. The sperm stories therefore illustrate that we need to develop and think along new lines of storytelling that draw on sociotechnical imaginaries that are neither technophobic nor technophilic. Instead I shall make a plea that, in the discussion of the technological and ethical dilemmas that emerge during practices of making life and kin, not only the technology as such, but also the implied sociotechnical imaginaries are discussed and challenged. As I have illustrated, they are part of the practices, exclusions, and occasional stigmatization; however, the narratives from The Alternative illustrate that sociotechnical imaginaries offer not only challenges but also potential and promises of subversive practices in the making of kin.

Notes

1 This chapter is an abbreviated, updated and revised version of the article: Adrian, Stine Willum. 2010. "Sperm Stories: Policies and Practices of Sperm Banking in Denmark and Sweden." *European Journal of Women's Studies* 17 (4): 393–411. © The Author(s) 2010. Reprinted by Permission of SAGE Publications, Ltd.

2 In 2002 there was only one large private sperm bank in Denmark. As an analytical point, I have renamed the bank to match the other anonymizations of the sites where I did my fieldwork. I only talk about the Viking Bank when I refer to the ethnographic fieldwork. Otherwise I refer to them as "the sperm banks," as the particularity of one or the other is not relevant for parts of the analysis.

3 Although the sperm banks and midwife-owned clinics have been able to conduct treatments without being regulated by the Danish law on ARTs, in terms of security and quality, they have nevertheless been regulated by the EU Cell and Tissue Directive (Adrian 2015).

4 A straw is a small plastic vial where the sperm is kept during cryopreservation.
5 See Waldby and Mitchell 2006.
6 I quote from a follow-up interview done in 2015, however, the same point was emphasized in the interview from 2013.
7 This practice was inaugurated on April 7, 2015.

References

Adrian, Stine W. 2006. "Nye skabelsesberetninger om æg, sæd og embryoner. Et etnografisk studie af skabelser på sædbanker og fertilitetsklinikker." [New Creation Stories of Eggs, Sperm and Embryos. An Ethnographic Study of Creations at Sperm Banks and Fertility Clinics]. PhD diss., Linköpings Universitet.

Adrian, Stine W. 2010. "Sperm Stories: Policies and Practices of Sperm Banking in Denmark and Sweden." *European Journal of Women's Studies* 17 (4): 393–411.

Adrian, Stine W. 2014. "Naturligvis? Når Lys, Hunde og Kønsceller Sætter Naturen til Forhandling på Fertilitetsklinikken." [Naturally? Negotiating Light, Dogs and Gametes]. *Kulturstudier* (1): 103–127.

Adrian, Stine W. 2015. "12. Subversive Practices of Sperm Donation: Globalising Danish Sperm." In *Critical Kinship Studies*, edited by Charlotte Kroløkke, Lene Myong, Stine W. Adrian, and Tine Tjørnhøj-Thomsen, 193–202. London: Rowman & Littlefield International.

Albæk, Erik. 2003. "Political Ethics and Public Policy: Homosexuals between Moral Dilemmas and Political Considerations in Danish Parliamentary Debates." *Scandinavian Political Studies* 26 (3): 245–267.

Aldridge, Gemma. 2015. "'I Want a Viking Baby': Single British Women Flocking to World's Biggest Sperm Bank in Denmark." *Mirror Online*, January 24. Accessed December 21, 2015. www.mirror.co.uk/news/uk-news/i-want-viking-baby-single-5037149.

Becker, Gay. 2000. *The Elusive Embryo: How Women and Men Approach the New Reproductive Technologies.* Berkeley: University of California Press.

Bryld, Mette 2001. "The Infertility Clinic and the Birth of the Lesbian: The Political Debate on Assisted Reproduction in Denmark." *The European Journal of Women's Studies* 8 (3): 299–312.

Callum, Pamela, Ludwine M. Messiaen, Peter V. Bower, Flemming Skovby, J. Iger, Susanne Timshel, Charles A. Sims, and Rena E. Falk. 2012. "Gonosomal Mosaicism for an NF1 Deletion in a Sperm Donor: Evidence of the Need for Coordinated, Long-Term Communication of Health Information Among Relevant Parties." *Human Reproduction* 27 (4): 1223–1226.

Christensen, Esben. 2014. "Staten Betaler for Retssag Mod Sædbank." [The State Pays For Lawsuit Against Spermbank]. *DR Nyheder.* Last accessed April 11. www.dr.dk/nyheder/indland/staten-betaler-retssag-mod-saedbank/.

Christensen, Louise. 2001. "Skarp Kritik af Sædbank." [Acute Critique of Spermbank]. *Politiken*, April 28. Accessed November 18, 2015. http://politiken.dk/indland/ECE20123/skarp-kritik-af-saedbank/.

Dahlgaard, Mette. 2013a. "Sædbank varsler sædtørke i Danmark." [Spermbank Warns Against Sperm Drought in Denmark]. *Berlingske Tidende*, January 2. Accessed November 22, 2015. www.b.dk/nationalt/saedbank-lukker-for-saed-til-danmark-0.

Dahlgaard, Mette. 2013b. "Bør én Mand Være Far til 100 Børn?" [Should One Man Father 100 Children?] *BT*, January 12. Accessed November 22, 2015. www.b.dk/nationalt/boer-en-mand-vaere-far-til-100-boern.

Franklin, Sarah. 1997. *Embodied Progress: A Cultural Account of Assisted Conception.* New York, London: Routledge.

Franklin, Sarah, Celia Lury, and Jackie Stacey. 2000. *Global Nature, Global Culture.* London: Sage Publications.

Inhorn, Marcia. 2003. *Local Babies, Global Science: Gender Religion, and In Vitro Fertilization in Egypt.* New York: Routledge.

Jasanoff, Sheila. 2015. "Future Imperfect: Science, Technology, and the Imaginations of Modernity." In *Dreamscapes of Modernity: Sociotechnical Imagianries and the Fabrication of Power*, by Sheila Jasanoff and Sang Hyun Kim, 1–33. Chicago: Chicago University Press.

Johnston, Jenny. 2015. "The Rise of the Baby Vikings: Why Single British Women Desperate for Children Are Turning to Sperm Donors in Denmark – Who'll Play No Part in Their Offspring's Lives." *Daily Mail Online*, January 20. Accessed November 22, 2015. www.dailymail.co.uk/femail/article-2917432/The-rise-BABY-VIKINGS-single-British-women-desperate-children-turning-sperm-donors-Denmark-ll-play-no-offspring-s-lives.html.

Kroløkke, Charlotte. 2009. "Click a Donor: Viking Masculinity on the Line." *Journal of Consumer Culture* 9 (7): 7–30.

Lade, Marie. 2001. "Design din Egen Superbaby." [Design Your Own Superbaby]. *Ekstra-Bladet*, November 18. Accessed November 22, 2015. http://ekstrabladet.dk/nyheder/samfund/article3199970.ece.

Lytken, Lærke Hviid. 2012a. "Etisk Råd efter Sædskandale: Stram Reglerne Endnu Mere." [The Ethical Council after Sperm Scandal. Tighten the Regulations More]. *DR Nyheder.* Last accessed September 24. www.dr.dk/nyheder/indland/etisk-raad-efter-saedskandale-stram-reglerne-endnu-mere.

Lytken, Lærke Hviid. 2012b. "Sædbank: Der er Fuldstændig Kaos i Lovgivningen." [Spermbank: The Legislation is in a Complete Chaos]. *DR Nyheder.* Last accessed September 25. www.dr.dk/nyheder/indland/saedbank-der-er-fuldstaendig-kaos-i-lovgivningen.

Lützen, Karin. 2000. "Nogle ideologiske-moralske rødder til velfærdsstatens familiepolitik." [Some Ideological-Moral Roots of the Family Politics of the Welfare State]. *Arbejder Historie, Tidsskrift for Historie, Kultur og Politik* 4: 4–16.

Ministeriet for Sundhed og Forebyggelse. 2015. VEJ nr 935. *Vejledning om sundhedspersoners og vævscentres virksomhed og forpligtelser i forbindelse med assisteret reproduktion.* [*Guideline on Health Persons and Tissue Centers Obligations Regarding Assisted Reproductive Technologies*]. Accessed November 22, 2015 www.retsinformation.dk/Forms/R0710.aspx?id=172755.

Mohr, Sebastian. 2014. "Semen: An Ethnography of Donating Sperm in Denmark." PhD diss., Københavns Universitet.

NFDanmark. 2015. "Dansk Forening for Neurofibromatosis Recklinghausen." [Danish Organization for Neurofibromatosis Recklinghausen]. Accessed November 22, 2015. www.nfdanmark.dk/index.php/omsygdommen.

Petersen, Michael N. 2009. "Fra Barnets Tarv til Ligestilling: En Queerteoretisk Undersøgelse af Folketingets Forhandlinger om Kunstig Befrugtning." [From the Best Interest of the Child to Equality: A Queer-theoretical Analysis of Danish Parliamentary Debates on Artificial Insemination]. *Kvinder, Køn og Forskning* 2: 30–42.

Polkinghorne, Donald. 1995. "Narrative Configuration in Qualitative Research." *Qualitative Studies in Education* 8 (1): 5–23.

Stormhøj, Christel. 2002. "Queering the Family: Critical Reflections on State-Regulated Heteronormativity in the Scandinavian Countries." In *Farväl heteronormativitet,* edited by Göran Söderström and Jan Magnusson, 38–56. Huddinge: Lambda Nordica Förlag.

Strathern, Marilyn. 1992. *Reproducing the Future: Anthropology, Kinship and the New Reproductive Technologies*. Manchester: Manchester University Press.

Sturken, Marita and Cartwright, Lisa. 2001. *Practices of Looking: An Introduction to Visual Culture*. Oxford: Oxford University Press.

Sundhedsstyrelsen [Danish Health and Medicines Authority]. 2012. *Kunstig Befrutning. Vejledning om Autoriserede Sundhedspersoners og Vævscentres Virksomhed og Forpligtelser i Forbindelse Med Kunstig Befrugtning*. [Artificial Conception. Guidelines on Autorised Health Persons and Tissue Centers Businesses and Obligations regarding Artificial Conception]. Copenhagen: Sundhedsstyrelsen.

Sundhedsstyrelsen [Danish Health and Medicines Authority]. 2015. "Information on Tissue and Cells." *Sundhedsstyrelsen*. Accessed April 28, 2015. http://sundhedsstyrelsen.dk/da/medicin/blod-og-vaev/vaev-og-celler.

Thompson, Charis. 2005. *Making Parents: The Ontological Choreography of Reproductive Technologies*. Cambridge: MIT Press.

Tjørnhøj-Thomsen, Tine. 1999. "Tilblivelseshistorier: Barnløshed, slægtskab og forplantningsteknologi i Danmark." [Conception Stories. Childlessness, Kinship, and Technologies of Conception in Denmark]. PhD diss., Københavns Universitet.

Vaaben, Line. 2012. "Sædbankens Nye tur Rundt i Mediemøllen." [The Sperm Bank Did the Rounds in the Media Again]. September 25. Accessed November 22, 2015. www.etik.dk/kunstig-befrugtning/s%C3%A6dbankens-nye-tur-rundt-i-mediem%C3%B8llen.

Waldby, Catherine, and Robert Mitchell. 2006. *Tissue Economies: Blood, Organs, and Cell Lines in Late Capitalism*. Durham: Duke University Press.

Williamson, Linda. 1989. *Hard Core: Power, Pleasure, and the "Frenzy of the Visible."* Berkeley: University of California Press.

21 Cellular Origins

A Visual Analysis of Time-Lapse Embryo Imaging

Lucy van de Wiel

On June 11, 2013, a baby named Eva was born in Glasgow. Nine months previously, her embryo had been selected for implantation in her mother's womb with the aid of time-lapse embryo imaging technology. Her birth made national headlines because she was the first person to be born from an IVF procedure that used "Early Embryo Viability Assessment" (Eeva) for embryo selection (BBC 2013). Although her parents insist that they intended to call their future daughter Eva before they ever heard about the test, the company that owns the Eeva technology, Auxogyn, boasts of the test's significance as "the most important breakthrough in IVF in recent decades" in a press release entitled "Baby Eva Named after Pioneering IVF Test" (BBC 2013; Kbhandal 2013b). The visual nature of this technology is emphasized by the press release's inclusion of a video of

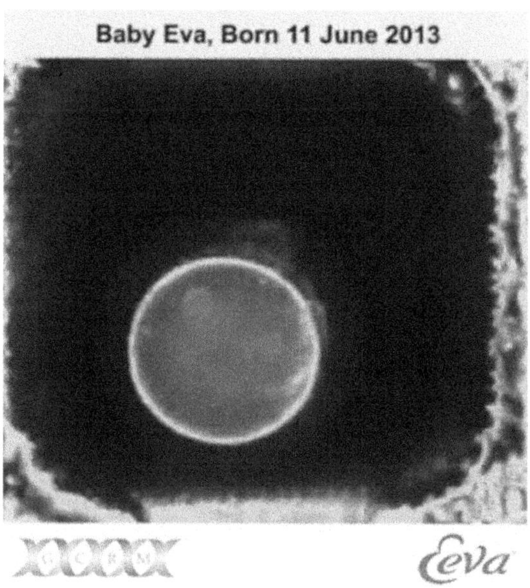

Figure 21.1 Embryo as individual. Still from Video "Baby Eeva Video – Eeva" (source: Kbhandal 2013a).

Eva's conception straight after the header (Kbhandal 2013a). The video shows a black-and-white image of the fertilized egg, which divides three times before the green-lettered word "HIGH" appears above it, referring to the embryo's quality. The video is framed by the logos of the Glasgow fertility clinic (GCRM) and Eeva below and the caption "Baby Eva, born 11 June 2013" above.

Two months prior to the Eeva news report, time-lapse embryo imaging had already been featured on BBC News as the latest breakthrough technology in IVF (Walsh 2013). This news item discussed a different embryo imaging technology, the EmbryoScope, which had followed 46 embryos through to birth.[1] The interviewed specialist, Dr Simon Fishel, managing director of the CARE Fertility Group, similarly claims that time-lapse embryo imaging is an important breakthrough: "In the 35 years I have been in this field this is probably the most exciting and significant development that can be of value to all patients seeking IVF." Notwithstanding the more or less groundbreaking technoscientific nature of these technologies, I will argue that they are also innovative in bringing into circulation a new set of images of early embryonic life.

As these news stories indicate, in 2013 several fertility clinics in the UK started marketing this method of embryo selection to patients as an alternative to conventional selection; it has since become widespread clinical practice.[2] Conventional selection is based on a daily visual examination of the embryos' static morphological appearance. In order to examine them, embryologists have to remove the embryos from their incubator into a suboptimal environment under the microscope. The time-lapse imaging technologies, by contrast, allow for continuous observation by taking photographs every five to 20 minutes while the embryos remain undisturbed in the incubator. The resulting videos not only give increased insight into the appearance of the embryos, but also visualize a temporal dimension that remained invisible in the conventional method: the timing of cell divisions and the movements of embryonic growth. By matching these videos with the growth patterns of embryos that developed into healthy fetuses, the time-lapse apparatus suggests which embryos are most likely to implant and grow in the woman's womb.

The time-lapse embryo imaging apparatus gives embryologists more visual and temporal information about the developing embryos, enabling them to avoid implanting those that are less likely to be viable while maintaining stable culturing conditions in the incubator. According to some biomedical studies, this approach results in increased implantation, pregnancy and live birth rates (Meseguer *et al.* 2012; Chen *et al.* 2013), while others – including a Cochrane review – hold that the current evidence of increased pregnancy or live birth rates is too limited to justify the routine adoption of time-lapse embryo imaging (Armstrong *et al.* 2015; Racowsky *et al.* 2015). Currently, three different time-lapse imaging systems, produced by two biotechnology companies, are used in fertility clinics: Auxogyn's Eeva and Vitrolife's EmbryoScope and Primo Vision.[3]

This alternative approach to embryo selection introduces moving images of embryonic development into the clinical experience of IVF. The resulting new set of embryo images circulates beyond the laboratory into the clinic, the patient's private sphere, and public discourses. Through these visual mediations, embryo selection becomes a more visible step in the IVF process – one that informs patient communication in fertility clinics and requires new decisions and financial investments from intended parents. As with other, existing medical imagery of prenatal life, it is hard to disentangle the medical and cultural meanings of these visual mediations of embryonic development (Van Dijck 2001, 103–104). As names like EmbryoScope and Primo Vision suggest, the observation and visualization of embryos play a key role both in the method and the marketing of time-lapse technology.

The visualization of embryos in time-lapse imaging is also instrumental in introducing temporal parameters as key indicators of viability in embryo assessment. The timing of the observed embryonic developmental process forms the basis for selecting which embryo(s) will be implanted in the woman's womb. Time-lapse embryo imaging thus brings together the innovations of visualized development, temporal assessment, uninterrupted incubation, increased digitization and standardization of selection. Although scholarly attention has been paid to the use of time-lapse microcinematography in a scientific research context – most notably by Landecker (2006, 2012) – the embryo videos produced in a clinical setting have not yet received critical reflection.

In this chapter, I draw attention to the visualization of embryonic development in time-lapse embryo imaging. I first explore how, and with what effects, embryos are visualized in time-lapse videos. Emerging in the wake of an increasingly visual interface with prenatal life, such as the iconic imagery of

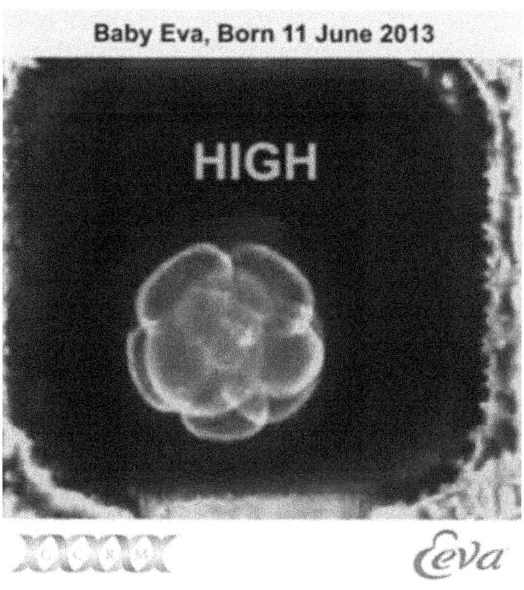

Figure 21.2 Embryo as individual. Still from Video "Baby Eeva Video – Eeva" (source: Kbhandal 2013a).

micro-injection and fetal ultrasound, both of which have had a profound impact on the public and private imagination of the reproductive process, time-lapse embryo videos add yet another visual dimension to the encounter with early human life on screen (Duden 1993; Van Dijck 2001; Franklin 2013). How can we position these embryo videos in relation to existing visual mediations of pre-natal life? What conceptualizations of embryos emerge from these videos and the ways in which they are framed by fertility clinics and biotechnology companies? How, and with what effects, do they engage human origin stories and the teleology of the reproductive process? In dialogue with scholarship on reproductive technologies in feminist technoscience studies, I engage with these concerns through a visual analysis of the framing of the time-lapse embryo videos – particularly Auxogyn's Eeva videos – that are publicly disseminated by fertility clinics, biotechnology companies and media outlets. In this reading of time-lapse embryo imagery, I will distinguish three approaches to visualizing embryos in the videos – as individuals, collectives, and populations – and consider what the implications may be if time-lapse imaging should become the "new normal" in embryo selection.

Baby Embryo: Watching Future Children

The first frames of Auxogyn's Eeva video, with which I opened this chapter, show a black-and-white image of a single cell (Kbhandal 2013a). The egg has a light-colored outline and is immersed in a dark gray background framed by a pronounced light border at the rectangular edges of the image. This ragged light border is a reminder of the apparatus through which the cell's image is produced, while the video's frame is branded by the logos of the company and the clinic, which reference the institutional context of its production. With the video's frame, and its inclusion in a press release, Baby Eva and the recording of her first cell divisions are publicly presented as the result of the ingenuity of the Eeva system and the expertise of the Glasgow Centre for Reproductive Medicine (GCRM). The "HIGH" inscription that follows the fertilized egg's cell divisions simultaneously signals the embryo's development, associates the institutions with success, and suggests a link between a HIGH prediction and a healthy baby. In this section, I will discuss the visualization of embryos in time-lapse videos and address how they become meaningful, both as individuals by association with the future child and as a collective to be scrutinized for selection.

Although moving images of dividing cells – and embryonic development in particular – are commonplace, time-lapse embryo imaging newly individualizes this scene through its clinical application. Here the link to the child is established in the Eeva video's departure from representing "everyembryo" to showing an individualized "Baby Eva" (Morgan 2009, 15). Quite literally, with its title "Baby Eva," the visualization of embryonic cell divisions is referred to as a baby and as a specific gendered individual named Eva. UK CARE Fertility similarly references a born individual to retrospectively ascribe meaning to the embryo depicted in the promotional video "Jaycie's Journey: Using Embryoscope Time

Lapse Imaging at CARE Fertility" (CARE Fertility 2015). In 37 seconds, the reproductive process is visualized in time-lapse embryo images of "Jaycie at fertilisation" and "Jaycie at 2 cells" to gray ultrasound images of "Jaycie at 3 months from fertilisation" and 3D ultrasound images of "Jaycie at 8 months," followed by a video recording of Jaycie as a newborn. Whereas in abortion and stem-cell debates, pro-choice and pro-research campaigners have employed images of early embryonic development to argue against the notion that an embryo is a small baby, here the emphasis on the reproductive continuum from embryo to fetus to baby reframes the cells' image as a recording of an individual's origin story.[4] The intensified association between images of embryonic development and born children is significant for its rhetorical function in reconfiguring the cultural imagination of human origin, motherhood, and the reproductive process.

More so than the static images of embryos that IVF patients could hitherto encounter in the clinical context (Lacey 2005), or the momentary peek *in utero* offered by moving ultrasound images of fetuses, the time-lapse embryo videos affirm the reproductive continuum by depicting prenatal development over an extended period of time. In their depiction of embryonic growth over the course of several days, these videos resemble the early scientific films of cellular development produced over a century ago, such as Julius Ries' 1907 recording of a sea urchin's fertilization and development. As Ries' films allowed "people other than scientists to participate visually in the sights of scientific work and the mode of experimental looking" (Landecker 2006, 123), so the novelty of time-lapse imaging technology follows from its clinical introduction, as the embryo videos allow intended parents to share in the embryologists' gaze and witness the cell divisions that become significant as depictions of a potential future child's origin story.

The compression of time in these videos further emphasizes the developmental progress of these embryos within a reproductive continuum. Much as Ries showed the sea urchin's cellular growth over 14 hours in a convenient two-minute film, so Baby Eva's and Jaycie's embryonic development over the course of days was compressed into a one-minute video (Landecker 2006, 124). If the recording and playback speed had been the same in the observation of human embryos, the cells would appear motionless, save for an occasional cell division. Sped up to an easily observable speed in time-lapse imaging, the embryonic cells' constant motion and sudden divisions represent the coming into existence of new human life by dramatizing a much slower, less spectacular process. In the early scientific films, the effect of watching these cells in accelerated motion was to convince audiences that "what they were seeing was really life" and had the effect of "making the subject more real … than still images" (Landecker 2006, 129). In the time-lapse videos, too, the acceleration of time has the effect of making the embryos appear more alive, as they move and divide in their microwells.[5] The increased speed imbues the cellular motions with a liveliness that is significant in the context of fertility clinics and intended parents' investment in the continued development of the embryos.

In keeping with the focus on the embryo-as-individual, the Eeva website frames the embryos for intended parents as expressly "yours." Auxogyn presents its technology to intended parents by pointing out that "your embryo's journey is captured in video form during the critical first days of development." The use of "your" emphasizes parental responsibility and a proprietary relationship to this "early human life" – one that can be met by employing the technology at the "critical time" of embryonic development (Auxogyn 2012). Similarly, CARE Fertility presents its EmbryoScope option as part of an IVF package that includes "a special download" of "a copy of the Time Lapse video of your embryo developing" (CARE Fertility 2013).

Described as "the ultimate home movie" (Wegner 2012), the embryonic time-lapse videos read like the earliest recording of the future child's existence; by locating a potential child's origin story in these images, they become instrumental in establishing the embryos as "yours." For example, Auxogyn's 2015 promotional video of the Eeva technology, in which a couple offers a testimonial of their successful experience of using time-lapse embryo imaging technology, concludes with two parents watching a video of their (now born) son's embryonic divisions within a domestic setting (Auxogyn 2015). Such videos of a single embryo's development, like this embryonic son's and Baby Eva's, therefore have a particular significance akin to that of fetal ultrasound imagery – a visual kinship that is affirmed in the video's mirroring of the ultrasound's traditional gray and blurry aesthetics. Like the ultrasound, and arguably to a greater extent because it shows human life at an even earlier stage of development, the video plays into a familiar "origin story," which functions as part of a narrative that locates the origin of an individual life at an observable moment (Morgan 2009, 8).

If the embryo video offers a new visual encounter with early prenatal life, it is also significant to note that – unlike the ultrasound – it positions the beginning of an identifiable life outside of the maternal body. While the ultrasound image presents the fetus as an interior other, with whom a relation can be established through the visual register, time-lapse embryo imaging externalizes the locus of new human life to the incubator. In this way, the embryo videos subscribe to a

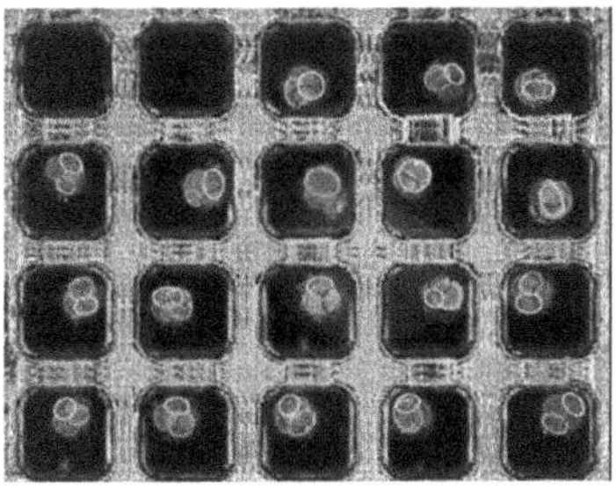

Figure 21.3 Embryo as collective. Still from "Eeva In Action (ASRM 2013)" (source: Auxogyn 2014).

broader visual convention in scientific and medical imagery of separating cellular entities from the body and depicting them as autonomous (Lie 2012, 478). In doing so, the embryo videos present a configuration of reproduction that was widely criticized in fetal ultrasound imagery, namely the presentation of a prenatal life as existing independently of its embodied uterine surroundings and the erasure of the maternal body from view (Petchesky 1987; Stabile 1992).[6] These embryo videos could similarly contribute to an understanding of reproduction that positions the locus of the beginning and the selection of future human life in technoculture rather than in the maternal body – particularly with reference to a second type of embryo image emerging with this technology.

Embryonic Collectives of Potential

When we zoom out from the single embryo frame in the "Eeva in Action" video (Auxogyn 2014), a second set of images emerges that shows a grid of several embryos developing at the same time. At the 2013 annual meeting of the American Society for Reproductive Medicine (ASRM), Auxogyn presented the merits of time-lapse imaging by showing this video footage of a grid of developing embryos recorded with the Eeva technology (Auxogyn 2014).[7] The video shows a collective of embryos growing side by side, each dividing their cells at different moments and wriggling independently within their squares. The grid visually juxtaposes the differences between the embryos and thereby invites a comparison: some move quickly, others remain still; some divide their cells steadily, while others lag behind. A valuation is attached to the active, inactive or seemingly erratic behavior of the embryos in the last seconds of the video, when a red "LOW" or a green "HIGH" appears underneath each of them.

This visualization of embryo selection naturalizes an approach to the reproductive process that involves the active choice of the "best" embryo to be implanted in the womb. While this is a seemingly common-sense approach, it presents the group of embryos in a vastly different way from the individual embryo that was celebrated as Baby Eva. Baby Eva's video situates the start of an individual's origin story at the first moments of conception. By contrast, the grid video depicts the potentiality of life that a set of embryos hold collectively – a potentiality that is not only reliant on the quality of the organic material and the culturing conditions, but also requires actualizing through an investment in the right technology for selection.

Time-lapse imagery thus visualizes an alternative organization of the reproductive process, which includes a moment of embryo selection analogous to the sperm selection that takes place prior to conception in the female body. Popular and scientific understandings of sperm selection typically present the female reproductive tract as the *in vivo* selection mechanism to prevent substandard sperm cells from interacting with the single egg released in ovulation (Martin 2001; Moore 2003). In these time-lapse images, the spatio-temporal organization of gametes and embryos differs from *in vivo* conception, with its single egg and multitude of sperm cells that may interact to become an embryo.[8] Rather than a single egg and a "winning" sperm resulting in a unique embryo, the time-lapse video presents in vitro embryos in groups that require selection to produce a healthy live birth. The time-lapse video shows eggs and embryos as visibly fallible and therefore, much like sperm, requiring selection mechanisms. By presenting the embryos as fallible, time-lapse embryo imaging visualizes embryo selection as a necessary and newly observable intervention in the reproductive process. "Natural" reproductive selection thus becomes a multifaceted techno-cultural selection that requires highly specialized technological apparatus.

Auxogyn's framing of a single embryo representing Baby Eva and the grid image of embryos in the time-lapse apparatus are thus indicative of two different origin stories. The first image, with its individualized embryo, appears to correspond to the origin story upheld in pro-life debates that "life begins at conception" (Franklin 2001, 348), and indeed the image could be employed to visualize that standpoint. However, the presentation of the single developing embryo in the Auxogyn press release does not ascribe personhood to every embryo, but specifically frames this image with the text "Baby Eva, Born 11 June 2013." This particular embryo is therefore ascribed personhood *because* it was born; only after June 11, 2013 did it retrospectively gain individuality as an embryo.

By contrast, Eeva's grid image of multiple embryos, with its weak and strong elements, does not individualize the embryos but visualizes the need for their selection in anticipation of a potential pregnancy and birth. Auxogyn's Eeva website presents its embryo selection method as the "difference you need for IVF success" and the test to "help reduce the risk of IVF failure" (Auxogyn 2012). This language of risk and success also characterizes the CARE Fertility clinic's presentation of its EmbryoScope and CAREmaps – with "maps" being an acronym for morphokinetic algorithms to predict success – as "a whole system designed to maximise the chances of success" (CARE Fertility 2013). This discourse of risk and success is matched in the grid image, which shows the embryos' observably arrested, erratic or active development and overlays them with "high" and "low" inscriptions. With this visualization of the fallible nature of the embryos, the time-lapse grid image may be employed to reframe reproduction as a technological achievement and the embryos as material that requires selection.[9] This textual and visual discursive construction of risk and success in the embryo grid, moreover, has a futural orientation as it references the embryos' potential for continued growth after the video ends. While textual framing of "Baby Eva" individualizes the embryo retrospectively, the "high" and "low" inscriptions are indicative of an anticipatory orientation toward the embryos in the grid image, in which they figure as a collective with weak and strong elements that holds the potential for a future live birth.

Time-lapse embryo imaging thus produces several representations of the embryo, including an individual embryo onto which ideas of personhood and individuality are bestowed and a collective of embryos that require selection prior to further development. What distinguishes these two framings of the embryo is less a matter of content – the former is simply a zoomed-in version of one of the embryos in the latter – and more a matter of temporality. While the image of the embryo grid signifies an *anticipatory* potential held by the collective throughout the process of selection, the single embryo *retrospectively* becomes meaningful as an individual once a birth, or even an ultrasound, has taken place that establishes individual personhood.

Embryo Populations

Time-lapse embryo imaging visualizes a third type of embryo: a population of embryos that is abstracted and superimposed over, or juxtaposed with, the image. The Eeva video concludes with a HIGH or LOW verdict by combining this visual analysis of the cells with data from earlier observations of embryonic development. In the EmbryoScope, the embryonic population that provided the basis for the embryo selection is visualized by graphs that juxtapose the embryo grid videos and provide a context for their interpretation. Depending on the observed growth patterns, the different frames in the embryo grid are colored a transparent red, blue or green to indicate predicted quality.

What these videos show, therefore, is a wider population of embryos translated into a body of visual and temporal information. As a result, the embryo videos depict not only a synchronous comparison between a particular group of incubated embryos, but also a diachronic one in relation to preceding populations. The time-lapse imaging systems watch through the lens of earlier observations caught in a database. In the incubator's eye, the statistically rendered embryonic population becomes visible, coloring the image of the developing embryo. This visualized data is a palimpsest of earlier observations: the translation of embryonic tissue growth into images, images into averages, averages into visible colors, shapes, and graphs that frame the embryo multiplying itself into existence.

Earlier I made a comparison between the cinematic scene of ICSI microinjection and time-lapse videos as images of technologized reproduction, yet the locus of what becomes recognizable as technology is significantly different in time-lapse imaging. Whereas the ICSI image features the injection needle as a visible technological actor, in the images of the time-lapse embryos the technology is located in the embryonic growth itself as the timing of cell divisions becomes the means for selection. In *Liminal Lives*, Susan Squier claims that the two forms of in vitro cellular growth of most interest in tissue culture research are organized growth and unorganized growth, which have been accessed with "iconic overdetermination" through the observation of, respectively, embryos and cancer cells (2004, 61). The temporal specificity of organized growth finds its clinical application – and is thereby rendered into a technology – in time-lapse embryo imaging. This approach synchronizes the embryo with a database from which temporal standards for the ideal type of embryonic development are deduced, as an indicator of anticipated growth and viability. Unlike ICSI or PGD, time-lapse imaging does not require or visualize invasive instruments that alter the cell's morphology. On the contrary, the apparatus functions to cause as little disturbance to the cellular tissue as possible. Giving new meaning to Franklin's "instrumental reframing of reproduction as technology" (2013, 40), the time-lapse apparatus transforms the temporal regularity of embryonic development, and its predictive value in anticipating future growth, into a technology.

In this way, the embryo videos visualize the double meaning of biology as the "thing itself" and the knowledge thereof; they make explicit how "biological knowledge, biotechniques and biology 'itself' reshape each other, and co-evolve" (Franklin 2006, 168). In time-lapse embryo imaging, the observation, translation and projection of past embryonic populations shape the value and destination of the embryos under current scrutiny, which in turn may affect future selections. In this way, time-lapse embryo imaging complements ICSI's scene of fertilization as, Franklin argues, an explicit visualization of Rabinow's (2008) argument that life " 'will become technique' in a manner that reverses the order of Darwinian evolutionary time and telos, by making culture the origin of biology" (2013, 40). The embryo videos visualize a model of technocultural selection that is based not only on the observed "survival of the fittest," but also on the calculated anticipation of future survival through the embryos' approximation to the population-based temporal norms of development.

Through the use of data from previous embryo populations in time-lapse selection, a different way of viewing the embryo emerges. Time-lapse embryo imaging entails a distancing and digitalization of the relation between the embryo and the embryologist, who increasingly touches and observes the screen rather than the petri dish. Whereas in conventional selection, the embryologist moves the embryos from the incubator to the optical microscope to analyze specific morphological markers, in time-lapse embryo imaging, they remain enclosed in the machine throughout the incubation period and become visible on the screen after digital image analysis. The increased reliance on automated analysis based on previous embryo populations also introduces new forms of standardization in knowledge production about embryos. As the maternal and the embryologist's bodies become further distanced from the embryos, they themselves become more intimately entangled in the time-lapse apparatus – to the extent that the academic community engages in debate about whether embryonic development is a natural occurrence or a proprietary, patentable part of the time-lapse method and machine (Cohen 2013; Reijo Pera 2013). Meanwhile, in light of the rapid implementation of time-lapse embryo imaging in places like the UK, the encounter with the developing embryo, and the origin stories implicit in its framing, are gaining influence in the IVF experience of intended parents, the clinical experience of embryologists and the conceptualization of the reproductive process for the wider public.

Conclusion

As IVF is now "included in the normal repertoire of getting pregnant" (Lie and Lykke, Editorial Introduction to this volume), attendant techniques such as time-lapse embryo imaging also emerge as "new normals" that could shift the cultural imagination of the reproductive process. Given the rapid introduction of time-lapse embryo imaging into fertility clinics, the use of moving images of dividing cells may become normalized in embryo selection. This shift toward analyzing visualized embryos with temporal indicators and population-based comparators should not only be considered for its effects on live birth rates, but also for its cultural implications in introducing a new set of images through which early human life may be imagined.

Three approaches to visualizing the embryo emerge from the time-lapse embryo videos: the retrospective image of the embryo-as-individual, the anticipatory grid view of a collective of embryos, and its layering with historical data about embryonic populations. The first presents an individualized embryo that bears a direct relation to the future child; the first embryonic divisions depicted in the video are here framed as the start of an individual human life. The second, zooming out to the grid level, offers a view of multiple, fallible embryos that require time-lapse technology to actualize their collective potential for "IVF success." While the time-lapse technology makes the footage of early embryonic development visible to the intended parents for the first time, and thereby offers a visual encounter with the earliest moments in the lives of their (potential) children, it simultaneously replaces an understanding of the embryo-as-individual by one of embryos as a group that collectively holds a potential for human life that is contingent on technocultural – as a variation on natural – selection. Third, the layering of visualized population data on top, to the side, or in the coloring of the images offers a reading of the incubated embryos in relation to earlier embryonic populations, whose temporal growth patterns have attained predictive value. Therefore, embryos, and their existence in time, not only function as material to be selected, but are themselves entangled as part of the technological tool. The temporal specificity of their development functions as a prism through which to observe other embryos and to determine viability through the recognition of organized growth. The clinical implementation of time-lapse embryo imaging should thus be considered instrumental in a contemporary rewriting of human origin stories, in which the timing of observing both the embryos and their videos affects the value ascribed to these cell divisions.

Notes

1 In a 2013 press release, Fertilitech, the company that produced the EmbryoScope, states that the system was cleared for clinical use in Europe in 2009. According to Fertilitech, it has been used by 275 clinics worldwide for 60,000 treatment cycles and they estimate that "more than 10,000 babies have been born using the EmbryoScope™ system" (Bahr 2013). Fertilitech was acquired by Vitrolife in 2014.

2 At the time of writing, it is offered by major clinics including CARE Fertility, Bourn Hall, the Bridge Clinic and the London Women's Clinic. According to biotechnology company Vitrolife's optimistic assessment, half the IVF treatments in the UK are done with time-lapse imaging (Vitrolife 2015, 3).

3 For detailed technical differences between the three systems, see Kovacs (2014, 124).

4 For example, proponents of embryo research have employed the embryo's image to argue against its individuality by pointing to its appearance as a cluster of cells that lacks recognizable human features (Williams *et al.* 2003, 801–803).

5 Microwells are small depressions in the culture dish. Each contains a single embryo.
6 Testifying to her foresight, the embryo videos literalize Duden's assertion that "the fetuses we live with today were first conceived not in the womb, but in visualizing technologies" (1999, 15).
7 Images of pairs or grids of embryos are also featured in patient-oriented videos by Auxogyn and fertility clinics.
8 More than one egg may be involved in the conception of fraternal twins or higher-order multiple births.
9 As "a special download" that intended parents may receive as part of their IVF cycle, these videos could function both as a desirable keepsake and as an affirmation of the value of including the extra step of time-lapse embryo selection as risk management (CARE Fertility 2013).

References

Armstrong, Sarah, Nicola Arroll, Lynsey M. Cree, Vanessa Jordan, and Cindy Farquhar. 2015. "Time-Lapse Systems for Embryo Incubation and Assessment in Assisted Reproduction." *The Cochrane Database of Systematic Reviews* 2: CD011320. doi:10.1002/14651858.CD011320.pub2.

Auxogyn. 2012. "Eeva – Early Embryo Viability Assessment Test." *Eeva*. Accessed November 8, 2013. www.eevaivf.com/.

Auxogyn. 2014. "Eeva In Action (ASRM 2013)." YouTube video, 2:06. Posted by "The Eeva Test," January 8. www.youtube.com/watch?v=hdL0kY5rPbM.

Auxogyn. 2015. "Patient Testimonial Video | Eeva Test." *Eeva*. Accessed October 18, 2015. www.eevatest.com/patient-testimonial-video.

Bahr, Francesca. 2013. "Unisense FertiliTech A/S to Present Large Scale Time-Lapse Data Analysis to Improve IVF Treatment – Unisense Fertilitech A/S." *Fertilitech*. July 4. www.fertilitech.com/en-GB/Information/Press-Releases/Recent-Press.aspx?PID=195&M=NewsV2&Action=1&NewsId=143.

BBC. 2013. "First Baby Conceived with Time-Lapse Imaging IVF Born in Glasgow." *BBC*. June 14. Scotland. www.bbc.co.uk/news/uk-scotland-22910864.

CARE Fertility. 2013. "Time Lapse Embryo Imaging, CAREmaps at CARE Fertility." *CARE Fertility*. Accessed November 4, 2015. www.carefertility.com/care-fertility-sc0/caremaps-and-time-lapse-embryo-imaging-maximising-success-sj39/.

CARE Fertility. 2015. "Jaycie's Journey Using Embryoscope Time Lapse Imaging at CARE Fertility." YouTube video, 0:37. Posted by "CARE Fertility," August 28. www.youtube.com/watch?v=vnm56Kiy4Jg.

Chen, Alice A., Lei Tan, Vaishali Suraj, Renee Reijo Pera, and Shehua Shen. 2013. "Biomarkers Identified with Time-Lapse Imaging: Discovery, Validation, and Practical Application." *Fertility and Sterility* 99 (4): 1035–1043.

Cohen, Jacques. 2013. "On Patenting Time and Other Natural Phenomena." *Reproductive BioMedicine Online* 27 (2): 109–110.

Duden, Barbara. 1993. *Disembodying Women: Perspectives on Pregnancy and the Unborn*. Cambridge, MA: Harvard University Press.

Franklin, Sarah. 2001. "Culturing Biology: Cell Lines for the Second Millennium." *Health: An Interdisciplinary Journal for the Social Study of Health, Illness and Medicine* 5 (3): 335–354.

Franklin, Sarah. 2006. "The Cyborg Embryo: Our Path to Transbiology." *Theory, Culture & Society* 23 (7–8): 167–187.

Franklin, Sarah. 2013. "Embryo Watching: How IVF Has Remade Biology." *TECNOSCIENZA: Italian Journal of Science & Technology Studies* 4 (1): 23–44.

Kbhandal. 2013a. "Baby Eeva Video – Eeva." *Early Embryo Viability Assessment Test*. June 14. www.eevaivf.com/video-of-eeva-conception/.

Kbhandal. 2013b. "Baby Eva Named after Pioneering IVF Test – Eeva." *Early Embryo Viability Assessment Test.* June 14. www.eevaivf.com/baby-eva-named-after-pioneering-ivf-test/.

Kovacs, Peter. 2014. "Embryo Selection: The Role of Time-Lapse Monitoring." *Reproductive Biology and Endocrinology* 12: 124. doi:10.1186/1477-7827-12-124.

Lacey, Sheryl de. 2005. "Parent Identity and 'Virtual' Children: Why Patients Discard rather than Donate Unused Embryos." *Human Reproduction* 20 (6): 1661–1669.

Landecker, Hannah. 2006. "Microcinematography and the History of Science and Film." *Isis* 97 (1): 121–132.

Landecker, Hannah. 2012. "The Life of Movement: From Microcinematography to Live-Cell Imaging." *Journal of Visual Culture* 11 (3): 378–399.

Lie, Merete. 2012. "Reproductive Images: The Autonomous Cell." *Science as Culture* 21 (4): 475–496.

Martin, Emily. 2001. "Body Narratives, Body Boundaries." In *The American Body in Context: An Anthology*, edited by Jessica R. Johnston, 257–272. Wilmington: Rowman and Littlefield.

Meseguer, Marcos, Irene Rubio, Maria Cruz, Natalia Basile, Julian Marcos, and Antonio Requena. 2012. "Embryo Incubation and Selection in a Time-Lapse Monitoring System Improves Pregnancy Outcome Compared with a Standard Incubator: A Retrospective Cohort Study." *Fertility and Sterility* 98 (6): 1481–1489.e10.

Moore, Lisa Jean. 2003. "'Billy, the Sad Sperm with No Tail': Representations of Sperm in Children's Books." *Sexualities* 6 (3–4): 277–300.

Morgan, Lynn. 2009. *Icons of Life: A Cultural History of Human Embryos*. Berkeley, Los Angeles: University of California Press.

Petchesky, Rosalind Pollack. 1987. "Fetal Images: The Power of Visual Culture in the Politics of Reproduction." *Feminist Studies* 13 (2): 263–292.

Rabinow, Paul. 2008. "Artificiality and Enlightenment: From Sociobiology to Biosociality." In *Anthropologies of Modernity*, edited by Jonathan X. Inda, 179–193. Oxford: Blackwell Publishing Ltd.

Racowsky, Catherine, Peter Kovacs, and Wellington P. Martins. 2015. "A Critical Appraisal of Time-Lapse Imaging for Embryo Selection: Where Are We and Where Do We Need to Go?" *Journal of Assisted Reproduction and Genetics* 32 (7): 1025–1030.

Reijo Pera, Renee A. 2013. "More than Just a Matter of Time." *Reproductive BioMedicine Online* 27 (2): 113–114.

Squier, Susan M. 2004. *Liminal Lives: Imagining the Human at the Frontiers of Biomedicine*. Durham: Duke University Press.

Stabile, Carol A. 1992. "Shooting the Mother: Fetal Photography and the Politics of Disappearance." *Camera Obscura* 10 (1 28): 178–205.

Van Dijck, José. 2001. *Het Transparante Lichaam: Medische Visualisering in Media en Cultuur*. Amsterdam: Amsterdam University Press.

Vitrolife. 2015. "Interim Report January–June 2015." Interim report. Gothenburg, Sweden: Vitrolife. http://mb.cision.com/Main/1031/9804468/401074.pdf.

Walsh, Fergus. 2013. "Time-Lapse Imaging 'Improves IVF.'" *BBC*. May 17. www.bbc.com/news/health-22559247.

Wegner, Carole. 2012. "Time Lapse Embryo Imaging: How It May Change IVF." *Fertility Lab Insider*. October 28. http://fertilitylabinsider.com/2012/10/time-lapse-embryo-imaging-how-it-may-change-ivf/.

Williams, Clare, Jenny Kitzinger, and Lesley Henderson. 2003. "Envisaging the Embryo in Stem Cell Research: Rhetorical Strategies and Media Reporting of the Ethical Debates." *Sociology of Health & Illness* 25 (7): 793–814. doi:10.1046/j.1467–9566.2003.00370.x.

Glossary

ARTs, Assisted Reproductive Technologies Technically assisted treatments for infertility, including many different procedures and technologies.

Cryopreservation A process in which cells or tissues are preserved at very low temperatures in containers of liquid or gaseous nitrogen.

Donor/donation The common term for providers of egg and sperm cells for other people. The notion of *provision* is a more apt term, insofar as economic compensation sometimes becomes a more significant factor than altruism, as noted in this volume.

Donor insemination The practice of using a syringe to place sperm from a sperm donor/provider into a woman's vagina with the aim of initiating a pregnancy.

Embryo The developing organism from the fourth day after fertilization to the end of the eighth week. At a later stage, it is usually referred to as a fetus.

Embryo transfer The insertion of one or more embryos into a woman's uterus after IVF fertilization.

Fallopian tubes Within a female body, the two tubes leading from the ovaries into the uterus.

Fertility travel Traveling abroad to obtain ART treatment, often because a particular treatment is not available in the home country, or because the individual wanting it is not eligible due to legal or other constraints. The term "fertility tourism" is also sometimes used, and the difference is discussed in this volume.

Fetus The stage from the post-embryonic phase until birth.

Gamete A mature male or female germ cell.

Gamete donation/gamete provision See **Donor/donation**.

Gestational surrogacy Surrogacy with egg and sperm donation/provision, usually from the intending mother and/or father. The embryo is created by IVF and the child is not genetically related to the surrogate.

Heterologous fertilization Fertilization takes place with gamete donation/provision, i.e., sperm and/or eggs from individuals other than the intending parent/s.

Homologous fertilization Fertilization takes place with an embryo created from sperm and/or eggs from the intending parent/s and inserted in the woman's uterus.

ICSI, intracytoplasmic sperm injection An IVF procedure in which a single sperm cell is injected directly into an egg cell.

Implantation The successful embedding of the embryo into the uterine wall, which usually occurs one to five days after embryo transfer.

Intending or intended parent/s Adults who engage in the use of donor eggs/sperm or enter into a surrogacy agreement under the terms that they will be the parent/s of the child intended to result from the procedure. The terminology "intended parent/s" and "intending parent/s" are used interchangeably in this volume.

IVF, in vitro fertilization In vitro, literally: in glass, i.e., in a glass dish. IVF is a process of fertilization external to the body. It involves stimulating a woman's ovaries, extracting mature egg cells, and combining egg and sperm in a laboratory dish. The fertilized egg cells are first cultured in a protected environment and then one (or more) embryo(s) is inserted into a woman's uterus.

Jus sanguinis Literally, "right of the blood." The right to citizenship is granted on the basis of the citizenship of one or both parents.

Jus soli Literally, "right of the soil." The right to citizenship is granted to individuals born in the territory of a state.

Morula An early stage in the development of an embryo. The stage of division into eight cells, 3–4 days after fertilization.

Oocyte An immature egg cell.

Ovum Egg cell.

PGD, preimplantation genetic diagnosis This procedure requires IVF to obtain oocytes or embryos for genetic diagnosis. An oocyte or a single cell, extracted from an embryo, will undergo the diagnostic procedure.

PND, prenatal diagnosis Prenatal screening and testing of pregnant women for diseases or risky conditions in the fetus or embryo.

Precocious menopause Premature or early menopause, i.e., before 40 years of age.

Pre-embryo A fertilized egg cell up to 14 days old, before it is implanted in the uterus.

Sui juris "In one's own jurisdiction." A legal term meaning that a person has full social and civil rights and has the capacity to manage their own affairs.

Surrogacy The process of carrying out a pregnancy for intending parents. The pregnancy is initiated by sperm injection or embryo provision. The latter is termed **gestational surrogacy**.

Zygote The cell formed after fertilization by the combination of an egg cell and a sperm cell.

Index

Page numbers in *italics* denote tables, those in **bold** denote figures.

Taylor & Francis eBooks

Helping you to choose the right eBooks for your Library

Add Routledge titles to your library's digital collection today. Taylor and Francis ebooks contains over 50,000 titles in the Humanities, Social Sciences, Behavioural Sciences, Built Environment and Law.

Choose from a range of subject packages or create your own!

Benefits for you

» Free MARC records
» COUNTER-compliant usage statistics
» Flexible purchase and pricing options
» All titles DRM-free.

REQUEST YOUR **FREE** INSTITUTIONAL TRIAL TODAY

Free Trials Available
We offer free trials to qualifying academic, corporate and government customers.

Benefits for your user

» Off-site, anytime access via Athens or referring URL
» Print or copy pages or chapters
» Full content search
» Bookmark, highlight and annotate text
» Access to thousands of pages of quality research at the click of a button.

eCollections – Choose from over 30 subject eCollections, including:

Archaeology	Language Learning
Architecture	Law
Asian Studies	Literature
Business & Management	Media & Communication
Classical Studies	Middle East Studies
Construction	Music
Creative & Media Arts	Philosophy
Criminology & Criminal Justice	Planning
Economics	Politics
Education	Psychology & Mental Health
Energy	Religion
Engineering	Security
English Language & Linguistics	Social Work
Environment & Sustainability	Sociology
Geography	Sport
Health Studies	Theatre & Performance
History	Tourism, Hospitality & Events

For more information, pricing enquiries or to order a free trial, please contact your local sales team: **www.tandfebooks.com/page/sales**

Routledge Taylor & Francis Group | The home of Routledge books

www.tandfebooks.com

For Product Safety Concerns and Information please contact our EU representative GPSR@taylorandfrancis.com
Taylor & Francis Verlag GmbH, Kaufingerstraße 24, 80331 München, Germany

www.ingramcontent.com/pod-product-compliance
Ingram Content Group UK Ltd.
Pitfield, Milton Keynes, MK11 3LW, UK
UKHW022010180926
475701UK00003B/284
* 9 7 8 0 3 6 7 3 5 0 8 2 6 *